TRIGGER FACTORS IN TRANSFUSION MEDICINE

DEVELOPMENTS IN HEMATOLOGY AND IMMUNOLOGY

Volume 31

The titles published in this series are listed at the end of this volume.

Trigger Factors in Transfusion Medicine

Proceedings of the Twentieth International Symposium on Blood Transfusion, Groningen 1995, organized by the Red Cross Blood Bank Noord-Nederland

edited by

C. Th. SMIT SIBINGA and P. C. DAS

Red Cross Blood Bank Noord-Nederland, The Netherlands

and

E. L. SNYDER

Yale New Haven Hospital Blood Bank, New Haven, CT, U.S.A.

KLUWER ACADEMIC PUBLISHERS

DORDRECHT / BOSTON / LONDON

A C.I.P. Catalogue record for this book is available from the Library of Congress.

ISBN 0-7923-4255-0

Published by Kluwer Academic Publishers,
P.O. Box 17, 3300 AA Dordrecht, The Netherlands.

Kluwer Academic Publishers incorporates
the publishing programmes of
D. Reidel, Martinus Nijhoff, Dr W. Junk and MTP Press.

Sold and distributed in the U.S.A. and Canada
by Kluwer Academic Publishers,
101 Philip Drive, Norwell, MA 02061, U.S.A.

In all other countries, sold and distributed
by Kluwer Academic Publishers Group,
P.O. Box 322, 3300 AH Dordrecht, The Netherlands.

Printed on acid-free paper

Printed in the Netherlands

Baxter

Acknowledgement

This publication has been made possible through the support of Baxter, which is gratefully acknowledged.

CONTENTS

Moderators and Speakers IX

Foreword XI

I. Demand and Supply

Customer-oriented Quality Systems in Transfusion 3
D.E. Nevalainen

Communication Mechanisms Between the Bedside and the Blood Bank .. 13
A.W.M. Koopman-Van Gemert

Informed Consent for Transfusion Recipients: How much is enough? 17
P.V. Holland

Factors That Influence the Demand for Transfusion 25
D.B.L. McClelland

The Process of Clinical Decision making in Blood Transfusion 35
L.T. Goodnough

Discussion 47

II. Product Qualities and Characteristics

Factors defining the clinical needs for supportive haemotherapy 57
J.Th.M. de Wolf

Factors Effecting the Clinical Efficacy of Blood Transfusion 65
W.G. Murphy

The Clinical Relevance and Biological Effects of Leukocytes Present in Cellular Blood Components 73
M. Blajchman

Platelets: What Qualities and Characteristics Do Justify the Need for Transfusion? 83
S. Murphy

The Clinical Relevance of Clotting Factor Characteristics 91
C.A. Ludlam

Discussion 103

III. Transfusion Policies and Clinical Pratice

Fears, Facts and Formulas About Blood Transfusion: On the Perception, Acceptance and Communication of Risks 113
C.A.J. Vlek

Surgical Criteria for Blood Transfusion: How Far Should We Go? 133
H.J. ten Duis

Transfusion Policies and Clinical Practice in a Tertiary Academic Medical Centre: The Role of Protocols and Documentation 143
M. Petrides and E.L. Snyder

Choice of Transfusing Single Donor Apheresis vs Random Pooled Platelets – Its Costs 161
A. Westerterp-Maas

Ethical Aspects of the Transfusion of Blood 169
C.R. Macpherson

What Triggers the Initiative of Developments in Transfusion Medicine: Advances in Ex Vivo Haematopoietic Cell Therapy and Next Generation Transfusion Products 177
D.E. van Epps

Discussion 193

IV. Evaluation and Feed-Back of Transfusion Policies

Evaluation of Bedside Transfusion Practice: Benefits vs Risks 199
R.S. Eisenstaedt

The Clinical Consultative Role of the Blood Bank in Transfusion Medicine 213
C.Th. Smit Sibinga

Audits in Transfusion Medicine: A Trigger Mechanism to Optimise Clinical Practice 219
Ch.H. Wallas

Legislative and Regulative Impact on Transfusion Medicine Practices 235
K. Sazama

Discussion 245

Index 253

MODERATORS AND SPEAKERS

Moderators

E.L. Snyder, chairman	–	Yale New Haven Hospital Blood Bank, New Haven, CT, USA
P.C. Das	–	Red Cross Blood Bank Noord Nederland, Groningen, NL
L.T. Goodnough	–	Washington University School of Medicine, St. Louis, MO, USA
W. Murphy	–	Royal College of Physicians, Edinburgh, UK
C.Th. Smit Sibinga	–	Red Cross Blood Bank Noord Nederland, Groningen, NL
H.J.C. de Wit	–	Red Cross Blood Bank Noord Nederland, Groningen, NL
J.Th.M. de Wolf	–	Academic Hospital Groningen, Groningen, NL

Speakers

M. Blajchman	–	McMaster University, Hamilton, Ontario, C
H.J. ten Duis	–	Academic Hospital Groningen, Groningen, NL
R.S. Eisenstaedt	–	Temple University, Philadelphia, PA, USA
D. van Epps	–	Baxter Healthcare Corporation, Round Lake, IL, USA
P.V. Holland	–	Sacramento Medical Foundation Blood Center, Sacramento, CA, USA
A.W.M.M. Koopman-van Gemert	–	Academic Medical Centre, Amsterdam, NL

C.A. Ludlam	–	Royal Infirmary of Edinburgh, Edinburgh, UK
C.R. Macpherson	–	U.C. Medical Center, Cincinnati, OH, USA
D.B.L. McClelland	–	Edinburgh & South East Scotland Blood Transfusion Service, Edinburgh, UK
S. Murphy	–	American Red Cross Blood Services, Philadelphia, PA, USA
D.E. Nevalainen	–	Abbott Quality Institute, Abbott Park, IL, USA
K. Sazama	–	Medical College Hospitals, Philadelphia, PA, USA
C.A.J. Vlek	–	University of Groningen, Department of Psychology, Groningen, NL
Ch.H. Wallas	–	American Red Cross Headquarters, Charlotte, NC, USA
A. van der Wiel	–	General Christian Hospital Eemland, Amersfoort, NL

Prepared Discussants

A. Westerterp-Maas	–	Red Cross Blood Bank Noord Nederland, Groningen, NL

FOREWORD

It is an honour and a pleasure to welcome you all at this 20th annual International Symposium on Blood Transfusion in the Netherlands. This year you celebrate its 20th anniversary and I congratulate the Staff of the Blood Bank Noord Nederland and especially Dr. Smit Sibinga for this great achievement. As most of you know, the name of the person of Dr. Smit Sibinga is unbreakably connected with the annual symposium in Groningen which he has organized each year from the very start, 20 years ago.

The reputation of any symposium depends heavily on the quality of the lectures. I think it is not possible to organize 20 symposia in a row if the topics lack actual relevance and the speakers are not of excellent reputation. Dr. Smit Sibinga has proven to have a keen eye for selecting interesting themes and eminent speakers. Although a lot of different topics have been dealt with in the past 20 years, which each attracted the attention of a different group in the field of blood transfusion, it is not surprising that after a tradition of 20 years several speakers but also a lot of attendees are not for the first time in Groningen to participate in this event. It gives the symposium a unique atmosphere of intimacy.

It is not hard to admit that most of the newer developments in transfusion medicine take place outside the Netherlands. Knowing that and in order to keep our position among the nations with the safest blood supply, we have to focus our view on the international field. Therefore, the Groningen symposium is of national importance. It not only established the extraordinary reputation of the Blood Bank in Groningen, but it also creates an international forum where the latest developments in Transfusion Medicine are exchanged.

For yet another reason this 20th symposium is a memorable one. Earlier this year the Red Cross Blood Bank Groningen-Drenthe, the organizer of the symposium over the last 19 years, merged with its neighbour, the Blood Bank Friesland to form the new Blood Bank Noord Nederland. It has a total of about 90.000 donations per year and is now one of the largest Blood Banks in the Netherlands.

I am sure that the medical knowledge of Dr. Smit Sibinga combined with the pharmaceutical knowledge of Mr. De Wit guarantee a winning team and a strong Blood Bank in the north of our country. This strong Blood Bank should co-operate in a cordial way with the other Dutch Blood Banks and with the Central Laboratory in Amsterdam. On the necessity of this co-operation I shall come back later.

The theme of this symposium "Trigger factors in Transfusion Medicine" puzzled me somewhat, so I had to consult my dictionary. I found: "a trigger is a movable catch or lever." Webster 1983 described a trigger as:

- a fingerpiece of gunlock;
- small lever or part, which, when pulled or pressed releases a catch spring.

I was already afraid that in the blood transfusion world guns had been introduced, but I was set at ease when I found in Longman's dictionary of contemporary English:

- Trigger: to start or cause a number of events, often of an undesirable kind, that happen one after another.

In the blood transfusion practice this start of a number of events is well recognized. The process from donation to transfusion consists of a considerable number of events that happen one after another. An undesirable event in the blood transfusion practice has almost always an excessive impact, far more than undesirable events in other fields of medicine.

In the past fifteen years, particularly after the introduction of HIV in the Dutch population, Blood Banks had to change considerably in order to guarantee the safety of their blood products. The concept of Good Manufacturing Practice was introduced in the processing of blood and its components. Also laboratory tests had to be improved in order to detect the presence of viruses in the donor blood.

Expensive manufacturing and laboratory equipment came and computer systems supported and safeguarded the process. The use of bag systems in stead of bottles made it possible to produce blood components in a closed system and guarantee the sterility of the product. In the last three years, each Blood Bank has been inspected by the Health Inspectorate. My inspectors could observe the improvement in quality level of blood banking in the Netherlands. Not all Blood Banks are yet at the same GMP-level, but the general impression is positive.

Besides the inspections by the Inspectorate, the Blood Banks themselves have developed a system of peer review which perfectly supplements our inspections. These efforts to improve the quality of blood banking have side effects. One of them is that Blood Banks will embrace more and more modern management strategies. Let us be aware that this could lead to a too commercial view on blood transfusion as a whole. Another side effect is, that there is a danger that blood transfusions are to be considered as a medicine, a pharmaceutically prepared product. In that view the blood donor is not more than "raw material". The motivation for the donor decreases substantially when donating his blood voluntarily and non-renumerated, and reading in the papers that blood transfusion is "big business".

Management of Blood Banks finds itself in a peculiar position with respect to finances. On the one side the Blood Banks have to provide a certain number of blood transfusions to achieve healthy financial situation but on the other side the Blood Banks have to propagate that the number of transfusions in the clinic should be as low as possible. Each Blood Bank director knows the potential of his products not only with respect to infections, but also in the field of the immunological effects of blood products and individual patients.

Maybe that these dualistic interests are the reason that a number of Blood Banks consider the moment that the blood product leaves the Blood Bank as the endpoint of the responsibility of the Blood Bank director. When blood is delivered to the hospital, the hospital Blood Transfusion Service (if present) or the clinical chemist is responsible for storage, distribution and delivery to the departments and transfusion is the responsibility of the physician in charge. In contrast to the small number of Blood Banks involved, the number of physicians in charge is enormous. All these doctors could have different opinions on the use of blood transfusion. Orthopedic and cardiac surgeons consider blood transfusion as an absolute necessity during their operations and they expect the Blood Banks to deliver the requested products without comment. Nowadays, a number of hospitals are using standard ordering lists of blood components potentially needed for the various operations, but still many doctors consider blood transfusion as a routine.

In the Netherlands we have nowadays the "Decree on the use of blood in hospitals" as a part of the Dutch Law on blood transfusion. Blood products should only be ordered by a physician with a signed prescription. Many telephone calls to my office were the result. In many instances, there was discussion about who was responsible for the transfusion in the operation room, the surgeon or the anesthesiologist. And why could they not order transfusions via the nursing staff? So, the formation of active Blood Transfusion Committees in hospitals is necessary. The best would be a consultation on a regular basis between the Blood Bank director and these active Blood Transfusion Committees. The construction could be that the Blood Bank director serves as an active member of the hospital committee or even an extraordinary member of the medical staff of the hospital. Only in good co-operation between the Blood Bank and the clinician a safe and economic blood transfusion practice is possible.

Blood Transfusion Committees should make protocols for the use of blood components in their hospitals in concordance with nationwide protocols. These protocols should specify the indication and use of blood transfusions but also a follow-up system for transfusions in the hospital. In most hospitals nowadays it is possible to trace the recipients of a certain blood donation. This system of traceability has proved to be very important in case of look-back procedures. Therefore in 1996 I consider to start an investigation into traceability of blood products in hospitals. The protocols for clinical indications should be based on national protocols developed by CBO or the Council for the Blood Transfusion and be accepted and subscribed by all the users of blood transfusion. My inspection considers these protocols as standards of the state of the art. In my opinion it is impossible to have SOP's for each procedure of donation and blood processing while there are no protocols on the clinical blood transfusion practice.

Patients ask for safe procedures from the donor to the transfusion. After the publication about the French blood scandal and other negative publicity patients became afraid of blood transfusion. Recently our "National Ombudsman" published a report on the HIV transmission via blood products in haemophiliacs and on measures taken by the government to prevent HIV transmission in the early eighties. This report contains a complete historic overview of the crucial years 1982–1987 and the responsibility of the government. In the press the information was rather negatively reported. When some weeks later a weekly journal pointed out disagreements between persons in the blood transfusion world, the negative publicity was complete, we have to realize that. The patient asks for assurance that blood transfusions are a clinically highly safe therapeutic tool. With all the safety measures Blood Banks take, they should now give information to the people about the safety of the blood products. Campaigns, like the blood donation campaigns in earlier years, could be considered to create understanding and public awareness.

Nowadays the physician must inform the patient about diagnostic and therapeutic procedures. In the Netherlands, recently the Wet op de Geneeskundige Behandelingsovereenkomst has come into force. This "Law on a medical treatment agreement" forces the physician to provide this kind of information. This means that he has to tell the patient or his representative that he intends to give transfusions with blood components and what the benefits and possible hazards are. It is not the intention of the Law that the patient is harmed and made uneasy about blood transfusion. To my opinion standard information for patients who receive a blood transfusion, should be developed nationwide. This standard information should be written down in information leaflets for the various medical interventions where transfusion is regarded necessary. Thus working, in the same way as the information to the donors, patients will be informed and may ask the physician specific questions. In these leaflets on blood (and blood component therapy) the benefits should also be emphasized, including a realistic demonstration of the potential hazards.

One of the subjects of this symposium concerns the ethical aspects of the transfusion of blood. I am concerned about the fact that these aspects of ethics are under pressure nowadays. Years ago the Netherlands Red Cross advertised the benefits of being a donor of blood. Still, up to now, the Dutch donor is willing to give his blood twice a year for the benefit of patients he does not know. The only reimbursement of the donor is a cordial reception and a cup of coffee and a limited medical check-up. The Dutch donor still is a real volunteer and gives his blood for free. The psychological factor is that the donor relinquishes a part of himself to help other people. Otherwise one can not explain why donors are even willing to submit themselves to plasmapheresis or even become potential bone marrow donors. One has to be very careful with this "donor feeling":

- Donors, whose blood is used for scientific purpose should be informed about that.
- Donors, whose red cells are exported, because of the fact that only their plasma is used for factor VIII production should be informed and give their consent.
- Donors, whose plasma goes to pharmaceutical firms should give their consent.

A special word I like to say about the guidelines for donor selection. Recently there was a new discussion on the exclusion of risk groups, and the Minister of Health intervened. Exclusion criteria should never hurt potential donors. The purpose should be to exclude donors with risk behaviour instead of excluding entire groups for a certain or even indefinite number of years. Therefore good communication skills of the physician who examines the potential donor are of utmost importance. The Federation of Blood Banks will bring out a manual, but we have to notice that practical exercise of these communication techniques is necessary. A manual is not enough, physicians should be trained in communication techniques. In their contacts with potential donors the individual responsibility of the donor should be stressed. The patients who receive the blood donation do not consider the donation as a gift. Possibly this is an aspect to be propagated more intensely.

In the Netherlands there are still sufficient blood donors to fulfill the need for erythrocytes and platelets. Blood Banks have the task to consolidate this.

Despite all efforts by the Council for the Blood Transfusion, the Federation of Blood Banks and the Central Laboratory there is no agreement in the Netherlands about the organization. The Minister of Health is consulting leading persons in the blood transfusion world. She asked a special adviser, the economist Professor Koopmans, how the blood transfusion world should be organized. Should we go for the Finnish system with one organization, consisting of a big centralized blood bank with subsidiaries in the country? Or should we go for the English system with a National Blood Authority? Should we go for the French system with a direct governmental responsibility?

In my advice to the Minister of Health, I stressed that the dichotomy between Central Laboratory of the Red Cross and the twenty independent Blood Banks does not work any more. In my opinion there should be an organizational form that includes Central Laboratory and Blood Banks. Above this organizational form there should be National Authority mandated by the Minister of Health who could take a final decision in the case of divided opinions. Blood Banks should co-operate more, especially in the efficient use of laboratory equipment, and they should get the possibilities to increase their plasma production.

With a nationwide transfusion system, we can prevent that an in itself healthy system dies because of mutual disagreements.

Mr. Chairman, blood transfusion practice in the Netherlands needs protection of all the workers in the field. I open this special symposium in the conviction that your efforts are directed to this protection.

J. Verhoeff, MD
Chief Inspector for Public Health
The Netherlands

I. DEMAND AND SUPPLY

CUSTOMER-ORIENTED QUALITY SYSTEMS IN TRANSFUSION MEDICINE

D.E. Nevalainen

Introduction

In the mid 1990s the blood banking environment can be characterized by challenge, consolidation, change, and competition. Blood organizations that meet these challenges successfully will survive into the future. The historical service oriented approach to blood banking is being replaced by integrated quality control systems with an emphasis on total process control. The process changes that are taking place in blood banks today are every bit as dramatic as those which occurred in most manufacturing industries in the 1980s. Success will require a significant investment in documentation, training, technology, and systems in order to achieve the benefits that a quality system can bring. Additionally, a change in organizational culture will be required by many in the blood banking industry in order to assure success and survival into the future. In light of all these changes it is worthwhile focusing on "Who Is The Customer".

Discussion

In the historical evolution of medical care, transfusion medicine developed as a medical service that was provided by professionally trained medical people. The health care service model relied on personnel training in a professional environment with focus on patient service. In general, after primary professional training was done, people went to work in various institutions and organizations with their primary training as a foundation of their activities for years to come. This naturally led to people performing essential procedures in different ways, based upon their previous training and experience. Today's environment requires careful attention to consistent and repeatable process outcomes to ensure the safety of the blood supply. To accomplish that end, a system of process control and accountability for outcomes must be in place. The United States of America is attempting to accomplish these objectives under the label of Good Manufacturing Practice (GMP) described in the Code of Federal Regulations part 211 [1] and 606 [2], coupled with more specific requirements outlined in the FDA *Guidelines for Quality Assurance in Blood Establishments* [3], the American Association of

Consolidation also results in high throughout systems which require good quality to operate. The benefits of technology and automation can then contribute to increased quality.Blood Bank's *Quality Program* [4] and *Quality Systems in the Blood Bank and Laboratory Environment* [5]. Elsewhere similar programs are defined by *Richtlijn GMP voor Bloedbanken* [11] (the Netherlands) modeled after the EU document called "*The Rules Governing medicinal products in the European Community Volume IV. Guide to good manufacturing practice for medicinal products, Luxembourg, 1989*" [12].

The blood bank environment in the 1990s can be described by several "C" words such as Competition, Consolidation, Costs, and Compliance. In the US, competition for market share is a very real issue in some regions. Pricing differentials are being used to gain market share in some regions, and even encouraging territorial expansion into areas previously served by other blood centers. New blood banks are starting up to serve markets previously served by other blood centers [6]. Those blood banks that can deliver good products and reliable services at the lowest price will increase their market share as hospitals continue to look for cost savings.

Consolidation in the blood screening environment is dramatically demonstrated on Table 1. Note that approximately 70% of the blood donations in the United States is being screened at eleven laboratories. In addition to those eleven laboratories, there are a handful of other large independent blood centers, and a large number of smaller, and small ones. While all blood banks will have to make the investment required to gain the cost advantages that quality systems provide. If they survive they will most likely be affiliated with some other regional blood bank for their testing and perhaps other services. The small community blood bank as we know it today will look much different in the future. Consolidation is beginning to accelerate as cost pressures continue to escalate. Compliance to standards and guidelines is receiving high profile attention as both the public and government officials increase their scrutiny of blood bank operations. In this cost containment environment, consolidation is one way to reduce costs and improve productivity. By consolidating activities into fewer locations the opportunities for error are also reduced, thus contributing to increased levels of quality production.

Table 1. Distribution of Blood Screening Laboratories in the United States.

Organization	**Donations ($\times10^6$)**	**Laboratories**	**Fraction of total**
ARC	5.00	9.00	0.50
NYBC	1.20	1.00	0.12
UBS	1.20	1.00	0.08
Other	3.00	200+	0.30
Total US	10.00	211+	1.00

US = United States; ARC = American Red Cross; NYBC = New York Blood Center; UBS = United Blood Services; Others = the rest of the group.

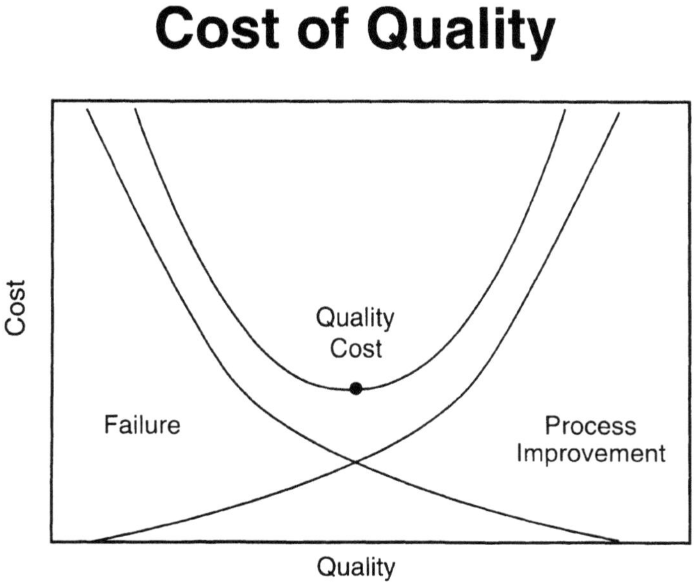

Figure 1. Minimum cost of quality.

Consolidation also results in high throughout systems which require good quality to operate. The benefits of technology and automation can then contribute to increased quality.

Compliance to standards implies more than just quality process standards, but also standards of practice in how blood and blood components are used. Studies have shown great variations in standards of practice within countries and within regions [13,14] and tracked mistakes and adverse outcomes [15–17]. Compliance to standards is the "new paradigm" of the 1990s. Clinical Practice pathways and standards are in development in many countries. Quality standards for the preparation of blood products include those set by regulatory agencies such as the Food and Drug Administration (FDA), Occupational Safety and Health Administration (OSHA), Environmental Protection Agency (EPA), professional associations (American Association of Blood Banks), State, regional and local authorities. Additionally, quality standards (ISO-9000) similar to those that are routinely used in manufacturing and service industries are beginning to be applied to blood banks [5,7–10]. High performance quality systems will be used by blood banks to improve productivity, lower overhead costs, and increase market share to ensure survival for those who implement it well. While it may be possible to run low volume operations with few process controls, it is almost impossible to run high throughput operations without good process controls and effective quality systems.

Understanding the cost of quality is the key to managing costs and provides a cost based rationale for redesigning production systems when coupled with process analysis [5]. A good activity based cost accounting system should be used

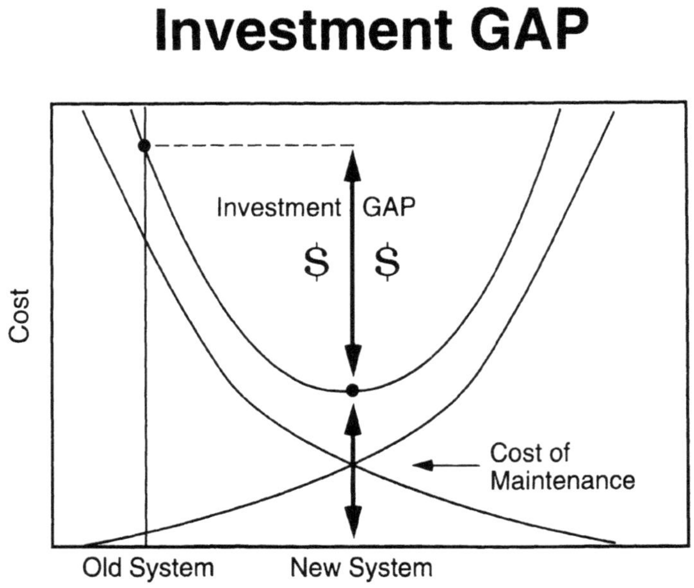

Figure 2. Investment gap. Old System - current blood bank organizations. New System = representative of a redesigned/highly productive blood bank of the future.

to fully assign costs to the point in production where they occur. Only then can process analysis focus on managing production cost. Prevention costs are defined as those costs incurred to prevent a failure from happening, making sure it will be done right before doing it. The fix is permanent and it is the least expensive way to operate. Appraisal costs are those costs incurred in checking, testing and evaluating products or services delivered, having someone check it after it is done. The fix is only temporary, for that one item checked, and is moderately expensive. Failure costs are those costs associated with understanding and resolving or correcting problems in products or services and includes lost time, rework, recalls, and related activities, or in short, doing it wrong, and then doing it over again.

The fix is too late, it is very costly, and may permanently damage customer confidence. Figure 1 shows that the lowest cost of quality is found at the point in which failure costs and process improvement costs are equal. At the point, further process improvement will again raise the cost of quality. Figure 2 demonstrates two hypothetical blood banks, one labelled "Old system" and one labelled "New System". The author believes that many blood banks are presently operating on the left side of the graph and incurring heavy failure costs due to poorly performing processes, products recalls, etc. With an appropriate investment in process improvement, it is possible to move the cost of quality to the right on the graph to achieve the lowest cost quality (New System). Looking at the graph it can be seen that the cost of maintaining the new system will be significantly less than the present cost of maintaining the old system. The difference between

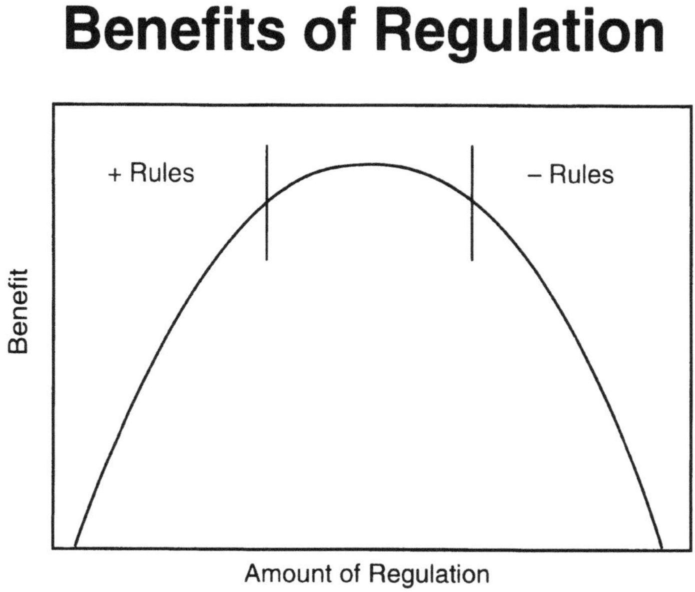

Figure 3. Benefits of regulation. Regulations are beneficial up to a point, beyond which we pay a price in cost, flexibility, or bureaucracy.

the two systems is called the "Investment Gap". It will take an investment in process improvement in order to move an organization to the right on the graph. That investment will be in some combination of people, money, documentation, training, technology, and infrastructure. Health care worldwide has been insulated from the quality movement that has swept the manufacturing sectors of the world economy. In today's environment, cost of quality is taking on an importance never before seen in health care. It is impossible to gain the benefits of quality without making an appropriate investment in the infrastructure of an organization to optimize and control all processes.

Compliance to standards goes beyond those standards promulgated by regulatory authorities, but includes appropriate voluntary quality standards as well such as ISO-9000 quality standards, the standards of the American Association of Blood Banks and the standards of the Federation of Dutch Red Cross Blood Banks. Compliance costs include costs associated with system audits and corrective actions (prevention cost), monitoring production for compliance to specifications (appraisal cost), and managing product failures with recalls, corrective action, regulatory responses, etc. (failure cost). A large part of the compliance costs can be seen to be associated with failure and appraisal costs due to poorly performing processes, weak document systems, and inadequate employee training. What is the failure cost of when measured in human life, or the transmission of hepatitis, HIV, etc? Complying with regulations is one built in cost that a regulated industry has to bear. Figure 3 compares the amount of regulation with the benefits gained from regulation. It can be seen that there is an optimum point

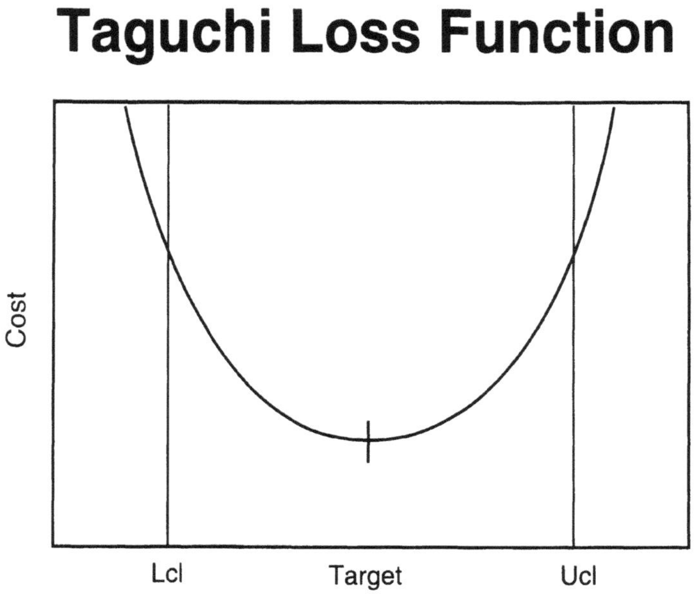

Figure 4. Taguchi loss function. All processes should be targeted to the center of their operational specifications/characteristics. Target the specification, not the range.

on the curve where regulation can maximize benefits, beyond which further regulation decreases benefits. It is the responsibility of the regulatory authorities, with input from the public and the blood bank community, to strive for optimization of regulation to ensure that the benefits of regulation are achieved. Over-regulation simply raises the cost and decreases the flexibility of the industry to adapt to new challenges. Another factor in the cost of quality equation and process control is characterized in Figure 4 (Taguchi loss function). Simply stated the cost of products and services, is minimum when processes are aimed at achieving specific targets for specifications or performance. Well defined and meaningful specifications and outcome objectives are necessary. When they have been defined, processes can then be designed to achieve those stated objectives. A process which operates at the target specification will be the cheapest to operate. As one moves in either direction towards the upper or lower specification limit, failure costs will go up. The medical device industry needs to target their manufacturing processes to provide the blood bank community with cost effective, rugged and reliable equipment. The blood bank community needs to design cost effective, reliable, high quality processes for the manufacturing of their products (blood and blood components). Doing so will help reduce, or keep cost of quality at the lowest possible levels.

In the grand picture, there is a balance that is necessary to achieve optimal quality at a reasonable price. Figure 5 shows the relationships between the public, the medical device industry, regulatory authorities, and the health care providers.

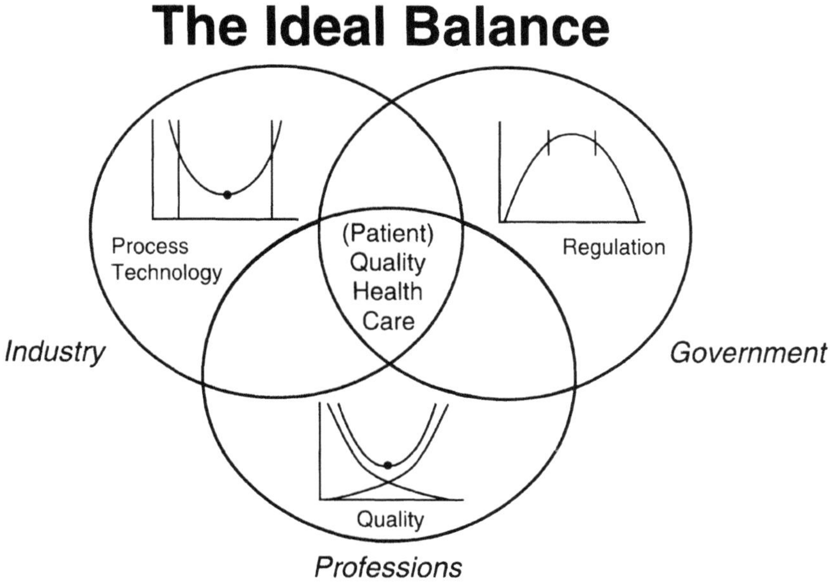

Figure 5. The ideal balance. Shared responsibilities between partners.

In an era of limited resources, it is necessary to optimize the cost of delivering quality health care. The overlapping circles in Figure 5 demonstrate the interdependence amongst the four groups mentioned. To the extent that the circles overlap and merge, we can see that the resources available for quality patient care can go up. To the extent that the circles have less overlap, there may be fewer resources available for patient care. Too much regulation increases costs to industry and to the health care providers. Poorly functioning equipment is not as cost effective as it could be for the health care providers, and tends to cause more regulatory oversight. Poorly designed and poorly performing processes in the blood bank industry tend to increase regulatory oversight, and high cost of quality due to persistent process failure.

The acceleration of consolidation and shared services requires increased use of validated computer systems for communication, information tracking, and data storage/retrieval. New systems are needed that are up to the task.

Conclusion

Implementation of high performance quality systems requires a focus upon good documentation, effective training, new technology, cost efficient processes, and a very good understanding of who our customer is? The next threshold of safety for the blood supply will come with effective implementation of process controls and quality systems. By doing this, all participants in the blood transfusion community will be renewing their commitment to the public that "quality of the blood supply" is still the number one objective of the blood industry. The public is the beginning and the end of the blood banking/transfusion process. It is necessary that we have good processes in place to manage the activities that occur from the pre-donation event through to the post transfusion monitoring of recipients and follow-ups as needed. Quality systems provide a pathway to follow in the quest for the safest blood possible. In the end analysis, quality in the transfusion community can be viewed as having "the right transfusion component, in the right place, at the right time, for the right clinical reasons, while maintaining safety within the parameters of biological limitations." With this definition as background perhaps we can now answer the question we raised in the beginning: "Who is the customer?" In a very real way we are all each others' customers. The recipient transfused is the ultimate customer or user of the transfusion product, but the public is also involved in the collection of the product. The rest of us are involved by the things we do and the decisions we make in processing, labelling, testing, and use of these products in therapeutic intervention. We can all look in the mirror and say thoughtfully, "I am the customer, and I am part of the solution." If I don't do it right, it won't get done.

References

1. Code of Federal Regulations. Food and Drug Administration. Current good manufacturing practice for manufacture, processing, packing or holding of drugs. CFR21-Part 210 and 211. August 1993.
2. Code of Federal Regulations. Food and Drug Administration. Current good manufacturing practice for blood and blood components. CFR21-Part 606. April 1992.
3. Center for Biologics Evaluation and Research. Food and Drug Administration. Guideline for quality assurance in blood establishments. Rockville, MD. 11 July, 1995.
4. The Quality Program. American Association of Blood Banks. Bethesda, MD, 1994.
5. Nevalainen DE, Callery MF. Quality systems in the blood bank and laboratory environment. American association of Blood Banks. Bethesda, MD, 1994.
6. Blood Bank Week. American Association of Blood Banks. 1 Sept 1995;33:12.
7. Nevalainen DE, Lloyd HL. ISO 9000 quality standards: A model for blood banking? Transfusion 1994;34:521-4.
8. Harvey H, Hewison C, Nevalainen DE, Lloyd HL. Maintaining quality in blood banking. Blood Reviews 1995;9:15-24.
9. Nevalainen DE, Callery MF. Quality systems and total process control in blood banking. Transfusion 1994;34:899-906.
10. Hoppe PA. Standards and external quality systems. In: Smit Sibinga CTh, Das PC, Heiniger HJ (eds). Good manufacturing practice in transfusion medicine. Kluwer Academic Publishers, Boston/Dordrecht/London 1994;177-94.
11. Richtlijn GMP voor Bloedbanken, College voor de Bloedtransfusie van het Nederlandse Rode Kruis, Amsterdam NL, September 1992.
12. The Roles Governing Medical Products in the European Community, Vol IV. Guide to Good Manufacturing Practice for Medicinal Products, Luxemburg, 1989.
13. The SANGUIS Study Group. Use of blood products for elective surgery in 43 European Hospitals. Transfusion Med 1994;4:251-68.

14. Sirchia G, Giovanetti AM, McClelland DBL, Fracchia GN. Safe and good use of blood in surgery (SANGUIS). European Commission, Luxembourg 1994.
15. Baele PL, De Bruyere M, Deneys V, et al. Bedside transfusion errors. A prospective survey by the Belgium SANGUIS Group. Vox Sang 1994;66:117-21.
16. Sazama K. Reports of 355 transfusions associated deaths: 1976 through 1985. Transfusion 1990;30:583-90.
17. Taswell HF. It's in the bag! (Or is it?) Transfusion 1991;131:386-7.

COMMUNICATION MECHANISMS BETWEEN THE BEDSIDE AND THE BLOOD BANK

A.W.M. Koopman-van Gemert, A. van de Wiel

Introduction

Transfusions of blood elements are important therapeutic procedures in daily medical practice which have contributed to the enormous expansion of possibilities in modern patient management. Larger and more complex operations have been made possible in surgery, while in non-surgical disciplines patients can be treated more intensively, for instance, in haematology and oncology. Transfusions have become part of a more total approach, which can be best described as supportive haemotherapy. This term is preferable over the term transfusion medicine since it is more adequately covering this entire area in modern patient care. It concerns a clinical discipline in which decisions on the nature and extent of therapy are mostly made at the bedside.

On the other hand, there has been an impressive increase in knowledge and technology within the blood banks, which have developed themselves from relatively small hospital departments into more or less autonomous institutes serving more than one hospital. Inevitably this often has resulted in an increased distance between the blood bank and the bedside. In order for the patient to have the full benefit of all the expertise accumulated thus far, good communication between all institutes involved is an absolute precondition.

Developments

Autonomous operation of blood banks on the one hand, and specific developments within clinical haematology on the other, have created a distance between blood bank and clinic.

The recruitment of donors, their medical examination, donation, processing and storage of blood products as well as all the safety aspects involved take place for the major part outside the scope of the hospital. Presently only a few clinicians fully realize the quality and safety demands made on blood products and the extent of tests done for this purpose. Also because of a more critical awareness of the population, there seems no end to this development and much of the time and work of blood bank employees is focused on the safety of their products.

In the clinical field another development concerning the safety of transfusions has taken place. Autologous blood transfusion programmes have been introduced to avoid the use of homologous blood as much as possible. To achieve the same goal new drugs have been developed, like growth factors and drugs improving haemostasis. However the most important development has been a more critical view on transfusions and the consciousness that transfusions are strictly not necessary under all circumstances.

Initially these developments seem to occur separately, but on careful examination they can only be successful when a close collaboration between the bedside and the blood bank has been established. A good example to prove this is the introduction of an autologous blood transfusion programme in a hospital. Although the wish to use autologous blood mostly comes from the patient or the physician, it can only be performed with the participation of the blood bank. The introduction of such a programme also illustrates the way several institutes involved have to communicate with each other.

Autologous blood transfusion programmes

An autologous blood transfusion implies that the patient is his own blood donor. Various forms of autotransfusion can be distinguished, for example, preoperative donation, the intra- and postoperative autotransfusion, and the preoperative hyper- and isovolemic haemodilution. Although the strictly medical indications for an autologous blood transfusion are limited, such as incompatibility, there is a growing demand for this form of transfusion from both patients and their physicians. This is for the most part based on arguments of safety, especially to avoid the transmission of viral infections and to prevent immunologic modulation. Particularly with a system like the preoperative blood donation, effective organization and communication are indispensable. Many initiatives have started enthusiastically but failed by lack of communication and logistical problems.

In the framework of an autologous blood transfusion programme the following persons, institutes and departments are involved:

- patient and physician;
- hospital organization i.e. the out-patient department, the administration of admissions and operating suites, surgical wards and the laboratory section;
- blood bank.

Upon acceptance of a patient for the programme at the out-patient department, the physician informs the administration of the hospital using a standard (green) form. This department plans the day of operation after consulting the operating rooms administration and informs both the surgical ward and the laboratory section.

The latter contacts the blood bank detailing all the information necessary, i.e. the day of operation, the number of units of blood to be collected and personal, medical and biochemical data of the patient. The blood bank schedules the patient for the phlebotomies, which occur in the blood bank. Since it concerns patients and not healthy donors, it is advantageous though not obligatory, when this blood bank facility is situated within or near the hospital.

A new development with a similar mutual dependency between bedside and blood bank is peripheral stem cell transplantation.

Communication

From this example of autologous blood transfusions, it can be concluded that communication between bedside and blood bank in daily practice is a communication between hospital laboratory and blood bank. The hospital laboratory is the area where blood products are temporary stored and from which they are distributed to the various wards. The clinician communicates with a representative of the laboratory staff rather than with the blood bank itself. A potential threat of this system is that clinicians take insufficient note of developments within the blood bank, while blood bank personnel are not in direct contact with the clinic and therefore loose sight of the developments at the bedside.

It is therefore strongly advisable to create within each hospital a blood transfusion team or committee including staff members from both surgical and non-surgical disciplines, representatives from the laboratory and hospital organization and at least one member of the blood bank staff. Such a team that meets at regular times should develop guidelines and protocols, advise members of the medical staff, communicate with the hospital organization and evaluate transfusion practice. In this manner, medical staff members are involved in transfusion practice and are regularly informed about progress in the blood bank world. The blood bank itself becomes again part of the hospital organization. Appointing a representative of the blood bank as a special member to the medical staff might even be considered.

Since, in the Netherlands, most if not all blood banks are responsible for delivering blood products to more than one hospital, they have a more or less regional function. This implicates that also on a regional level communication takes place between blood bank, physicians and hospital representatives. The instrument for this is a regional medical advisory committee that assists and advises the blood bank. This committee will especially control the quality aspects of the work performed by the blood bank and seek to implement national guidelines in the various hospitals.

Conclusion

While, on the one hand, certain developments within the blood bank world and clinical medicine have created a greater distance between the two, other developments have shown clearly that a close collaboration and reduction of this distance is necessary. Today's patients demand excellent, safe products with maximal expertise from both clinician and blood bank involved. This can only be achieved with efficient communication between the institutes.

Representatives of the blood bank have to possess and strive to gain insight into clinical developments, while clinicians have to be continually informed concerning the essentials of the blood bank. Such a communication can be best established by the institution of a blood transfusion team or committee in every hospital with representatives from medical staff, laboratory and hospital organization, and blood bank. Such a team approach with insight and respect for each other's needs and knowledge is essential to be able to anticipate new developments and to allow optimal haemotherapeutic support.

Acknowledgement

The authors wish to thank Ms. M.A. Kopecky for critical review of the text.

INFORMED CONSENT FOR TRANSFUSION RECIPIENTS: HOW MUCH IS ENOUGH?

P.V. Holland

Introduction

Transfusion of blood and blood components is usually performed to help patients with illnesses where there is an acute or chronic need for one or more elements of the blood. However, like all medical and surgical therapies, blood transfusions carry both potential benefits and possible risks. Patients need to be informed of the reasons for their impending transfusions, along with the expected benefit and potential risks of this form of therapy. True informed consent is only possible for elective or planned transfusions for blood and components, which are not given in emergency or urgent situations [1]. When there is insufficient time to explore the rationale and alternatives, as well as potential harm from the transfusion, or where the patient is unable to comprehend the process of informed consent, then, it may be deleted or, when time permits, provided to a parent or guardian who is acting on behalf of the patient [2,3].

Definition of informed consent

To properly provide informed consent, e.g., for a transfusion, a patient must be informed and consent [4,5]. "Informed" means that the patient, or guardian, has been given sufficient information to make an intelligent choice. "Consent" means that the patient is competent and free to consent, or to agree to the transfusion. Informed consent may be an oral or written process. An oral process is preferred, i.e., a dialogue with patients to ensure that they are properly informed, their questions are answered, and they truly give consent to the procedure. However, written informed consent is useful for documentation and legal proof, whether this is a form or a chart note. The most important point of informed consent is that it is a "process, not a single event in time, marked by the patient's signing of a formal document." [6] The dialogue, which goes on between the patient and the knowledgeable individual seeking informed consent, is the important process. A formal document which provides proof of informed consent is just that, evidence that it has been obtained.

While blood transfusion used to be considered merely incident to medical and surgical therapies, it is clear that it is a treatment in and of itself. As such, it can be considered an "invasive procedure" [7]. Therefore, it should merit its own procedure-specific consent process, which is separate from any blanket authorization covering routine measures provided to hospitalized patients. Thus, it should not be incident to the consent for a surgical procedure, or for a course of chemotherapy. Transfusion consent should be a separate process covering its own benefits, risks and alternatives. Further, this process should be documented, e.g., by a form, or some notation in the patient's chart, that the process has been carried out and the patient has consented (or refused) transfusion therapy.

The process of informed consent has a number of important elements [6]. These are detailed in Figure 1. The process begins with providing information to the patient about the need for transfusion of blood, blood components, or blood derivatives. The second element is an explanation of what the expected effect will be with the transfusion, along with the potential, significant risks. In effect, the patient needs to know why the transfusion is being recommended or ordered, as well as the anticipated effect, hopefully a beneficial one, for the patient. As for the risks, patients do not need to know each and every risk of the transfusion [8]. However, they do need to know about those which are frequent (1% or greater), or "significant." "Significant" means those risks which carry serious morbidity or mortality. Patients should be given time to consider these risks and how they may be minimized. Only in an emergency, may this process be deleted, where it is deemed the patient may not survive without blood transfusion therapy. The patient should have an opportunity to ask questions about any and all aspects of the anticipated transfusion. They should be told of all alternatives, including the alternative of not being transfused, by the physician or person providing the information; this person should reinforce the expected benefit by pointing out the potential risk to the patient if transfusions are not given. Certainly, advice without coercion should be given to the person needing a transfusion. Finally, there should be documentation of the consent, or the refusal of the patient to consent, to the type of transfusion available.

1. Providing information
2. Expected benefits and potential risks
3. Time for consideration (except in emergencies)
4. Opportunity to ask questions
5. Offering alternatives
6. Advice (without coercion) re treatment
7. Documentation of consent/refusal

Figure 1. The process of informed consent.

Change in elements of transfusion consent

For years, the major risks of transfusion were viral hepatitis and haemolytic transfusion reactions. The former was relatively common, but the latter could result in an immediate fatality. Most other risks were unappreciated, or quite remote. Thus, in the early 1980's, telling a patient about viral hepatitis and a haemolytic transfusion reaction could be the essence of the risk discussion for blood transfusions. Patients were advised of the reasons for the transfusion, and any alternatives which were reasonably available. This process was relatively simple and straightforward and would often be completed as part of the overall medical or surgical treatment plan.

When the acquired immune deficiency syndrome (AIDS) became accepted as a risk of a transfusion, especially with its potential of death, then, this risk, albeit rare, was added to the informed consent process for blood transfusions. Certainly, for elective, surgical procedures, options impacting the risk of transfusion-associated AIDS (TAA), such as autologous or patient-designated blood, should also have been provided, along with the expected outcome if the patient refused transfusions altogether. The anticipated transfusion risks were provided, but placed in the context of the overall risks of the patient's medical or surgical treatment.

In the later 1980's, it became clear that recommendations were being made regarding obtaining a *separate* informed consent before transfusion. This was recommended by the American Association of Blood Banks in 1986, even if they could not address it in their *Standards* [9]. The primary reason for this is that *Standards* applied to blood banks and transfusion services, and not to physicians who ordered transfusions and were deemed mainly responsible for obtaining informed consent.

In our regional blood centre, where we provide out-patient transfusions, or use transfusion therapy as part of other procedures, e.g., therapeutic apheresis, we elected to have an abbreviated transfusion consent, in addition to whatever informed consent process the patient's primary physician had performed. In March of 1987, we added to our consent that, "the risk of AIDS, although very remote, cannot be completely eliminated, with current testing and blood screening methods." While we believed the risk to be minute with the multiple means we had in place, nonetheless, patients were concerned about this risk. If infected with the virus of AIDS, the human immunodeficiency virus (HIV), there was a high likelihood of significant morbidity and eventual mortality. We periodically revise our informed consent and try to make it as up-to-date and appropriate as possible. In addition, we have a witness verify that information has been provided to the patient about to undergo an elective transfusion.

To make sure that patients understand, we also provide a notice to them about receiving transfusions, so that they have something in writing to refer to, should there be some complication of the transfusion. We provide a list of the signs or symptoms which may occur during, or following, the transfusion, as well as the possibility that hepatitis may develop within six months subsequent to the transfusion. Patients are asked to notify their own physician, as well as the blood centre, if any of these occur after the transfusion.

Alternatives to transfusion

The major alternative to a transfusion is the lack of one. Thus, it should be clearly explained to patients, what their anticipated risk would be, if the transfusion of blood or blood components is not given. For example, in major surgical procedures, the risk of anaemia or blood loss may be marked and result in increased mortality in the perioperative period for those patients who refuse transfusions [10]. The risk of mortality increases with the degree of anaemia and the amount of blood loss in the perioperative period. Patients who undergo similar major surgical procedures, but who receive transfusions, have much lower risks of dying in the perioperative period [11]. In many cases, the risks of the procedure, including anaesthesia and the disease for which the patient is undergoing surgery, far exceed the minute risks of transfusions today.

For elective, upcoming surgery with anticipated blood loss, autologous transfusions (AT) are an important option for patients and a viable alternative to allogeneic (homologous) blood. If there is time, and they have sufficient haemoglobin, they may donate one or more units of blood for upcoming, elective surgical procedures with anticipated significant blood loss. This is clearly the safest option for patients, but it is not entirely risk free [12]. Intraoperative and postoperative salvage of shed blood are other means of AT, returning patient's blood to them.

Many patients believe that they can select safer donors than can a blood centre. Thus, they may request that their relatives or friends be their donors, i.e., patient-directed or patient-selected donors. There is no evidence that these individuals are any safer that the volunteer, unpaid, altruistic individuals recruited by blood centres. In fact, there is some evidence that these individuals may actually increase risk for their own selected patients, especially if they are relatives [13, 14]. There is pressure on such individuals to donate, especially if they have not been a regular volunteer donor previously. In addition, persons who sell their blood, so called "paid donors," also present a higher risk for transfusion recipients, for example, in the transmission of viral hepatitis [14]. They may not be as truthful about revealing risk factors for HIV infection and hepatitis, for example. To help patients with these different transfusion choices for elective, surgical procedures, we prepared a video for use in surgeons' offices. The video, entitled "An Informed Choice," has an accompanying brochure; in about ten minutes, the video explains the benefits and risks of allogeneic, autologous, and patient-directed blood transfusions.

Significant risks of a transfusion

The patient should be told about transfusion risks which occur with a reasonable degree of frequency, for example, one percent or greater ($\geq 1\%$). Patients may be told that about 1% of transfusions may cause fever, chills, or urticaria (hives). These are common, and usually not life-threatening; but if the patient is aware of them ahead of time, when they do occur, they are not fearful of these minor risks. Certainly, a haemolytic transfusion reaction is always a possibility, especially if the wrong blood is given to a patient. Even though this risk is remote, approximately 1 in 12,000 transfusions in the USA, if it is not recognized, about 1 in 10 patients may die due to this complication [15]. Viral hepatitis is certainly a much lower risk than it was 15 or 20 years ago [14]. At the moment, the current risk of viral hepatitis of any type (—)B, C, as well as non -A, B and C(—) is no more than 1 in 5,000 per unit of volunteer blood.

Patients fear most the risk of AIDS from transfusions. With our recruitment of volunteer donors, screening procedures and excellent tests in place, this risk of HIV infection is really quite remote today. The current estimate in the United States is that about 1 in 450,000 units of blood may, nonetheless, transmit HIV despite all of our efforts. To further reduce this chance, blood banks in the United States will soon be performing HIV-antigen testing. The rationale for this is that we will identify a proportion (approximately one-quarter) of those individuals who are in the "window" period of HIV infection, and may not be detected by the very sensitive HIV antibody tests in place. However, it is also possible that more individuals at risk of AIDS will come into blood centres to seek "the new AIDS test" and may actually increase the risk of HIV in the blood supply.

Neither the risk of transfusion-associated AIDS nor any of the other risks of a transfusion can be made zero. One cannot reduce all risks of anything to zero. "Life is not and cannot be free of risk" [2]. One intent of the process of informed consent for transfusions is that patients will understand the minute not zero risk of this beneficial, and actually very safe, form of therapy.

Medical/legal considerations

Unfortunately, one of the main reasons today why people seek informed consent for transfusion is to prove, in any subsequent legal action, that it has been obtained [3]. The reason should really be to provide the patient with information about anticipated transfusions, their benefits, alternatives and potential risks. Today, however, there must be proof that this has been done, so that in a future, legal suit, the physician, as well as others involved in providing transfusions, have given the patient appropriate informed consent before the transfusion was performed.

A number of legal cases in the United States have been filed on the basis of the failure of transfusion informed consent, or failure of full informed consent. If there is documentation in the record, whether it is a form being signed, or a notation in the chart, then this is an excellent defense for health care providers [3].

The element of informed consent, which is of most concern to the courts, is whether or not the risks were disclosed to the patient. While, in general, the disclosed risks must be relevant, i.e., have a reasonable chance of resulting in severe morbidity or mortality, a recent ruling has proven to be of help to defendants in these cases. In a case entitled, Gibson v. Methodist Hospital, a transfusion-associated AIDS case, the Texas Supreme Court, in 1993, stated that, "the undisclosed risk must be material enough to influence a reasonable person to withhold consent to the procedure" [16]. This is often difficult to prove in hindsight, but is an important point to make. Would the patient have proceeded with the transfusion, or the medical/surgical therapy with the need for transfusion, if the risk were remote? Would knowledge of a minute risk have made any difference? Further, in this same case, the Texas Court stated that the plaintiff must show that the injury was caused by the failure of informed consent.

Many physicians to this day do not get "formal" informed consent for transfusion [17]. This includes individuals who provide many transfusion therapies, such as haematologists and oncologists, as well as surgeons [18]. While a formal informed consent may not be necessary, there needs to be a *process* of informed consent, a discussion of the risks and benefits plus alternatives of transfusion, with documentation in the chart. In Figure 2 is a summary of what the informed transfusion recipient should expect as part of the informed consent process before transfusion of blood, blood components or blood derivatives.

1. Description of procedure in lay terms
2. Expected benefit: Outcome without transfusion
3. Reasonably foreseeable adverse consequences
4. Opportunity to ask questions
5. Time to provide information
6. Ability to comprehend

Figure 2. "Informed" transfusion recipient.

Conclusion

Like all medical and surgical therapies, blood transfusions carry both potential benefits and risks. Patients about to undergo elective transfusions should be properly informed about, and consent to, this treatment option. For emergency or urgent transfusions, there usually is not time to obtain full informed consent (appraisal of all alternatives and the beneficial attributes and risks of each); further, patients may not be able to be truly informed or give consent in such situations. For patients unable to provide consent because of their age or mental status, a parent or guardian should be informed of the transfusion options and be given the opportunity to ask any questions.

The informed consent process, when feasible, should be performed by a knowledgeable individual, preferably by the treating physician, and should be documented in the patient's chart. For non-emergent transfusions, patients should be simply told the benefits and risks of allogeneic blood (from volunteer, paid or patient directed sources) versus autologous donations, as well as the option of other alternatives, including refusing transfusions altogether (as do some Jehovah's Witnesses). Only with sufficient knowledge of the various transfusion options and alternatives, their anticipated need and benefits, plus the current risks of each, can a patient, or a guardian, make an intelligent and informed decision regarding transfusions of blood, blood components, or blood derivatives.

Patients do not need to know *every* risk of each transfusion option, but they do need to know about frequent (1% or greater) and significant ones (those carrying a risk of serious morbidity or mortality) plus the risks involved in *not* being transfused. When the benefits of transfusion outweigh the risks of anaemia or the risks of the disease without benefit of blood components, patients should be encouraged to receive the safest blood or blood component that is reasonably available. If provided enough information, in a timely and understandable fashion, patients will be informed about (understand) their need for transfusions and can then properly consent to them.

References

1. Rennie D. Informed consent by "well-nigh abject" adults. N Engl J Med 1990;302:917-18.
2. Keeney RL. Sounding board: Decisions about life-threatening risks. N Engl J Med 1994;331:193-96.
3. Piper A. Truce on the battlefield: A proposal for a different approach to medical informed consent. J Law Med Ethics 1994;22:301-17.
4. Drane JF. Competency to give an informed consent: A model for making clinical assessments. JAMA 19 1984;252:925-27.
5. Ingelfinger FJ. Informed (but uneducated) consent. N Engl J Med 1972;287:465-66.
6. Curran WJ. Forward. In: Rozovsky FA (ed). Consent to treatment: A practical guide. 2nd ed Boston: Little, Brown & Co., 1990
7. Rozovsky FA. Consent to treatment: A practical guide. Supplement 1.12.4, 1991:4.
8. Curran WJ. Law-medicine notes. Informed consent in malpractice cases: A turn toward reality. N Engl J Med 1986;314:429-31.
9. Holland PV, Schmidt PJ (eds). Standards for Blood Banks and Transfusion Services. 12th ed Arlington, VA: AABB, 1987.
10. Carson JL, Spence RK, Poses RM, Bonavita G. Severity of anemia and operative mortality and morbidity. Lancet 1988;i:727-29.
11. Busch ORC, Hop WCK, Hoynck van Papendrecht MAW, Marquet RL, Jeckel J. Blood transfusions and prognosis in colorectal cancer. N Engl J Med 1993;328:1372-76.
12. Haditsch M, Binder L, Gabriel C, Muller-Uri P, Watschinger R, Mittermayer H. *Yersinia enterocolitica* septicemia in autologous blood transfusion. Transfusion 1994;34:907-9.
13. Ohto H, Yasuda H, Noguchi M, Abe R. Risk of transfusion-associated graft-versus-host disease as a result of directed donations from relatives. Transfusion 1992;32:619-92.
14. Aach RD, Lander JJ, Sherman LA, et al. Transfusion-transmitted viruses: Interim analysis of hepatitis among transfused and non-transfused patients. In: Vyas GN, Cohen SN, Schmid R (eds). Viral hepatitis: A contemporary assessment of etiology, epidemiology, pathogenesis and prevention. Philadelphia: Franklin Institute Press, 1978:383-96.
15. Linden JV, Paul B, Dressler KP. A report of 104 transfusion errors in New York State. Transfusion 1992;32:601-6.

16. Gibson v. Methodist Hospital. Texas Supreme Court, 1993. Texas Medicine 1993;89: 55-56.
17. Capen K. Informed consent and blood transfusion: What does Krever's interim report mean to doctors? Can Med Assoc J 1995;152:1663-65.
18. Faber-Langedoen K. Testimony before FDA Panel on June 6, 1995; CCBC Newsletter, June 23, 1995:9.

FACTORS THAT INFLUENCE DEMAND FOR TRANSFUSION

D.B.L. McClelland

Definitions

It may be helpful to start by defining two conventions that will be used in this paper.

Demand: The products and services that the provider of blood is called on to supply.

Need: The products and services that are needed for the effective care of the patient population concerned.

Demand is broadly equal to the sum of need and inappropriate or ineffective requests, including the effect of inefficiencies due to the supply system.

Constituents of demand – a classification

The elements to be considered are the patient, the clinician, the supply system and the providers and purchasers of health care.

The *patient* has expectations and fears that may vary with the individual's age, culture, education and experience. A prime influence on the patient's views is the mass media coverage of transfusion, especially safety issues.

The *clinician* is motivated by the professional wish to do the best for the patient in the light of knowledge, experience, the prevailing authority systems and fear of litigation. Influences on the clinician's decisions include the effect of continuing professional education, commercial marketing, clinical guidelines, peer group comparisons and values and in some instances, pressure exerted by patients.

The *supply system* will deliver according to factors that include: the availability of donors and other essential resources, the presence or absence of incentives within the payment system that create pressure to sell more product and the marketing efforts of certain commercial suppliers.

The *health care provider* who uses blood and the *health care purchaser* influenced increasingly by economic constraints and output target. Providers may also be strongly influenced by their assessment of exposure to risk of litigation arising from real or supposed errors and accidents during treatment episodes.

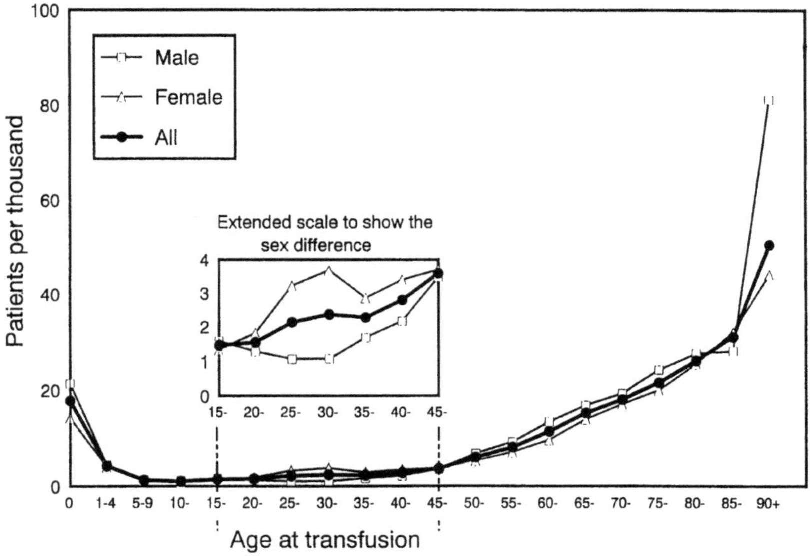

Figure 1. With increasing age above 45 years, there is a steady upward trend in the proportion of the population who receive one or more red cell transfusions in a given year. The implications are illustrated in Figure 2.

Influences on both need and supply

Demographic change

This affects both donor and patient populations. As the population continues to age for the next decade or more, we should anticipate increasing difficulties in maintaining adequate numbers of donors. Furthermore, as Figure 1 illustrates, the utilization of red cell transfusion increases progressively with advancing age so that the per capita use will inevitably continue to rise with population ageing, unless there are substantial changes in prescribing practice for these elderly patients.

Safety expectations

The progressive introduction of more stringent criteria for donor selection has the effect of increasing the refusal or deferral of volunteers. Another, less obvious consequence, but one which may have even more profound effect on the blood supply is the de-motivating effect of intrusive questioning and frequent deferral. Previously committed volunteers may conclude that it is no longer a good experience to attend. Secondly one result of new safety tests on blood that is donated is to increase the losses of donations in the production process, further threatening the adequacy of future supplies (Figure 2).

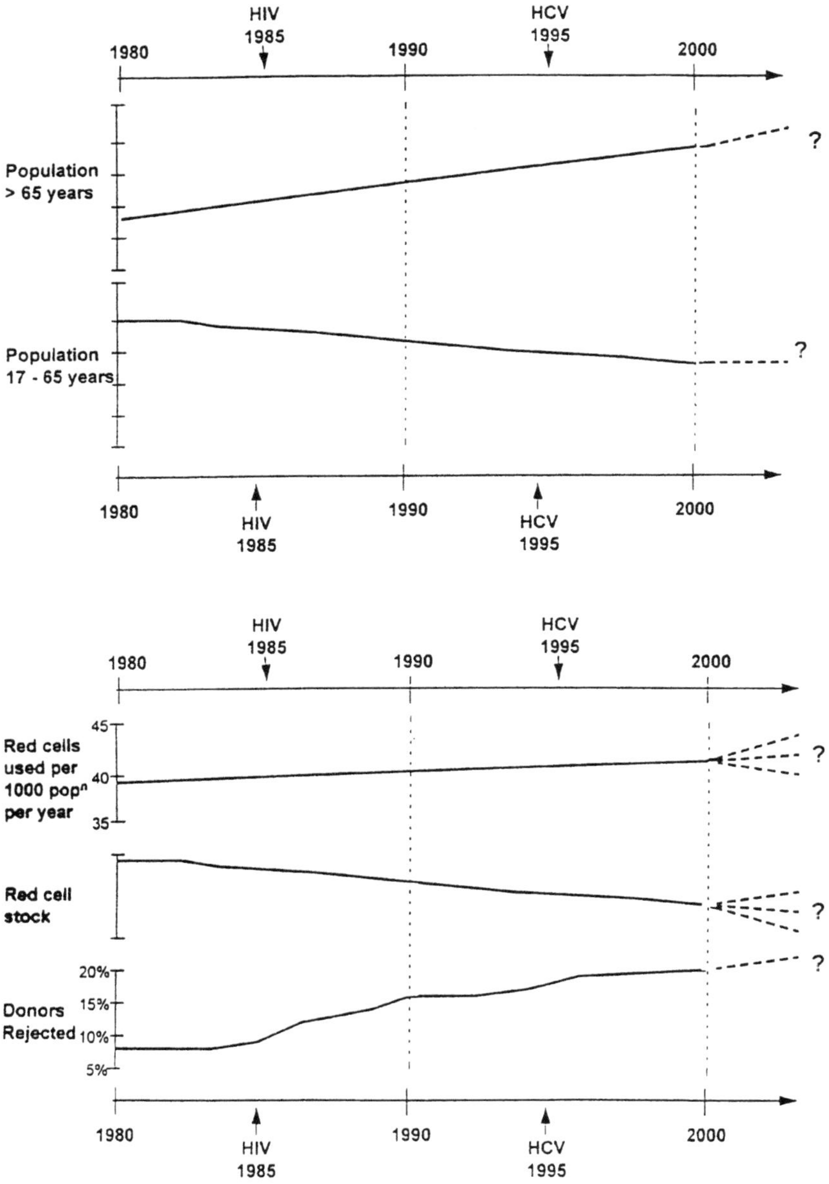

Figure 2. This figure summarizes the critical trends in projecting red cell supply and demand. Population change will increase need and reduce supply. Donor rejection rates will increase. Combined with a slow upward trend in red cell need due to demographic change, the overall result will be shortage, reflected in falling stock levels.

Together these trends suggest strongly that the clinical need for red cells (and for adjunctive interventions such as autologous transfusion and erythropoietin) will continue to increase in the face of a declining availability of donated blood. Supply will decline in relation to need and shortage situations, where need exceeds supply will become more common even in countries where supplies have traditionally been adequate.

Defining clinical need

How much do we really know about clinical need? There are few if any reports describing the clinical epidemiology of red cell transfusion for large, representative patient populations. The study from which Figure 1 [1,2] is taken records the actual transfusion of red cells in a population of 2.4 million over a period of four years and provides the first comprehensive picture of the age and gender related consumption of red cells, reflecting current patterns of practice in a Northern European setting. Data such as these will be required as a basis for future planning.

However, this will only tell us about the overall use of blood by a large population of prescribers, and we already know that there are very large variations in clinical practice among different hospitals and clinical teams or individual clinicians [3]. Chalmers [4] and other authors have pointed out that of all clinical interventions, only about one third have actually been proved to be effective in terms of offering real improvements in clinical outcome as demonstrated by well conducted randomized controlled clinical trials.

Red cell transfusion is just like many other commonly practised interventions – there are no trials that tell us what is the most effective practice in most of the commonest clinical situations in which the treatment is used.

This topic is further considered in Dr Murphy's paper in this volume[1], so only two further points are made here. Firstly, we face a major challenge in designing, funding and carrying out the trials needed to provide a firm basis of evidence for red cell transfusion practice guidelines. Secondly, there is no prospect of the results of definitive trials being available for several years. In the meantime, there is still a great deal that we can do to improve the match between clinical demand and clinical need and in doing so to improve care *and* reduce demands on the scarce resource of volunteers donors.

Variations in practice

It is an uncomfortable fact that if one was awaiting for an elective operation such as hip replacement, one could choose from teaching hospitals in the EU where the chance of receiving a perioperative transfusion of donor blood was 100%, one where the chance of transfusion was 30%, or anything in between these two extremes (Table 1). Also one would discover that there are hospitals where most

1. Murphy WG. Factors effecting the clinical efficacy of blood transfusion. pp. 65-72.

the chance of receiving a perioperative transfusion of donor blood was 100%, one where the chance of transfusion was 30%, or anything in between these two extremes (Table 1). Also one would discover that there are hospitals where most patients can and do pre-deposit their own blood for surgery and others where this is never done. Figure 3 illustrates the first statement [3].

This interesting situation persists even though all the clinicians concerned have access to clinical guidelines and many other sources of information about current practice and about the range of options available to support blood conservation. While it is important to stress that the available clinical guidelines do not reflect the strictest standards of evidence, there can be little doubt that if they were widely followed, the present wide variations in blood use could be drastically reduced towards the lower end of the range. At the present time, there is no evidence to suggest that conservative use of transfusion according to current guidelines would lead to less good clinical outcomes [5-10].

Changing practice patterns

It is well known that the simple dissemination of information is unlikely to produce changes in clinicians' practice [11], so if we are serious about moving towards a more optimal pattern of blood prescribing, a serious and sustained campaign will be needed. Indeed we might do well to re-define the product of

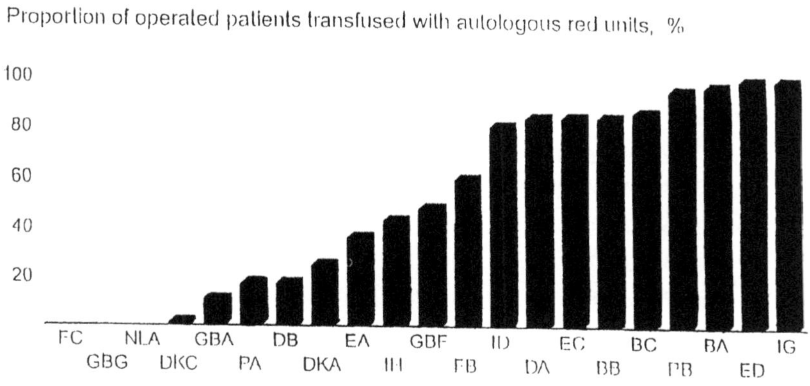

Figure 3. Corronary artery bypass grafts – the use of autologous transfusion. Hospitals vary greatly in the extent to which autologous transfusion is used. This figure is modified from Figure 5.9 (p. 143) of reference 3.

the transfusion services. Our product in future should be *the optimal use of blood* and we should be prepared to market this product drawing on all the skills and techniques of the marketing profession to identify those that will help to achieve and sustain the changes in practice that are needed.

The next section mentions one approach that may contribute to such a campaign. This and other ways of attempting to change practice patterns will require to be carefully evaluated, since there is little merit in interesting initiatives that fail to achieve the required result, and at a reasonable cost.

Practice indicators

Since clinicians may be expected to take an active interest in how their own practice compares with that of their peers, they may be motivated by the regular availability of concise, relevant and up to date information on transfusion in their own unit as compared to those of their colleagues. In the case of surgical units these data may be quite challenging since it may well be considered that the typical amount of blood transfused for a given type of procedure is one important marker of the overall quality of practice of the surgical team.
The main characteristics of a serviceable practice indicator are:

- Constructed from data that are regularly recorded in routine process of care and are quantitative and reliable;
- Clinically relevant.

From the experience of the SANGUIS study [3], it is possible to derive several potentially useful indicators of red cell transfusion practice using only the information routinely recorded for haemoglobin or haematocrit value and the record of all red cell units transfused. These are:

- Units of red cells transfused per patient operated (Table 1).

Table 1. The extremes of variation in the use of red cell transfusion for 5 elective surgical procedures in European teaching hospitals [3].

	Transfused % of operated patients	**Red cell units per transfused patient**	**Red cell units per operated patient**
Colectomy	0- 79 (41)	1-4 (2)	0.3 (1)
TURP	0- 46 (17)	1-3 (2)	0-1 (0,5)
CABG	17-100 (88)	1-5 (4)	0-6 (3)
AAA	64-100 (83)	2-7 (3)	1-7 (3)
THR	29-100 (81)	2-5 (3)	0-5 (2)

– "Avoidable" red cell transfusion (Table 2).

Table 2. The concept of a practice indicator for "avoidable" red cell transfusion and the extreme values of this indicator found in the SANGUIS Study [3].

"Avoidable" red cell transfusion	Red cell units given that result in a discharge Hct >33% (or any other chose value)	
"Avoidable" red cell transfusion in total hip replacement (43 hospitals)	"Avoidable" red cells (1 or more units)	
	Lowest 23%	Highest 82%

This is based on the last haematocrit recorded for the patient and the total number of red cell units transfused. Taking a chosen value of haemoglobin, say 11 g/dl, as an acceptable level for that patient prior to discharge from hospital, it is simple to estimate the number of units red cells that were probably given unnecessarily. Using this approach, Goodnough [12] found that about 25% of patients had received one or more units of red cells than were required. Data from the SANGUIS study show that up to 50% of red cell recipients had been transfused to a level above 11 g/dl.

– "Big bleed" indicator (Table 3).

Table 3. The concept of a practice indicator to show the consistency/inconsistency of red cell use for a particular procedure in a given hospital. The lower panel shows the range of variation for this indicator, for hip replacement operations. On the SANGUIS Study [3].

"Big bleeds"	Number of operated patients who receive more than twice the median number of red cell units for that procedure and hospital	
SANGUIS "Big bleed/big transfusion" in THR	% of patients receiving >2 x median number of red cell units	
	Lowest 62%	Highest 10%

This is based on the variability of red cell use for patients undergoing a given procedure. In the SANGUIS data we found that there were some hospitals in which the number of red cell units used for a given procedure was very uniform, with no patients ever receiving more than twice that hospital's median transfusion for that operation. In contrast, there were hospitals where a substantial proportion of patients received more than twice the hospital's median quantity of blood. This type of variation is probably more indicative of differing approaches to the conduct of surgery than of differences in transfusion policies.

– Change in haemoglobin haematocrit (Table 4).

Table 4. Fall in Hct from preoperative to discharge (Delta Hct). Peri-operative change in haematocrit or haemoglobin provides a part of the picture for the red cell loss and support of a surgical patient. The table shows the extent to which different hospitals achieved different values for this indicator [3].

	Smallest	**Greatest**
AAA	−2	− 9
Colectomy	+1	− 6
CABG	−4	−11
THR	−3	−10

One measure of the overall haemoglobin balance of the patient during an episode of surgery is the change in haematocrit or haemoglobin from the time of admission to the last recorded value. It is evident that different surgical teams achieve very different results in this respect, whether according to explicit guidelines or not we do not know. Together with the other indicators, this information provides a broad picture of the transfusion behaviour of a surgical team, ranging from those who transfuse little and yet achieve only a small drop in haemoglobin to the other extreme of those who transfuse a lot, and whose patients still experience a large drop in haemoglobin.

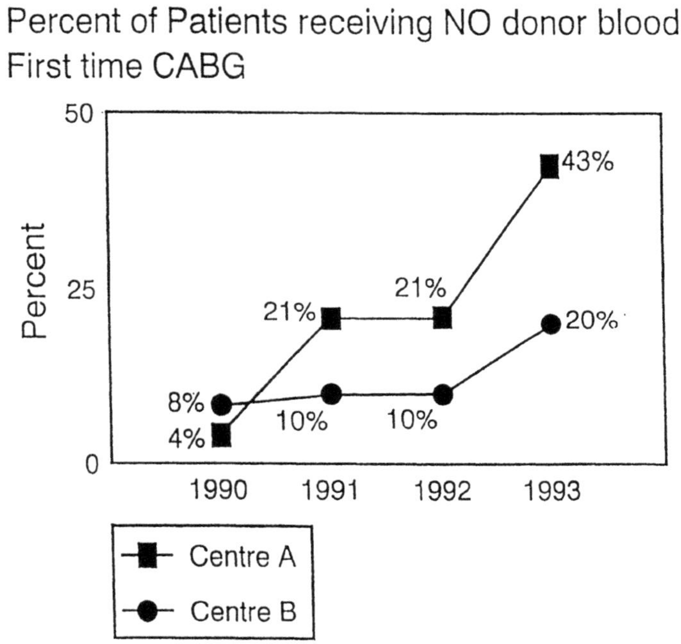

Figure 4. Changing use of red cells for CABG in two centres.

Can change in transfusion practice be achieved?

Striking changes in the use of red cell transfusion *can* be achieved. Figure 4 shows data from two similar units serving a uniform population for coronary artery bypass grafting. Over the four year period, one has progressively increased the proportion of patients who received no blood at all during the episode, whereas the other has maintained a rather constant pattern of red cell uses. Unfortunately, although there are many cross-sectional studies on the variations in transfusion practice between centres, there appear to be few longitudinal studies that document the year on year trends for individual units. These studies are essential if we are to develop a better understanding of the factors that lead to the achievement of *sustainable* changes in practice.

References

1. McClelland DBL, Moores HM, Phillips P. Demography of recipients of red cell transfusion in eastern Scotland, 1991-94. (1996, in preparation).
2. Phillips P, Moores M, Picken M, McClelland DBL. Who gets red cells? Abstract of presentation. Surgical Audit Meeting, London (1996, to be completed).
3. Sirchia G, Giovanetti AM, McClelland DBL, Fracchia GN. Safe and good use of blood in surgery (SANGUIS). Use of blood products and artificial colloids in 43 European hospitals. Luxembourg, European Commission, 1994.
4. Chalmers I, Enkin M, Keirse MJNC. Effective care in pregnancy and childbirth: A synopsis for guiding practice and research. In: Chalmers I, Enkin M, Keirse MJNC (eds). Effective care in pregnancy and childbirth. Oxford University Press, Oxford 1989:1465-77.
5. Carson JL, Willet LR. Is a haemoglobin of 10 g/dl required for surgery. Med Clin of North America 1993;77:335-47.
6. Peri-operative red blood cell transfusion. Consensus Conference. JAMA 1988;260: 2700-3.
7. Lunn JN, Elwood PC. Anaemia and surgery. Brit Med J 1970;3:71-3.
8. Rawstron ER. Anaemia and surgery. A retrospective clinical study. Aust NZ J Surg 1970;39:425-32.
9. Johnson RG, Thurer RL, Kruskall MS, et al. Comparison of two transfusion strategies after elective operations for myocardial revascularization. J Thorac Cardiovasc Surg 1992;104:307-14.
10. Consensus statement on red cell transfusion. Proceedings of a consensus conference held by the Royal College of Physicians of Edinburgh. Brit J Anaest 1994;73:857-59.
11. Russell I, Grimshaw J. The effectiveness of referral guidelines: A review of the methods and findings of published evaluations. In: Roland M, Coulter A (eds). Hospital referrals. Oxford General Practice Series no. 22. Oxford University Press, Oxford 1992:179-211.
12. Goodnough LT, Vizmeg K, Riddell J IV, Soegiarso RW. Discharge haematocrit as clinical indicator for blood transfusion audit in surgery patients. Transf Med Rev 1994;4:35-44.

THE PROCESS OF CLINICAL DECISION-MAKING IN TRANSFUSION MEDICINE: INCORPORATING GUIDELINES AND ALGORITHMS INTO TRANSFUSION PRACTICES

L.T. Goodnough

Introduction

Guidelines for transfusion practice have had limited impact in altering physician transfusion behaviour in patients undergoing surgery. This may be due to:
- a lack of consensus on the relative risks and benefits of blood in these patients who are anaemic;
- limited access to timely data that are necessary on which to base transfusion decisions;
- the recognition that empiric haemoglobin/haematocrit thresholds are limited clinical indicators of the need for blood;
- or a combination of these.

Medical practice guidelines are being promoted as a means to improve the effectiveness of the health care system. Guidelines for medical practice in general, and transfusion practices in particular, can contribute to improved care only if they change physician transfusion behaviour. However, guidelines are unlikely to change behaviour unless there are incentives for physicians to do so [1]. Examples of such incentives that have helped make autologous blood procurement a standard of care include:
- patient satisfaction (autologous blood predeposit is popular with patients);
- physician convenience (the availability of autologous blood makes regional blood inventory shortages less relevant for the elective surgical patient);
- better patient care (fewer allogeneic blood exposures in autologous blood donors) and, in some instances,
- lower medical costs (autologous blood procured by acute normovolemic haemodilution is less costly than allogeneic blood purchased from the regional blood centre).

In the absence of such incentives, there is wide-spread scepticism about the value of guidelines or recommendations from consensus conferences [1]. One promising approach is to guide the decision-making process by coupling the use of algorithms for the transfusion of blood and blood components with readily-available clinical information obtained from point-of-care testing, rather than laboratory-based assays. An overview of published information relevant to transfusion guidelines, along with possible approaches for the surgical patient that can be used effectively by physicians in order to improve transfusion outcomes, will be discussed.

Guidelines and utilization review

Medical practice guidelines have been promoted as a way to improve the cost effectiveness of medical care [1]. However, there is scepticism about the effectiveness of guidelines or of recommendations from consensus conferences [2]. For example, in one report in an intensive care setting, transfusion guidelines could successfully alter blood ordering practices, but they were not able to reduce over-all blood use [3]. A recent review concluded that transfusion audits can improve transfusion practices if they are performed in a timely manner and are combined with education of the individual ordering physician [4]. Plasma and platelet products are particularly amenable to this approach. Two studies using concurrent education or consultation reduced plasma usage by 46% and 77%, respectively [5, 6]. Another study using a retrospective audit was able to reduce inappropriate plasma use from 53% and 22% of units transfused [7]. Similarly, use of platelet transfusions were reduced by 56% and 14% in two studies that used consultation [8] and audit [9], respectively. Another study followed all requests for transfusion with a nonrequested consultation and was able to reduce transfusion of platelets by 44%, plasma and cryoprecipitate by 57%, and red blood cells (RBC) by 19% over a four year period [10]. However, other studies cast doubt on whether utilization review is really an effective process. Hoeltge [11] used a combination of indicators to evaluate transfusions on medical and surgical services, and concluded that nearly 96% of transfusions were justified. Renner {12 found the percentage of unjustified transfusions to be 1.4% before and 0% after an educational intervention. The percentages of transfusions that failed initial screening were only 0.5% and 3.2%, with and without the intervention, respectively. At our own institution in 1994, in which 23,002 RBC units were transfused, 46 transfusion events underwent peer review by the transfusion committee and only 2 cases (or a rate 1 in 10,000) were felt to be unjustified.

These extraordinary low rates of "inappropriate" transfusions may be a consequence of several factors. Firstly, RBC transfusion audits in circumstances of haemorrhage are difficult, if not impossible, to evaluate. These would include the emergency room/trauma unit, the operating rooms, and the medical intensive care units (patients with gastrointestinal bleeds). At our own institution, our process of utilization review excludes transfusions administered intraoperatively. Yet, retrospective studies of transfusion practices in orthopaedic surgery indicate that at least 25% of RBC transfusions in this setting are inappropriate [13]. Secondly, the clinical indicators that define "appropriate" transfusion practice may be too generous. In one study that concluded that 96% of transfusions were "appropriate", a post-transfusion Hgb level of 11 gm% was used as a threshold to distinguish "appropriate" from "inappropriate" [11]. Thirdly, the medical chart audit has substantial limitations. Clearly documented information as to why the transfusion was administered is commonly unobtainable. We found in a previous study that only 68% of transfusion events in orthopaedic surgical patients on postoperative days had documentation of blood loss and/or change in vital signs [14]. Furthermore, the rationale for transfusion was recorded in only 16% of day-of-surgery transfusions and in only 27% of transfusion administered on postoperative days. At our institution, 9 of 29 cases reviewed by the transfusion committee over twelve months were felt to have inadequate documentation for the reason for transfusion at chart audit.

With these limitations, one alternative approach to retrospective chart audit is the prospective use of transfusion algorithms, in which the decision process is coupled with clinical information that serves as clinical indicators for transfusion. The cardiac surgical patients can serve as a paradigm in order to illustrate this approach. The rationale for the incorporation of transfusion guidelines into algorithms that can be used by physicians in order to improve transfusion outcomes for the surgical patients, will be reviewed.

Transfusion practices

The evolution of cardiac surgery has been accompanied by blood conservation interventions that combined blood salvage techniques [15] along with acceptance of postoperative normovolemic anaemia [16]. This resulted in a single institution report of allogeneic red blood cell transfusions in as few as 10% of patients undergoing elective CABG [16]. However, a later study from the same institution reported allogeneic blood transfusions in 40% of patients, largely as a result of changing patient demographics such as increasing age and redoes [17]. Considerable variation in transfusion practice among institutions has been identified. A multicenter audit of 18 institutions demonstrated a wide range in allogeneic red blood cell transfusion requirements for patients undergoing simple, first-time CABG [18]. The variability has been confirmed in two subsequent studies [19, 20]. Follow-up studies of transfusion outcomes in cardiac surgical patients indicate that a substantial number of blood components in patients are transfused inappropriately [21].

Issues of blood safety in transfusion medicine have renewed interest in blood conservation and alternatives to blood transfusion. Practice guidelines have been summarized by the National Institutes of Health (NIH) consensus conferences on perioperative transfusion of red blood cells [22], plasma [23], and platelets [24]. Yet, as guidelines have suggested haemoglobin (Hgb) thresholds as low as 70 gms/L for transfusion in surgical patients [22], concern has been raised over whether the pendulum has swung too far [25]. This realization, along with the understanding that Hgb is a poor clinical indicator of RBC mass and tissue oxygen delivery [26], has focused attention on the importance of more physiologic indicators for blood transfusion.

Clinical indicators for blood transfusions

Critical haemodilution has helped define the physiologic threshold in humans at which oxygen consumption starts to decrease because of insufficient oxygen delivery: Hgb of 40 gm/L, an oxygen extraction ratio of 0.44, a mixed venous PO_2 of 34 mmHg, and a mixed venous oxygen saturation of 56% [27]. Haematocrit levels of 18% have been described to be as well tolerated as 27% during CPB [28]. Yet, patients have been reported to be at risk for perioperative ischaemic injury in the setting of substantial postoperative haemodilution to haematocrit (Hct) levels of 21-24%, with a delay on myocardial metabolic recovery [29]. Haemoglobin levels have been suggested as clinical indicators for transfusion in patients undergoing coronary bypass:

- Hgb 60 gm/L for well-compensated chronically anaemic patients; healthy (ASA Class I and some Class II) patients undergoing intentional haemodilution; and patients undergoing hypothermia.
- Hgb 80 gm/L for most postoperative bypass patients excepting those with left ventricular hypertrophy, incomplete coronary revascularization, low cardiac output, poorly controlled tachycardia, or sustained fever.
- Hgb 100 gm/L for patients unlikely to increase cardiac output, patients with symptomatic cerebrovascular disease, and elderly (age >65) patients.

Others emphasize that it is unlikely that one Hgb number can be universally applicable [31]. More physiologic indicators of the adequacy of oxygen delivery have been proposed [32]. The routine placement of a thermodilution pulmonary artery catheter in CABG patients enables regular assessment of mixed venous oxygen saturation (SVO_2), along with haemodynamic variables such as cardiac index (CI), heart rate (HR), and blood pressure. SVO_2 is an indicator of the relative balance between the total body oxygen supply and demand. As a sensitive but non-specific indicator, SVO_2 represents a weighted balance from all perfused vascular beds. When arterial oxygen saturation is adequate (SaO_2 >0.90), the SVO_2 inversely reflects the oxygen supply-demand balance. Mixed venous oxygen saturation SVO_2, provides continuous quantification of global oxygen extraction, in which a mixed venous oxygen tension (PVO_2) greater than 40 mmHg (SVO_2 approximately 75%) is believed to indicate adequate tissue oxygenation in most clinical states, and PVO_2 less than 20 torr (SVO_2 approximately 30%) suggests inadequate tissue oxygenation [33].

In a recent study of critically ill patients with sepsis, a goal to optimize oxygen delivery ($V^{\bullet}O_2I$ of >600 ml/min/m2) in a series of interventions including fluid boluses, administration of blood products, and the use of inotropes was evaluated [34]. While the intervention group was found to have the same number of complications, number of days on ventilator and in intensive care, and hospital charges compared to a standard therapy group, analysis of the subset of patients from both groups who had $V^{\bullet}O_2I$ in excess of 600 ml/min/m2 showed that these patients had a much lower mortality rate (14%) compared to patients who could not achieve this level of oxygen delivery (mortality of 53%). This study illustrates the paradigm that patient-specific physiologic clinical indicators can be associated with better clinical outcomes [32].

In addition to clinical indicators for RBC transfusion (tachycardia, hypotension, oliguria, etc.), physiologic indicators of clinically significant impairment of the oxygen supply-demanded balance include SVO_2 <0.60 and/or PVO_2 <30 mm Hg. When the Hgb level falls below "acceptable" values, these indicators indicate a potential benefit from transfusion. However, the precise "acceptable" haemoglobin concentration range is unknown. The NIH consensus conference concluded that most patients with Hgb levels >100 gm/L do not require blood, whereas most patients with Hgb <70 gm/L benefit from blood [22]. Silent perioperative ischaemia has been identified as a significant clinical problem in noncardiac [35] as well as cardiac [36] surgical patients, emphasizing that the heart is an organ at risk with regards to tissue oxygenation. A recent case report illustrated that in a surgical patient with a haematocrit level of 27%, silent myocardial ischemia was corrected with the transfusion of two red blood cell units [37]. Haemoglobin levels from 70 gm/L to 100 gm/L, a range in which physiologic indicators may identify patients who can benefit (or not benefit) from blood, therefore need to be the most closely scrutinized.

Blood conservation practices

The evolution of cardiac surgery has been accompanied by a wide variety of techniques and equipment available for blood conservation, along with identification of preoperative risk factors for subsequent need for transfusion [16, 38]. The complementary relationship between blood conservation and blood transfusion practice may explain the lack of consensus regarding the effectiveness of conservation strategies. In a study by Ward et al. [39], the autologous reinfusion of 619 to 1,159 mL of postoperative chest tube drainage in 18 patients was accompanied by allogeneic red cell transfusions in six patients, no different than 6 of 17 patients in a control group in which 438 to 779 mL of postoperative mediastinal drainage was discarded. A conservative red cell transfusion protocol was used, so that mean red cell transfusions were less than two units per patient for both groups. The lack of efficacy of single blood conservation techniques has been found in other controlled prospective trials for intraoperative as well as for postoperative settings. On the other hand, a recent study of postoperative autotransfusion of shed mediastinal blood showed efficacy in reducing the need for blanked blood [40]. To a greater or lesser extent, the reports cited above incorporated criteria for blood transfusion in their blood conservation protocols, so that modification of physician transfusing practices became uncredited interventions. Thus, defined transfusion triggers and standardized blood conservation practices are important contributors to outcomes in cardiac surgery patients [41].

Previous studies have found that while the RBC needs of these patients are substantial, a combination of conservative transfusion practice and blood conservation that could provide the equivalent of four blood units, might avoid allogeneic blood exposure in up to 75% of CABG patients [19]. Since 80% of RBC trans-

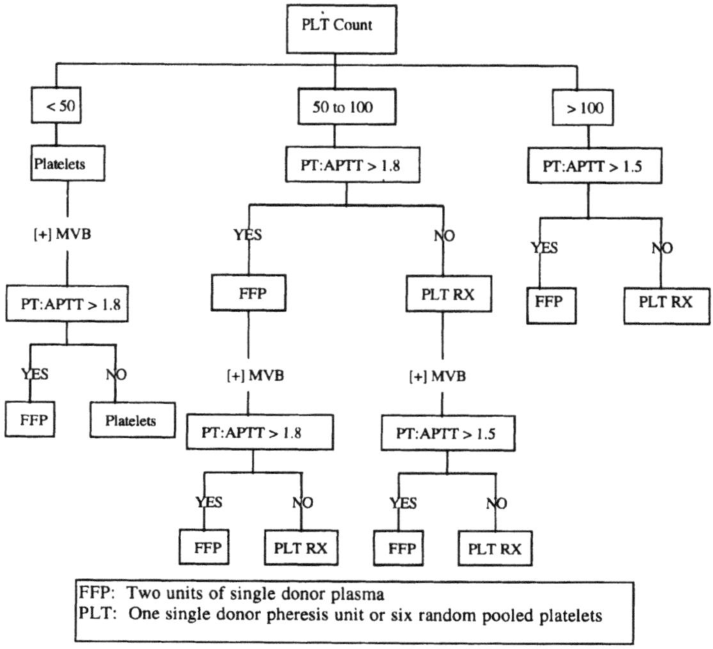

Figure 1. An algorithm approach for haemostatic therapy in cardiac patients determined to have microvascular bleeding after heparin neutralization. Platelets = platelet transfusion (6 units of random-donor or apheresis unit equivalent); PLT RX = platelet therapy (platelet transfusion and/or DDAVP therapy at physician's discretion); FFP = plasma therapy (2 units of fresh-frozen plasma); [+] MVB = continued MVB; PT:APTT = whole blood prothrombin time and activated partial thromboplastin time control values (values/mean values from a normal reference population); PLT count = platelet count ($\times 10^3/mm^3$). Reprinted, with permission, from Despotis et al. J Thor Cardiovasc Surg 1994; 107:271-39.

fusions are received on the postoperative (PO) day and 90% by end of PO day 1, the effectiveness of interventions focused on these two days would be substantial. Patients have been found to be transfused in excess of their needs if decisions to transfuse are made on a clinical indicator, such as estimated blood loss, that is poorly quantifiable [42]. Transfusion algorithms therefore may be especially useful if they incorporate point of care information that is both physiologic and patient-specific for transfusion decisions.

Transfusion algorithms

While the discharge Hct level is useful in a retrospective understanding of transfusion outcomes [42], transfusion guidelines utilizing concurrent clinical indicators are necessary if physician transfusion behaviour is to be altered. We have conducted studies to evaluate the impact of point-of-care testing [43,44], in which intraoperative assays (on-site evaluation of whole blood prothrombin

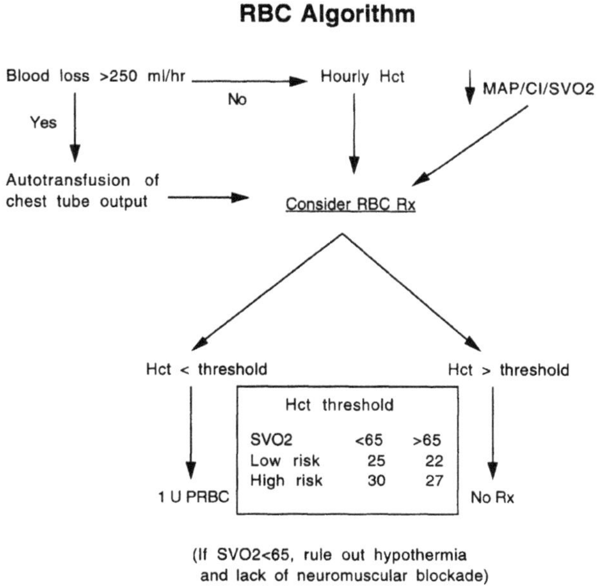

Figure 2. An algorithm approach for red cell transfusion, in cardiac surgical patients postoperatively. After establishing that the patient's volume status is adequate, decisions to transfuse would be based on haemoglobin/haematocrit level, rate of blood loss, and haemodynamic parameters. Thresholds for transfusion would differ for patients determined to be at "low" risk and "high" risk for perisurgical complications. Mixed venous oxygen percent saturation (SVO_2) could serve as a physiologic indicator of the balance between oxygen supply and demand for transfusion decision-making. Reprinted, with permission, from Goodnough et al. Ann Thorac Surg 1995;60:473-80.

time, activated partial thromboplastin time and platelet count with results available within four minutes) were linked with a transfusion algorithm (Figure 1) for plasma and platelet transfusions in cardiac surgical patients.

This algorithm approach reduced blood component transfusions for the algorithm treated patients group, compared to patients who were treated under standard practice using laboratory-based testing. Sixty six patients with a diagnosis of microvascular bleeding (MVB) were randomized to either standard therapy (n=36), in which blood products were transfused at the discretion of the physician according to any laboratory-based test results requested; or to an algorithm group (n=30), in which on-site platelet count, PT, and aPTT results were available within 4 min. Platelet and plasma therapy were given according to an algorithm, according to on-site results. The three decision pathways of this algorithm where based initially on platelet count measurements, followed by branch pathways determined by PT and aPTT results. Both intraoperative and initial postoperative chest tube drainage were less in the algorithm group, indicating that haemostatic therapy was more successful in treating MVB in the algorithm group. Point-of-care testing and patient-specific (i.e., targeted to each patient's lab test results) blood component therapy may have better distinguished haemostatic vs surgical bleeding for the surgical team at the close of the procedure, as suggested by the fact that only one patient in the algorithm group required later surgical re-exploration, compared to five patients in the standard group. Eight of 36 (25%) standard therapy patients received different blood component therapy from what would have been designated by our algorithm [44]. The more effective therapy in the algorithm group was reflected in the lower RBC transfusion needs in the algorithm group compared to the standard therapy group (5.9±3.8 vs 9.8±8.4 units, respectively). The improved patient care along with reduced blood transfusions resulted in substantial economic savings [44]. This approach has been described as a "powerful engine of change" [45].

Decisions to transfuse the surgical patient should acknowledge that patients are heterogeneous for risks related to anaemia. One prospective approach to risk stratification for cardiac surgical patients has been published recently [46], in which clinical variables determine whether a patient is considered as a "standard" or as an "increased" risk for cardiac surgery. While complications related to anaemia represent only one aspect of morbidity/mortality in this setting, the physiologic changes known to accompany acute anaemia [36], and the potential for myocardial tissue injury [37], suggest that risk stratification for RBC transfusion decisions would be prudent. A recent analysis of over 2,000 cardiac bypass patients has led to a model that calculated a transfusion risk score, which was then validated prospectively in over 400 additional patients [38]. Now that cardiac surgery patients can be prospectively stratified not only for surgical risk but also for transfusion likelihood, the role of algorithms may be especially productive in the standardization of blood transfusion and blood conservation practices.

An algorithm that incorporates the balance between oxygen delivery and oxygen consumption as reflected by changes in SVO_2 within a range of haematocrit level, may be effective as a clinical indicator for RBC therapy. Such an approach is illustrated in Figure 2 [47]. With the recognition that transfusion support is dependent on both rate of blood loss as well as Hgb level, the decision to transfuse each unit of RBC could be based on Hgb level, the quantity (rate) of blood lost, and haemodynamic parameters. Each patient would achieve adequate pulmonary capillary wedge pressures (PCWP) filling pressures with crystalloid/ colloid therapy before entering a transfusion algorithm. Controlled clinical trials comparing this approach to current, unmonitored transfusion practices are needed.

Conclusion

Guidelines for transfusion management in surgical patients are most effective when a decision algorithm can be coupled with clinical information that assists the physician in management. Cardiac surgery can serve as a paradigm for this approach. Blood component therapy can be improved when administered according to physiologic indicators for transfusion that are based on patient-specific, point-of-care test results.

References

1. Audet AM, Greenfield S, Field M. Medical practice guidelines: Current activities and future directions. Ann Int Med 1990;113:709-14.
2. Lomas J, Anderson GM, Domnick-Pierre K, et al. Do practice guidelines guide practice? N Engl J Med 1989;321:1306-11.
3. Littenberg B, Corwin HL, Gettinger A, Leichter J, Aubuchon JP. A practice guideline and decision aid for blood transfusion. Immunohematol 1995;11:88-94.
4. Toy PTCY. Effectiveness of transfusion audits and practice guidelines. Arch Pathol Lab Med 1994;118:435-37.
5. Ayoub MM, Clark JA. Reduction of fresh frozen plasma use with a simple education program. Am Surg 1989;55:563-65.
6. Shanberge JN. Reduction of fresh-frozen plasma use through a daily survey and education program. Transfusion 1987;27:226-27.
7. Barnette RE, Fish DJ, Eisenstaedt RS. Modification of fresh-frozen transfusion practices through educational intervention. Transfusion 1990;30:253-57.
8. McCullough J, Steeper TA, Connelly DP, Jackson B, Huntington S, Scott EP. Platelet utilization in a university hospital. JAMA 1988:259:2414-18.
9. Simpson MB. Prospective-concurrent audits and medical consultation for platelet transfusions. Transfusion 19 1987;27:192-95.
10. Lichtiger B, Fisher HE, Huh YO. Screening of transfusion service requests by the blood bank pathologist: Impact on cost containment. Lab Med 1988;19:228-30.
11. Hoeltge GA, Brown JC, Herzig RH, et al. Computer-assisted audits of blood component transfusion. Cleve Clin J Med 1989;56:267-69.
12. Renner SW, Howanitz JH, Fishkin BG. Toward meaningful blood usage review: Comprehensive monitoring of physician practice. QRB Qual Rev Bull 1987;13:76-80.
13. Goodnough LT, Verbrugge D, Vizmeg K, Riddell J. Identification of elective orthopaedic surgical patients transfused with blood volumes in excess of blood needs: The "transfusion trigger" revisited. Transfusion 1992;32:648-53.
14. Audet AM, Goodnough LT, Parvin CA. Evaluating the appropriateness of red blood cell transfusions: The limitations of retrospective medical record reviews. Inter J Qual Health Care, In press.
15. Cosgrove DM, Thurer RL, Lytle BW. Blood conservation during myocardial revascularization. Ann Thorac Surg 1979;28:184-89.
16. Cosgrove DM, Loop FD, Lytle BW, et al. Determinations of blood utilization during myocardial revascularization. Ann Thorac Surg 1985;40:380-84.
17. Loop FD, Lytle BW, Cosgrove DM, et al. Coronary artery bypass graft surgery in the elderly. Cleve Clin J Med 1988;55:23-34.
18. Goodnough LT, Johnston MFM, Toy PTCY and the TMAA Study Group. The variability of transfusion practice in coronary artery bypass graft surgery. JAMA 1991;265: 86-90.
19. Surgenor DM, Wallace EL, Churchill WH, Hao SHS, Chapman RH, Collins JJ. Red cell transfusions in coronary artery bypass surgery. Transfusion 1992;32:458-64.
20. Stover EP, Siegel LC, Parks R, et al. Variability in transfusion practice for coronary artery bypass surgery despite national consensus guidelines. Anest 1995;81:1223A (abstract).
21. Goodnough LT, Soegiarso RW, Birkmeyer JD, Welch HG. Economic impact of inappropriate blood transfusions in coronary artery bypass graft surgery. Amer J Med 1993;94:509-14.

22. National Institutes of Health Consensus Conference. Perioperative red cell transfusion. JAMA 1988;260:2700-5.
23. National Institutes of Health Consensus Conference. Fresh frozen plasma: Indications and risks. JAMA 1985;253:551-53.
24. National Institutes of Health Consensus Conference. Platelet transfusion therapy. JAMA 1987;257:1777-80.
25. Faust RJ. Perioperative indications for red blood cell transfusion: Has the pendulum swung too far? Mayo Clin Proc 1993;68:512-14.
26. Spence RK, Costable JP, Young CS, et al. Is hemoglobin level alone a reliable predictor of outcome in the severely anemic surgical patient? Am J Surg 1992;58(2): 92-95.
27. Van Woerkens ECSM, Trauwborst A, van Lanschot JJB. Profound hemodilution: What is the critical level of hemodilution at which oxygen delivery-dependent oxygen consumption starts in an anesthetized human? Anesth Analg 1992;75:818-21.
28. Lilleaasen P. Moderate and extreme hemodilution in open heart surgery: Blood requirements, bleeding, and platelet counts. Scand J Thor Cardiovasc Surg 1977;11:97-103.
29. Weisel RD, Charlesworth DC, Mickleborough LL, et al. Limitations of blood conservation. J Thor Cardiovasc Surg 1984;88:26-38.
30. Robertie PG, Gravlee GP. Safe limits of isovolemic hemodilution and recommendations for erythrocyte transfusion. Int Anesth Clin 1990;28:197-204.
31. Leone BJ, Spahn DR. Anemia, hemodilution, and oxygen delivery (editorial). Anesth Analg 1992;75:651-53.
32. Nelson LD. All goals are not the same (editorial). Crit Care Med 1993;21:815-16.
33. Bryan-Brown CW, Baek SM, Makabali G, Shoemaker WC. Consumable oxygen: Availability of oxygen in relation to oxyhemoglobin dissociation. Crit Care Med 1973;1:17-21.
34. Yu M, Levy M, Smith P, Takiguchi SA, Miyasaki A, Myers SA. Effect of maximizing oxygen delivery on morbidity and mortality rates in critically ill patients: A prospective, randomized, controlled study. Crit Care Med 1993;21:830-38.
35. Mangano DT, Browner WS, Hollenberg M, London MJ, Tabau JF, Tateo IM. Association of perioperative myocardial ischemia with cardiac morbidity and mortality in men undergoing noncardiac surgery. N Engl J Med 1990;323:1781-88.
36. Rao TLK, Montoya A. Cardiovascular, electrocardiographic and respiratory changes following acute anemia with volume replacement in patients with coronary artery disease. Anest Dev 1985;12:49-54.
37. Parksloe MRJ, Wuld R, Fox M, Reilly CS. Silent myocardial ischemia in a patient with anaemia before operation. Brit J Anaesth 1990;64:634-37.
38. Magovern JA, Sakert T, Benckart DH, et al. A model for predicting transfusion after coronary artery surgery. Ann Thorac Surg. In press.
39. Ward HB, Smith RRA, Landis KP, Nemzek TG, Dalmasso AP, Swaim WR. Prospective, randomized trial of autotransfusion after routine cardiac operations. Ann Thorac Surg 1993;56:137-41.
40. Morris JJ, Tan YST. Autotransfusion: Is there a benefit in a current practice of aggressive blood conservation? Ann Thorac Surg 1994;58:502-8.
41. Goodnough LT. Blood conservation and blood transfusion practices: Flip sides of the same coin. Ann Thor Surg 1993;56:3-4.
42. Goodnough LT, Vizmegk, Riddell J, Soegiarso RW. The discharge hematocrit as a clinical indicator for blood transfusion in surgery patients. Transf Med 1994;4:35-44.

43. Despotis GJ, Grishaber JE, Goodnough LT. The effect of an intraoperative treatment algorithm on physician transfusion behavior in cardiac surgery. Transfusion 1994;34: 290-96.
44. Despotis GJ, Santoro SA, Spitznagel, et al. Prospective evaluation and clinical utility of on-site coagulation monitoring in cardiac surgical patients. J Thorac Card Surg 1994;107:271-79.
45. Reinersten JL. Algorithms, guidelines, and protocols: Can they really improve what we do? Transfusion 1994;34:281-82.
46. Higgins TL, Estafanous FG, Loop FD, Beck GJ, Blum JM, Paranand L. Stratification of morbidity and mortality outcome by preoperative risk factors in coronary artery bypass patients. JAMA 1992;267:2344-48.
47. Goodnough LT, Despotis GJ, Hogue CW, Ferguson TB. On the need for improved transfusion indicators in cardiac surgery. An Thorac Surg 1995;60:473-80.

DISCUSSION

P.C. Das and L.T. Goodnough – moderators

K. Sazama (Philadelphia, PA, USA): Dr. Holland, thank you very much for a very interesting presentation about informed consent. I just have one comment and one question. The first is that I would like to make the audience aware of the fact that there is a very fine videotape that has been distributed through the American Medical Association on the topic of informed consent, which I think is worth looking at. It relates to the troubling aspects of informed consent which has had a very checkered history in transfusion medicine and other aspects of medicine. What is troubling to us is that very often we discover that the treating physicians do not have the knowledge to have an effective informed consent discussion with relation to transfusion. The discussion should be on the information relevant to the transfusion. We find that a number of our colleagues simply are not informed. They do not have the correct information about risks, benefits and alternatives which should include what is going to happen if no transfusion is given. Then I will share just briefly what we have undertaken in our hospitals to involve the transfusion committee in helping to elucidate correct information which then can be distributed to the medical staff so that they are more comfortable in actually having a knowledgeable discussion.

P.V. Holland (Sacramento, CA, USA): Thank you dr. Sazama. You may know that Dr. Sazama is both a physician and a lawyer, so she has two reasons for asking these questions. I think it is up to us first of all to keep our colleagues up-to-date on what we think are the most current risks. We have to constantly tell them about where we stand based upon our donor selection and testing (and whatever) at every conference, every medical staff meeting and also transfusion committees. So, I think we do have means to get that information out.

The other part is more difficult. I really think physicians should have learned, and when they have not, should be learning why they are doing things. I mean I cannot believe the haematologist who is giving tons of platelets did not have some idea why he was giving the platelets. So you may not know all the reasons or we may not know the complete spectrum. But, I think within our scope of practice, if we do not know, we should learn and we should be really telling our patients why they are getting the transfusion and what we think is going to happen with and without that particular component that we are likely to transfuse. But,

I think we have to work more in medical school and residency, and every avenue you can, to educate so that within their area physicians can know what they are doing.

K. Sazama: One additional comment, because you alluded to the legal side. I think current wisdom among the legal community about informed consent, at least in the United States, is that the discussion should involve any risk of death. Any risk, which means one in a million, one in two million or whatever. I think that has come about particularly in the transfusion practices by virtue of the fact that AIDS is also transfusion transmitted.

D. van Epps (Round Lake, IL, USA): A question for dr. McClelland and dr. Goodnough related to the introduction of erythropoietin into the field. Do you anticipate any impact on the demand for red cells as a result of the in vivo use now of erythropoietin. The second part of the question is: Two or three years away I would anticipate the introduction of a thrombopoietin. Do you anticipate that it will have a significant impact on the demand for platelets?

L.T. Goodnough (St. Louis, MI, USA): I think that the emerging pharmacologic agents that serve as alternatives to blood include erythropoietin, to stimulate red cell production, but also haemoglobin solutions as blood substitutes and agents to reduce blood loss like aprotinin. I think that a whole family of pharmacologic agents will have an impact on the use of red cells in surgical patients. It will be a substantial number in part depending on cost considerations. Our own blood service is raising the price of red cell units between 15 and 25% per year. So right now there is not much of a cost equivalence between red cells and the alternatives to red cells, but I think in the very near future there will be cost equivalence between red cells and alternatives to red cells. So I think there will be a substantial impact of pharmacologic agents as alternatives to red cells.

D.B.L. McClelland (Edinburgh, UK): Dr. Goudnough has written most of the papers on clinical application. My perspective from the UK is that the impact, at least as far as perioperative red cell use goes, is likely to be fairly small for a while. I have the impression that only a small proportion of the total patient group undergoing the major common red cell using procedures, will actually be enroled for EPO use in the UK over the next few years. Thrombopoietin I think is anybody's guess; if it is safe (and it is certainly effective), it is going to make a big impact. However, it is very interesting that in some parts of the world, notably Australia, there are very big changes, down-swings in platelet utilisation without any influence of thrombopoietin at all. So there is a lot going on there.

R.S. Eisenstaedt (Philadelphia, PA, USA): Some comments for dr. Goodnough. I am worried about dr. Littenberg's work[1], which sounds to me was done under the assumption that too much blood was being transfused in the ICU and that the 7 gram transfusion trigger, that has been discussed often for perioperative patients, was reasonable to aim for in that group of patients. There is a lot of evidence that suggests that they do not have many of the adaptive mechanisms that would make that reduction of oxygen content reasonable to be satisfied with. I wonder what are you going to make of dr. Nelson's work[2] that you just showed about increased mortality. Along that same theme I was struck by dr. Holland's estimation of transfusion risks these days with hepatitis C now being 1 in 6,000 range or so. That is an incredible reduction in what I have always discussed as the most important downside of blood transfusion. I think we have to re-write this whole analysis of benefits and risks.

L.T. Goodnough: Your point is well taken. I think that the presumption that somehow very sick, critically ill patients in the intensive care unit could be successfully treated at a lower haemoglobin threshold of seven is probably naïve. The transfusion was given from one haemoglobin threshold to something else for the very reason that the patient was sick enough to need blood based on blood loss, ischaemic events or oxygen transport. What I learned the most from Nelson and especially from you is that maybe we ought to free ourselves up completely from the haemoglobin threshold. Critically ill patients who commonly have invasive lines in, where you could do more physiological measurements of oxygen transport and oxygen consumption, may have clinical outcomes that are independent from red cell issues yet important with respect to morbidity and mortality.

R.S. Eisenstaedt: If those invasive lines are already in, you might use them for that purpose. But the risk of putting them in may be greater than the risk of the transfusion, if you do not need them for any other reason based upon some of the information that we already heard.

L.T. Goodnough: If you successfully show that mortality was significantly associated with maximal oxygen delivery mortality then you could justify the risk of an invasive line.

D.B.L. McClelland: Just a couple of comments. I think what Littenbergh's study shows is that the clinicians did exactly the same thing, but they filled in the forms differently, which is what people do. People are sensible. If you pressure them not to transfuse for anaemia then they would not write anaemia on the request form when they ask for the blood. They did not want to hassle, but they know

1. Littenberg B, Corwin HL, Gettinger A, Leichter J, Aubuchon JP. A practice guideline and decision aid for blood transfusion. Immunohematol 1995;11:88-94.
2. Nelson LD. All goals are not the same. Crit Care Med 1993;21:815-16 (editorial).

the patient needed a transfusion so they just behaved like sensible clinicians. Two comments about invasive monitoring. If you are going to have the lines in anyway then you should use the data that you can get from them and that has got to be sensible. The oxygen delivery is really important because the risks of anaemia may be high. However, for most of the people transfused for most surgery, it is just not available. So, you need so much simpler measuring tools than the ones they are talking about if you really want to make an impact.

L.T. Goodnough: It is also unclear whether oxygen delivery is a parameter that you want to look at or whether oxygen uptake and utilization on a tissue or cellular basis is a critical number.

B. Justiça (Oporto, P): Dr. Holland, is it obligatory for all physicians to get informed consent for transfusions and how much do they comply; how frequently do they actually do this.

P.V. Holland: I do not believe that it is obligatory in most of the United States. I do not believe it is required. However, in California some elements of transfusion informed consent are the law. Now, the compliance with that is very difficult to monitor. Hospitals are trying to monitor this, but they are finding very poor, very low compliance, but I think it is too late then to find out whether or not they have gotten the informed consent. The informed consent, meaning the patient must know the alternatives, and the main alternatives, are autologous, patient selected, patient directed, and allogeneic and the risks and benefits of each, must be provided for elective or anticipated medical or surgical procedures with a reasonable possibility of a blood transfusion. That is the current wording of the law. So, it means that only for procedures that are elective – hip operations and certain procedures planned ahead – is it even required and it should be documented. It should be given to the patients during the office visit, not in the hospital, because it must be done ahead of time. At the moment, even though it is required we have no idea how often it is actually being done by the physician ahead of time. My job is to help them to do this ahead of time, so that the patient has time, especially for autologous and directed units; but I have no idea how often, how low or high, they are actually complying. In the rest of the United States, to my knowledge, there is no such requirement.

A. Lust (Aalst, B): Dr. Nevalainen, I am probably in a good position to say that being tall or being big is not always the best of all. You should remember that major disasters occurred in major organisations, be it national or commercial. It is the way you work, that is an assurance of total quality commitment. You were speaking about cost containment in doing the same job with less people. However, people that are not on the job any more are costing as much for the social security as they were costing before.

D.E. Nevalainen (Abbott Park, IL, USA): I am still collecting data on that point. Recently I started to work with one blood bank. We started to focus on indirect costs and to look at what their cost structure is internal to their operation. I am looking for a quality metric to track between countries and between blood banks, because I think it is going to tell us an awful lot about how efficient the internal processes are in each given blood centre. I will be particularly interested in comparing United States blood banks with the FDA prospective to some of the European blood banks that have slightly different regulatory profile. I do not know what it means at this point of time. My suspicion is that there is lot of indirect cost that is probably not valued as a cost due to compliance efforts, lack of efficient processes, which causes look backs that would not have to be done, where you have to trace all the records back to the hospitals with the labour and time involved. There are many horror stories when you start to add up all of these things in terms of what that financial impact is and that is all failure cost. So, I cannot tell you exactly what the norm is, I do not know but I think it is a very general useful number to look at just to get some general comparisons.

A. Lust: The first was meant as a comment that growing larger is not always an advantage as major transfusion disasters occurred in major organisations already. It is the way you are working in your total quality, not so much if you are a big organisation or not.

D.E. Nevalainen: I agree big is not necessarily beautiful. You can have a big disaster in a very short time in a large organisation because of the volume. That is one of the reasons that you have got to have a good quality system in place, because you cannot have high volume consistent performance without good process control and good quality, whereas in a low volume operation you can do it one by one. It costs more money, it is more expansive but you can have output; so that is part of the differences between the two processes. With volume you will get the economies of scale, you will get lower per unit costs. All of this is starting to happen, but is does need to be controlled very well; no question about it.

K. Sazama: Dr. McClelland, a question related to some of the studies that dr. Goodnough shared with us as well, which is about the question of appropriateness. I noticed you were showing blood use by age and gender and there was a striking finding. I am sure you are not unaware that men over the age of 90 are being transfused at a huge rate relative to the females in that age group. I just wondered whether that was something of interest to you or is there an explanation for why that it is so strikingly different.

D.B.L. McClelland: The explanation is very simple. There is an extremely small number of patients and I do not think the comparisons up there are really important. I think the important part of the data is really the ramp up to patients aged 85. By normalizing for the size of the population within each age band then you can see much more clearly what you already know, that the men are dying off earlier. They start to get transfused more at a younger age, and then you can see the effect of earlier mortality in the males. It did not show very well in that presentation, but the 90's is just a small number problem.

K. Sazama: I regret I cannot recall the exact literature that looked at transfusion in terms of cardiac bypass procedures (probably published in 1992 or 1993[1]), in which there clearly is a difference in the transfusion rate based on the gender; the likelihood of being transfused was much, much greater for males than for females. I raise the question only in the context of saying when we are looking at appropriateness of transfusion there may be variables in addition to the ones that already have been described that also need to be kept in mind.

D.B.L. McClelland: You are absolutely right. If you look at the data there are some quite clear differences between transfusion patterns for males and females. The other interesting thing is the preoperative haematocrit range. Of course the women tend to be a bit lower, but after transfusion males and females converge on a common value. So what was a physiological difference preparatively is obliterated in the postoperative implicit target value, which is quite interesting. So there are some pretty irrational things in there.

K. Sazama: What is your concern about the age of your donor group? Is consideration being given to increasing or permitting donation at an older age among the donors?

D.B.L. McClelland: No, we actually go up to 70; we need the individual to have an independent certification from their own physician to continue donation between 65 and 70, but I certainly would not at all advocate extending the age beyond that for a number of reasons. One is that I think there maybe a real risk of morbidity. I think there is enough evidence of ischaemic events associated with quite modest levels of blood loss in that age group with ischaemic heart disease. The other reason is we have to understand the population dynamics of the younger people and revise our motivation strategies to deal with that problem.

K. Sazama: Do you have the same age restrictions for autologous donors?

D.B.L. McClelland: Yes, although autologous predeposit donation in the United Kingdom to my knowledge remains a minority activity, so the amount of data about it is minimal. But there is a national guideline which has similar age restrictions.

---

1. Goodnough LT, Soegiarso RW, Geha AS. Blood lost and blood transfused in coronary artery bypass graft operation as implications for blood transfusion and blood conservation strategies. Surg Gynaecol Obstet 1993;177:345-51.

K. Sazama: Well, part of the basis for the questioning is of course that in the US we have different practices and unless things have changed dramatically in most blood centres that I am aware of, there is no upper age limit. Donors, allogeneic and autologous over the age of 70, are regularly accepted, obviously with attention to their medical and clinical indications. I am not aware of any new data that suggest that there is an excess morbidity beyond what would be anticipated for the disease conditions. So I am curious about the data to which you are alluring.

D.B.L. McClelland: There is quite a substantial amount of data. I have reviewed some of them and I am happy to share this with you. Other members of the panel I think are also conversant to this literature. Dr. Holland was talking about it recently.

P.V. Holland: We already have double standards for autologous donors with respect to haemoglobin levels and how often you can donate, because we understand that when you donate autologously it is for your own benefit as opposed to somebody else's. I have no problem with the double standard for age. When you are doing one thing for your own benefit, you might have a higher threshold for age than when you are doing it for somebody else's benefit.

D.B.L. McClelland: I would have a problem. How do you obtain properly informed consent from an individual to whom you are offering the option of autologous donation versus an allogeneic donation from a well organized centre with good data on safety? Particularly, in view of that really interesting survey report published recently by the AABB[1] what advice would you give them with regard to the intrinsic safety of the procedure. I would be scared since from these data, autologous transfusion looks absolutely out of control.

P.V. Holland: I would like to speak on two aspects of that. With all due respect to my colleague dr. Nevalainen I think you actually misinterpreted the data that dr. McClelland just referred to. It was 23 hospitals is my recollection that said that they had at least one error, one out of those 1800. Now you extrapolated that to the millions. We do not know exactly how many thousands of units those hospitals handled. So this is not quite the same. The second point is what dr. Sazama illustrated. I think we have learned a lot from taking autologous patients as donors. We have learned that we can take a unit of blood from them every week for several weeks, lower their haematocrit down to 33 or below. It is quite a safe procedure, so why are we so reticent about taking healthy people who have no symptoms. That is a double standard. So, I think, in fact, that our autologous experience has taught us a great deal about the safety of blood donations and we have some wonderful, very regular 20, 30 gallon donors who are well in their seventies, into their eighties, who are donating quite regularly. Now we have a

---

1. Mackey J, Lipton KS. AABB position on testing of autologous units. Association Bulletin 1995;4, Bethesda, MD, American Association of Blood Banks.

long history of them and we feel quite comfortable with them. But I think the autologous practices have really taught us a great deal. It is relatively safe to take a unit of blood from people that are much beyond the age of sixty-five. Of course it is not age per sé, but it is the physiological condition that is really more important.

D.B.L. McClelland: I think this is a really interesting discussion and your choice of words intrigues me: "relatively safe". To me as a director of a blood donation programme this does not mean that it is safe enough. I mean if there is one bit of our business where we have to say risk must be zero, it is in the process of taking blood from healthy donors and I am not satisfied with the data about very elderly donors' safety.

P.V. Holland: Well, let me give my definition of relatively safe. In fact we have evidence that for perfectly healthy normal donors, it is no more risky in terms of whatever you want to measure: morbidity, mortality. For these people we have about the same risk of a vaso-vagal reaction; that is a minor reaction, who cares? We have no significant difference in the number of individuals who have some cardiac ischaemic episodes, so I believe that we have comparable safety for each of them.

D.B.L. McClelland: There was a very good article in the British Medical Journal[1] recently by a distinguished statistician whose name I have forgotten entitled "The absence of evidence is not the same as the evidence of absence". If you look at the denominator of the number of 85 year old regular donors that you have got data on and the number of 40 year old donors that you got data on worldwide I am still not convinced, I am sorry.

P.V. Holland: No, I agree with your quote; we have been drawing on the order of 12 to 14,000 units of autologous blood each year for almost ten years now, since the AIDS crisis. But, knock on wood, something may happen tomorrow; this is about 7,000 autologous donors a year (we take an average of two units from each) and we have the same complication rate of minor reactions in them as with our other allogeneic 100,000 plus donations. We have not recorded that; we have not published that. Nonetheless, I think that experience is duplicated by actually many people.

D.B.L. McClelland: I think you should publish it; but I bow to your greater experience with this group of donors.

---

1. Altman DG, Bland JM. Absence of evidence is not evidence of absence. BMJ 1995; 311:485.

A. W.M.M. Koopman-van Gemert (Amsterdam, NL): In the Netherlands we have not that much experience with autologous donation like my colleague dr. Holland, but we have the same experience, we have also no age limit.

K. Sazama: I want to make a comment about the informed consent question that dr. McClelland mentioned and also that dr. Holland did before. The first is that the new 1996 requirements by the Joint Commission on Accreditation for Healthcare Organizations[1] requires informed consent for transfusion. So beginning January 1st, 1996 all accredited JCAHO institutions must have informed consent explicitly for transfusion. The second point that dr. McClelland made is that the content of the information being described should be addressed to the exact intervention treatment prevention or whatever is going on. In studying blood collection settings, this would mean the additional risks, e.g. of the autologous patient, who is having blood collected and/or the additional risks if you are using an automated collection device in addition to the risk of just the donation itself, so that is a very important point.

H. Hambley (London, UK): I wanted to make a comment about the last exchange between dr. McClelland and dr. Holland. I must be one of the minority UK autologous blood transfusers and it is a very, very small part of my practice. We see a lot of patients. To some extent the patients if they want to donate then I will do it, but I do it in a very careful way and I will see the patient and examine or have examined by an other physician and the blood will be taken of under very careful circumstances. I think the autologous transfusion is probably safe, but I think the circumstances got to be very carefully controlled. I think that is one of the reasons for such a minority in the United Kingdom. The point I want to make about informed consent is, I agree with dr. Holland, it has to be the physician who is using the blood. I think it also has to be seen as part of the whole business of the procedure that is taking place. I do not think you can take the blood transfusion issue out and put the spotlight on that. I think he is very right, you have to put that in the context of perhaps saying yes, my mortality from open heart surgery is 10%. I think it is very, very important that all of that is actually given to the patient and the last thing I just wonder if it is a good idea to actually video these conversations where informed consent is actually being given, so that in later times if there is a question of litigation the court and the jury will actually see how much information was given and how much understanding the patient really did appear to have.

1. Comprehensive Accreditation Manual for Hospitals. Joint Commission for the Accreditation of Healthcare Organization, Oakbrook Terrace, Il, 1996.

II. PRODUCT QUALITIES AND CHARACTERISTICS

FACTORS DEFINING THE CLINICAL NEED FOR SUPPORTIVE HAEMOTHERAPY

J.Th.M. de Wolf

Introduction

There should be no difference between the factors defining the clinical need for supportive haemotherapy and other forms of clinical therapy. In general the choice of a therapy must be based on the present balance of efficacy, adverse effects and costs. Efficacy focuses on the benefit achieved when medical technology, for instance the transfusion of blood products, is applied under ideal conditions for specific individuals having a particular medical problem. Effectiveness emphasises what a technology actually does. It reflects performance of a medical technology under ordinary conditions when applied by an average practitioner, to a typical patient. In order to make rational choices we depend on relevant literature. As there are thousands of articles published each year, the first we ought to do is to decide what is relevant literature. Sackett et al. [1] and Guyatt et al. [2,3] made suggestions for the use of articles concerning therapy or prevention. The guides, readers might use for an article on therapy or prevention can be very well applied to evaluations on the use of blood products.

There are three main items (Table 1):

1) are the results of the study valid;
2) what are the results; and
3) will the results help me in caring for my patients.

The question concerning the validity of the study focuses on the methodology: do these results represent an unbiased estimate of the treatment effect, or have they been influenced in some systemic way leading to a false conclusion.

The question "what are the results" emphasises the magnitude and precision of the estimated treatment effect. The treatment effect can be presented as an absolute or relative risk reduction, which can be calculated as follows: suppose from 100 treated patients 5 patients died, whereas in 100 non-treated patients 10 died. The risk in the non-treated arm (X) = 10/100 = 0.10 or 10%. The risk in the treatment arm (Y) is 5/100 = 0.05 or 5%. The absolute risk reduction (X-Y) is 0.10-0.05 = 0.05. The relative risk is Y/X = 0.05/0.10 = 0.5. The relative risk reduction (RRR) will then be $[1-(Y/X)]\times 100\% = 50\%$. If another 100 patients

Table 1. Readers' Guides for an article about therapy [2].

Are the results of the study valid?

Primary guides:

- Was the assignment of patients to treatments randomized?
- Were all patients who entered the trial properly accounted for and attributed at its conclusion?
- Was follow-up complete?
- Were patients analyzed in the groups to which they were randomized?

Secondary guides:

- Were patients, health workers, and study personnel "blind" to treatment?
- Were the groups similar at the start of the trial?
- Aside from the experimental intervention, were the groups treated equally?

What are the results?

- How large was the treatment effect?
- How precise was the estimate of the treatment effect?

Will the results help me in caring for my patients?

- Can the results be applied to my patient care?
- Were all clinically important outcomes considered?
- Are the likely treatment benefits worth the potential harms and costs?

will be studied not exactly the same figures could be expected. The precision of the estimated treatment effect will be obtained from the confidence intervals (CI). Usually the 95% CI is used: reporting the range that includes 95% of the studied parameter if the study will be repeated in a lot or number of aselectively chosen samples. The narrower the CI the more precise the reported estimated treatment effect will be, and the larger the sample size the narrower the CI. An RRR of 0% means no effect of the experimental treatment. A negative percentage means a possibly unfavourable effect. An RRR of 25% in a relatively small sample might have a CI of -8% to +58%, meaning a chance of harm of the experimental treatment.

With the CI we can judge if the study was big enough to justify the conclusions. In positive studies (studies claiming a positive result) the lower limit must be above the level we consider to be clinically relevant. If we consider an RRR of 7% not relevant, then despite a statistical significance the study is to small to be considered definitive. On the other hand if in a negative study the upper limit of the CI is higher then the percentage we consider relevant than the study has failed to exclude a clinically important effect of the studied treatment.

Are the results relevant for the treatment of my patients?

Important in this matter are the targets which are studied. Required is an improvement of outcomes that are relevant to the patient. Often intermediate or substitute targets are studied like improvement of blood pressure or a laboratory end point in stead of relevant issues such as survival, hospitalization or decreasing risk on myocardial infarction. Another question is, whether it is worth the effort to change to another treatment or product. Illustrative might be the number needed to treat (NNT) to obtain benefit or, if the treatment has adverse effects harm. The inverse of the absolute risk reduction equals the number of patients we have to treat to prevent one event or to obtain one patient experiencing an adverse effect. If there is a risk reduction (X-Y) of 50% of an adverse effect which occurs without the new treatment in 1% of the cases, the absolute risk reduction is 50% of 0.01 = 0.005. The inverse (1/absolute risk reduction) is 200. We would have to treat 200 patients in order to prevent one adverse effect. Whether this is worth doing depends on aspects like costs, adverse effects and ease to perform the new treatment.

Clinical need in daily practice

We now have outlined the criteria to be used for the evaluation of standard and new blood products. How does this relate to daily practice.

The most important clinical requirement for blood products is their effectiveness. The primary goal of the transfusion of red blood cell concentrate is to restore or maintain an adequate supply of oxygen. The most important reason to transfuse platelet concentrates is to maintain or restore haemostasis as far as platelets (by deficiency in number or function) are held responsible for the defect in haemostasis, or to prevent thrombopenic or thrompathic bleeding. The primary goal of the transfusion of plasma is to maintain or restore haemostasis as far as a deficiency of clotting factors is held responsible for the defect in haemostasis. Traditionally the standard products red blood cell concentrate (RBC) buffy coat included, platelet concentrate (PC) not leukocyte-depleted and fresh frozen plasma (FFP) are used. In recent years a number of modified products has been introduced. For instance buffy coat depleted RBC, RBC resuspended in a medium containing saline-adenine-glucose-mannitol (SAGM), leukocyte-depleted PC, PC resuspended in a conditioned medium. From these products one might expect, as for other therapies that the value has been demonstrated according to the criteria mentioned above. A modified product should not be propagated or introduced because it is supposed to be better for the patient for theoretical or pathophysiological reasons. As the use of these blood products is to improve oxygen carrying capacity and haemostasis, the question arises in what way these modifications provide important benefits to the patients. The answer has to come from the literature which should meet the criteria shown in Table 1.

Important in the review of the literature are the targets studied: are these really clinically important issues or intermediate/substitute end points? It could be possible to prevent HLA-alloimmunization in surgical patients by using leukocyte-depleted products. However, if these patients are not considered to be candidates for platelet transfusions then for the patient there is no clinically relevant benefit to be expected from leukocyte depleted blood. Another important point is the question if the modification is worth the effort. The removal of the buffy coat from RBC has been justified by its ability to prevent febrile non-haemolytic transfusion reactions (FNHTR), the most frequently reported adverse reaction of blood transfusions.

Again, what is the benefit of buffy coat depleted RBC for my patient? Menitove et al. [4] reported an incidence of FNHTR of 0.5% in 43,724 RBCs transfused, Decary et al. [5] mentioned an incidence of 1.06% in 10,277 RBC transfusions. If the removal of the buffy coat would decrease the incidence by 50% 200-400 patients should be transfused with buffy coat depleted RBC to prevent 1 FNHTR.

What about the bedside practice? If a patient develops a FNHTR he will get an antipyretic. After three or more FNHTRs the patient has developed a more then usual chance of getting reactions in the future. Important for the clinical relevance is the study of Vamvakas et al. [6] who showed that 75.3% of the patients transfused will not receive further transfusions in the coming 10 years. In my opinion we can stay with the standard RBC and for the small subgroup of patients with recurrent FNHTRs we should use leukocyte-depleted RBC. Another point of consideration is the local situation. The incidence of an adverse reaction caused by a particular blood product might differ from one country or part of the country to another. A preventive measure might be useful when the incidence is high but this might be hardly effective in another situation.

Remarkable is the difference in reported febrile reactions due to platelet transfusions which ranges from 0 to 70% [7]. Heddle et al. [8] recently reported febrile reactions in 20% of the platelet transfusions given to 12 premedicated mostly acute myeloid leukaemia patients; 9 of these 12 patients experienced more than one adverse reaction of which 43% was graded as severe. The platelets were stored for 4-5 days before transfusion. In our centre[1] we perform a study on the effect of non-leukocyte depleted but stored blood products on the incidence of HLA-alloimmunization. Until September 1995 63 acute leukaemia patients received during induction chemotherapy 25 ± 11 units of RBC, buffy coat included and stored before transfusion for 3 weeks at 4°C, and 16 ± 10 platelet transfusions consisting of a pool of 6 donor units stored for 3-5 days at 20-24°C. The incidence of febrile reactions was 2.1%. One patient received leukocyte depleted RBC because of recurrent febrile reactions after RBC, that did not occur after platelet transfusion. In an other haematology centre in the Netherlands the incidence of febrile reactions is estimated between 0-30% despite leukocyte depletion [9]. Striking was the observation of two different estimates of febrile reactions in hospitals using platelets from the same blood bank: 0.35 and 30% respectively. It seems that a lot of researche needs to be done before a generalized conclusion and justified advise for prevention, for instance by modifying the product, can be made. Until now we pointed out the important role of the medical literature in order to define the clinical need for supportive haemotherapy.

---

1. Department of Haematology, University Hospital Groningen, NL.

Table 2. Guidelines for How to Use Articles Describing Clinical Practice Guidelines.

Are the recommendations valid?
Primary guides:
- Were all important options and outcomes clearly specified?
- Was an explicit and sensible process used to identify, select, and combine evidence?

Secondary guides:
- Was an explicit and sensible process used to consider the relative value of different outcomes?
- Is the guideline likely to account for important recent developments?
- Has the guideline been subject to peer review and testing?

What are the recommendations:
- Are practical, clinically important, recommendations made?
- How strong are the recommendations?
- What is the impact of uncertainty associated with the evidence and values used in the guidelines?

Will the recommendations help you in caring for your patients?
- Is the primary objective of the guideline consistent with your objective?
- Are the recommendations applicable to your patients?

What about guidelines and does all the evidence have the same value?

Hayward et al. [10] presented guidelines for how to use articles, describing guidelines for clinical practice (Table 2). One of the important issues for expert committees generating recommendations for the preparation and/or use of blood products is: what rules of evidence should be applied. Cook et al. [11] described several levels of evidence ranging:
- Level I: randomized trials with low false positive and low false negative errors (statistically significant and high power).
- Level II: randomized trials with high false positive and high false negative errors (statistically non-significant and low power).
- Level III: non-randomized trials with a concurrent cohort (comparison between two contemporaneous groups).
- Level IV: non-randomized trials with an historical cohort (comparison between an historical and a contemporaneous group).
- Level V: case series without control subjects.

Sometimes randomized controlled trials have not yet been carried out, or other high level evidence is not available. In those situations recommendations should come from clinical observations and expert opinions. However, it must be clear on what scientific evidence or subjective judgement the recommendations are based. This represents the strength of the guideline, and by that the difference between yes or no in implementation of the recommendation.

Conclusion

When conventionally used standard blood products are modified, the benefit for the patient must appear from scientific evidence and not only from theoretical considerations. If recommendations are made concerning the preparation and/or use of blood products it is a great comfort to the practising physician when the basic evidence is available and the strength of the recommendations obvious.

References

1. Sackett DL, Haynes RB, Guyatt GH, Tugwell P. Clinical epidemiology. A basic science for clinical medicine. Little, Brown and Company. Boston/Toronto/London 1991.
2. Guyatt GH, Sackett DL, Cook DJ. Users' guides to the medical literature. II. How to use an article about therapy or prevention. A. Are the results of the study valid? JAMA 1993;270:2598-601.
3. Guyatt GH, Sackett DL, Cook DJ. Users' guides to the medical literature. II. How to use an article about therapy or prevention. B. What were the results and will they help me in caring for my patients? JAMA 194;271:59-63.
4. Menitove JE, McElligott MC, Aster RH. Febrile transfusion reaction: What blood component should be given next? Vox Sang 1982;42:318-21.
5. Decary F, Ferner P, Giavedoni L, et al. An investigation of nonhemolytic transfusion reactions. Vox Sang 1984;46:277-85.
6. Vamvakas EC, Taswell HF. Probability of red cell transfusion in an unselected population. Transfusion 1994;34:1014-15.
7. Brand A. Passenger leukocytes, cytokines, and transfusion reactions N Engl J Med 1994;331:670-71.
8. Heddle NM, Klama L, Singer J, et al. The role of the plasma from platelet concentrates in transfusion reactions. N Engl J Med 1994;331:625-28.
9. Novotny VMJ. Personal communication.
10. Hayward RSA, Wilson MC, Tunis SR, Bass EB, Guyatt GH. Users' guides to the medical literature. VIII. How to use clinical practice guidelines. A. Are the recommendations valid? JAMA 1995;274:570-74
11. Cook DJ, Guyatt GH, Laupacis A, Sackett DL. Rules of evidence and clinical recommendations on the use of antithrombotic agents. Chest 1992;102:305S-11S.

FACTORS AFFECTING THE CLINICAL EFFICACY OF BLOOD TRANSFUSION

W.G. Murphy

For the purposes of this paper clinical efficacy as it describes a therapeutic product or manoeuvre is meant very specifically to mean the ability of that product or manoeuvre to benefit in a clinically meaningful way the patient who receives or undergoes it. For example a red blood transfusion may be ordered by a surgeon to raise the patient's postoperative haemoglobin level to a figure that the surgeon feel comfortable with, but the patient will probably interpret the action, quite reasonably, as intended to improve well being or to prolong or maintain life [1]. The patient's trust may be misplaced in this case, for several reasons. A raised haemoglobin level is not acceptable as an endpoint of relevance in discussing clinical efficacy until such time as studies equate it with real benefit in terms of morbidity and mortality, and refute extant evidence to the contrary [2,3]. Clinically meaningful endoptions are confined to endpoints that would be valued by the patient and include saving life, prolonging life, decreasing morbidity, discomfort or pain, and increasing well-being, without doing anything that will undermine these valued gains. This definition excludes efficacy measured by many endoptions that are commonly accepted in the literature; however, endoptions such as a raised platelet count, avoidance of alloimmunization, even prevention of haemorrhage cannot be assumed to be of overall clinical value unless they have been shown to improve clinically important endpoints such as morbidity and mortality. For example, platelet transfusions have been associated with improved haemostatic care in patients with malignancy, but their role when administered uncritically in improving survival has never been shown, and comparative studies that back up assumptions of applicability of in vitro measures to clinically valuable outcomes have never been done. This makes it difficult, but not impossible [4] to compare the clinical efficacy of different platelet preparations or transfusion regimens. Given that the results of Gmur's study [5] were applicable to the general picture of care of thrombocytopenic patients the clinical efficacy of a vast number of platelet transfusions given today would at best be zero. The factors that affect the clinical efficacy of a transfusion episode are listed in Table 1. Primary factors are taken to include the patient, the prescriber, the bedside caregiver and the blood component itself. Secondary factors are the transfusionist, the health care system and the depth and availability or penetration of the knowledge base in regard to the clinical circumstances pertaining.

Table 1. Major factors influencing the efficacy of a transfusion.

The patient The prescriber	The transfusionist	The healthcare system
The caregiver The component		The knowledge base

To what extent commercial interests affect clinical activities in a way that influences clinical efficacy is probably worthy of separate analysis.

The patient

Patients contribute to clinical efficacy in several ways. Apart from individual clinical factors, which are discussed in detail below, the patient's knowledge or understanding of the need for or alternatives to blood transfusion have the ability to play an important part in the transfusion process. Patient-led demand has a remarkable ability to influence transfusion decisions and transfusion efficacy - the demands of Jehovah's Witnesses have contributed considerably to reappraisal of the need to transfuse blood at certain haemoglobin levels [2]. In addition, patients' perceptions of the benefit of autologous blood transfusion programmes can be a major factor in determining the success of these programmes. While these factors (reduction of transfusion triggers, autologous transfusion) may not be globally applicable if transfusion strategies become to some degree more indication specific they will probably have an impact on clinical efficacy in many patients.

Other features of the patient may have an important influence on the efficacy of blood transfusion. The consequence of an adverse effect such as infection with hepatitis will depend to some extent on the life expectancy of the recipient: for children the consequences could be considerably greater than for an adult.

The prescriber

Different doctors do different things. Practice varies with the seniority and location of the clinician [6-8]. The reasons for these differences have not been systematically studied in relation to blood transfusion, but their existence provides grounds for reasonable doubt of efficacy. They do not prove that there are variations in efficacy: several different systems may produce clinically indistinguishable results, but in general some useful pointers should be gained from comparative studies. However, studies of comparative practice may simply lead to regression outcomes. It is not clear how or why differences in transfusion practice arise or persist [8]. We undertook studies of surgical blood transfusion practices throughout Scotland [6,11]. For hip surgery and elective aortic aneurysm surgery differences in mean blood use per operation existed between and within different regions. These differences did not depend on the use of blood ordering schedules (consistent with lack of transfusionist influence) but were strongly suggestive of an effect of individual surgeons' practices.

Understanding the evolution of current practice might lead to understanding how to optimise practice in the future (assuming we knew what optimum practice was). Several studies have attempted to do this in relation to blood transfusion [9,10]. though it may be too early to determine whether these will have a long lasting effect, or too difficult to identify the causes for any changes observed. For many years it was common practice (for no very good reason) to transfuse platelets in pools of ten units in North America; in some areas at least this practice is in decline, though the clinical evidence has not changed; whether papers in influential journals [9], consensus statements [12], local practice guidelines, increased numbers of transfusion medicine physicians or threat of litigation have brought this about is impossible to know. Perhaps a necessity to extract consent to transfusion may have an effect in improving clinical efficacy, although presumably informed consent is obtained for the many thousands of useless surgical procedures performed annually. Programmes of undergraduate and postgraduate education of physicians in training may help improve clinical efficacy in transfusion; perhaps the advent of serious contenders for alternatives to allogeneic blood transfusion will be the major agent of change.

The bedside caregiver

The nurse is responsible for several important components of the transfusion process that have an impact on the clinical efficacy of the event. For example the majority of ABO disasters, the commonest identified cause of transfusion-induced death, are due to mistakes in patient or sample misidentification at the bedside [13-15]. In addition the nurse is responsible for the post-issue care of the blood component, such as proper storage on the ward and proper use of bedside filters, and for peritransfusion monitoring of the patient. Furthermore it is to the nurse that the patient will often turn to for information and advice on blood transfusions. Finally, it is quite conceivable that in the future the role of nurses in transfusion medicine will increase, and well designed and tested programmes will need to ensure the maximum contribution of this professional group to clinical efficacy of transfusion.

The blood product

The design, the specification, the manufacture and the availability and delivery of a blood product may have major consequences for the clinical efficacy of a transfusion. It is not possible at present to conduct a comparative analysis to determine which features of supply or delivery have an effect on clinical efficacy. The area of manufacture that has been addressed most intensively in recent years has been leukodepletion. An effect on clinical outcomes of significance has yet to be defined [16-19] or found to be applicable to all blood product manufactures. For example the results of the Dutch study [16] found that there was not a definable difference in outcome when standard blood product was used compared to leukodepleted blood. However the standard blood product tested in this trial was buffy coat reduced, so that the findings cannot be extrapolated to blood centres using non-buffy coat reduced product. In addition filters are not identical, and starting material is not identical, so that products derived from a filtration process may vary considerably in terms of real clinical efficacy, particularly if soluble factors play an important role in causing events of consequence [20,21]. Applying the results of a comprehensive and definitive study of a manufacturing process such as the Dutch study discussed above, or a study of the comparative efficacy of leukodepleted and CMV-screened blood in preventing transmission of CMV [22] to other similar manufacturing processes or plants may not be valid, particularly where the effective part (if any) of the process is as poorly understood as it is in the two examples given (and overall outcome data are unavailable from the CMV study as yet).

Product design has tended in the past to be approached from the manufacturer's point of view rather than from the patient's. There are good reasons for this, mainly the impositions of the source of the material and to a lesser extent the need to limit donor exposures in recent times. As an illustration of the limitations that are imposed by the source material, it is unlikely that if and when tissue oxygen delivery is managed by soluble rather than cellular pharmaceuticals the units of dose will be in RBC unit equivalents, i.e. 250+/-75mls of RBCs of age between 1 and 42 days of variable O_2 delivery capacity and variable electrolyte content. Equally importantly the clinical efficacy of blood transfusion has been influenced by several prevailing concepts in blood component design. These are the concepts of *unit equivalence*, *indication equivalence*, and *surrogate equivalence*.

Unit equivalence in relation to red cells dictates that a unit of blood at the end of its shelf live is clinically equal to a week 1 or 2 unit. There are generally accepted exceptions in neonatal transfusion practice, but in spite of considerable data indicating impaired in vitro performance of stored blood, the absence of clinical data is taken to indicate the absence of clinical effect in adults. However, the study on which this concept could be based has never been done, and would be exceedingly difficult to do, not least because any effect would be most likely seen in the setting of acutely ill patients where the impact of a single factor such as age of blood transfused would be very difficult to demonstrate and even more difficult to refute. A study of tissue oxygen delivery in response to blood transfusion in septic patients raises considerable doubts about the concept of unit equivalence [23]: patients receiving blood greater than 15 days old developed paradoxical splanchnic ischaemia (attributed to microvascular occlusion from rigid stored red cells), while even patients receiving younger blood failed to demonstrate increased oxygen uptake. Were the findings of this study to be extended to a well defined clinically important outcome the implications to the blood supply would be enormous, and the implications for autologous blood transfusion programmes could also be very important. Perhaps the concomitant use of oxygen delivery solutions, erythropoietin and stored blood will ultimately circumvent the problem, if it exists.

The concepts of *indication equivalence* and *surrogate equivalence* require that the patient needing transfusion for one indication is, from the point of view of clinical transfusion efficacy, the same as the patient with a different indication. Thus a patient with a haemoglobin level of 8 gm/dl following a gastrointestinal haemorrhage may be considered as requiring essentially the same transfusion as a postoperative patient or a patient with hypoplastic anaemia with similar haemoglobin levels. The patients are the same if a surrogate marker such as haemoglobin level are the same. In addition measures such as haemoglobin level or oxygen delivery are taken as measures of important outcomes such as survival and morbidity. That these concepts cannot be universally applied is demonstrated by the study of Blair et al. [3] where transfusion in a group of patients where there would have been little serious debate as to its necessity was show in a prospective randomized trial to have a detrimental impact on important measures of outcome, for reasons that are far from clear. Fifty patients presenting to a single unit with gastrointestinal haemorrhage who were stable, and who's haemoglobin without transfusion was greater than 8 gm/dl were randomized either to transfusion or not transfusion. The rebleed rate was 36% in the transfused arm and 4% in the non transfused arm, with mortality limited to rebleeding transfused patients. The authors proposed one potential mechanism for this phenomenon; others are possible, not least an effect of splanchnic ischaemia for transfusion of old blood as described by Marik and Sibbald [23]. Blair's study is one of the very few attempts to *randomize* patients to transfusion or no transfusion and provides a basis for extending this approach to other stable groups of patients.

In the design of plasma preparations for transfusion the major factors influencing clinical efficacy have been the limitations in manipulating the specifications of the source material, and the limited data about the requirements for the treatment of thrombotic thrombocytopenic purpura (TTP), which after multiple factor replacement is one of the most important residual indications (although the widespread variations in plasma use suggest that plasma may be used frequently where no indication exists [7]). For complex acquired coagulopathies there are no data to indicate that any variable of the product other than dose has any influence on overall outcome. For TTP, while plasma is probably better than other therapies, the relevant constituent in the plasma is not known [24] and may be a combination of several factors. Indeed the relevant factor in plasma may be different in different patients.

For platelet transfusions product design has concentrated on surrogate markers of clinical efficacy such as dose, *in vivo* recovery and survival in stable patients and in vitro markers for these *in vivo* surrogates such as pH and a host of other markers of probable and improbable utility. However, efficacy in improving real health outcomes from design specifications derived from such studies is difficult to measure, or more importantly the results of such *in vitro* and *in vivo* studies are difficult to apply to patients for whom the surrogate readouts were not optimised. These include unstable refractory patients, who constitute a significant proportion of those with thrombocytopenia-related morbidity [5,25].

For prophylactic platelet transfusions in patients with circulating platelet counts at levels above 10×10^9/l most transfusions will be unnecessary [25], even if within current guidelines [12,26]. Design factors of relevance to clinical efficacy in this setting would be monumentally difficult to demonstrate, needing approximately 500 transfusion events in each arm of a well designed and conducted study to demonstrate effect or lack of it with acceptable power. While an incrementing platelet transfusion may be more haemostatic than a non-incrementing one a variable effect of platelet age has never been proved or disproved in spite of widespread assumption to the contrary. These features of product design will become increasingly important as platelet substitutes enter clinical trial and claim equivalence or superiority.

The transfusionist

The blood transfusion community contributes to clinical efficacy of blood transfusion through product design and development, and product and service provision. Product design is currently a balance between operational contingencies and therapeutic requirements. Service provision embraces products, education, and service development.

Do these activities have a measurable impact on clinical efficacy of blood transfusion that extends noticeably beyond that derived from product provision alone? Do different transfusionists' beliefs and practices lead to differences in morbidity and mortality and other valuable endpoints in patient care? Since the effect if any of transfusion practice other than product supply on patient care would be difficult to measure surrogate markers would be needed; this approach is likely to be fraught with difficulties. A negative effect of transfusionists and their practice on patient care is possible, and not without precedent that has been considered in court of law. Markers of clinical efficacy of transfusionists might include uptake of well-validated changes in practice, or survival of well-discredited ones in the clinical communities serviced by the transfusionists, number of surgical procedures postponed or delayed through non-availability of blood, residual rates of Rhesus sensitisation in the community. But even these are influenced by other factors well outside the sphere of influence of the transfusionist.

Conclusion

Many of the factors influencing clinical efficacy of blood transfusions and of transfusion medicine practice are unknown and even undefinable. In the coming years effects of transfusion on overall outcomes that are not currently recognised may come to light with a shift towards reduced use of fresh or plasma-derived products. With increasing capital interest in biotechnology the borders between commercial interest and patient interest may become indistinct, and the possibilities for defining therapies of real value may become even more slender. Prospective randomized controlled trials in blood transfusion have proved difficult to do, but the necessity to establish a firm evidence-based core for transfusion practice has never been greater.

References

1. Gray A, Murphy WG. A study of patients' perceptions and experiences of blood transfusion. Transf Med 1993;3(Suppl 1):81.
2. Carson JL, Rees Willett L. "Is hemoglobin of 10 g/dL required for surgery?" Med Clin North Am 1993;2:335-47.
3. Blair SD, Janvrin SB, McCollum CN, Greenhalgh RM. Effect of early blood transfusion on gastrointestinal haemorrhage. Brit J Surg 1986;73:783-85.
4. Murphy S, Litwin S, Herring LM, et al. Indications for platelet transfusion in children with acute leukemia. Am J Hematol 1982;12:347-56.
5. Gmur J, Burger J, Schanz U, Fehr J, Schaffner A. Safety of stringent prophylactic platelet transfusion policy for patients with acute leukemia. Lancet 1991;338:1223-26.
6. Murphy WG, Phillips P, Gray A, et al. Blood use for surgical patients: A study of Scottish hospital transfusion practices. JR Coll Surg Edinb 1995;40:10-13.
7. Sirchia G, Giovanetti AM, McClelland DBL, Fracchia GN. Safe and good use of blood in surgery (SANGUIS), European Commission, Luxembourg, 1994.
8. Nicols MD, White G. Red cell, plasma and albumin transfusion decision triggers. Anaesthesia & Intensive Care 1993;21:156-62.
9. McCullough J, Steeper TA, Connelly DP, et al. Platelet utilization in a university hospital. JAMA 1988;259:2414-18.
10. Thomson A, Contreras M, Knowles S. Blood component treatment. A retrospective audit in 5 major London hospitals. J Clin Pathol 1991;4:734-37.
11. Milne AA, Murphy WG. Current blood transfusion practice in aortic aneurysm surgery in Scotland. JR Coll Surg Edinb 1995;40:104-8.
12. Consensus Conference. Platelet transfusion therapy. JAMA 1987;257:1777-80.
13. Honig CL, Bove JR. Transfusion associated fatalities: Review of bureau of biologies reports 1976-1978. Transfusion 1980;20:653.
14. Murphy WG, McClelland DBL. Deceptively low mortality from failure to practice safe blood transfusion: An analysis of serious blood transfusion errors. Vox Sang 1989;57:59-62.
15. Phillips P, McClelland DBL. Errors in blood transfusion in Britain. Survey of hospital haematology departments. Brit Med J 1994;308:1205-6.
16. Houbiers JGA, Brand A, van de Watering LMG, et al. Randomized controlled trial comparing transfusion of leucocyte-depleted or buffy coat depleted blood in surgery for colorectal cancer. Lancet 1994;344:573-78.
17. Jensen LS, Andersen AJ, Christiansen PM, et al. Postoperative infection and natural killer cell function following blood transfusion in patients undergoing elective colorectal surgery. Brit J Surg 1992;79:513-16.
18. Busch ORC, Hop WCJ, Hoynck van Papendrecht MAW, et al. Blood transfusions and prognosis in colorectal cancer. N Engl J Med 1993;328:1372-76.
19. Heddle NM, Klama L, Singer J, et al. The role of the plasma for platelet concentrates in transfusion reactions. N Engl J Med 1994;331:625-28.
20. Heddle NM. The efficacy of leucodepletion to improve platelet transfusion response: A critical appraisal of clinical studies. Transf Med Rev 1994;8:15-28.
21. Kluter H, Mullersteinhardt M, Danzer S, et al. Cytokines in platelet concentrates prepared from pooled buffy coats. Vox Sang 1995;69:38-43.
22. Bowden RA, Cays S, Schoch G, et al. Comparison of filtered blood (FB) to sero-negative blood products (SB) for prevention of cytomegalovirus (CMV) infection after marrow transplant. Blood 1993;82(Suppl 1):204a.

23. Marik PE, Sibbald WJ. Concepts in emergency and critical care. JAMA 1995;273: 1439-44.
24. Murphy WG, Moore JC, Warkentin TW, et al. Thrombotic thrombocytopenic purpura. Blood Coagulation & Fibrinolysis 1992;3:655-59.
25. Murphy WG, Palmer JB, Green RHA. The management of haemorrhage in the refractory non-alloimmunized thrombocytopenic patient. Vox Sang 1994;67(Suppl 1): 99-103.
26. British Committee for Standards in Haematology, Working Party of the Blood Transfusion Task Force. Murphy MF (Convener) Brozovic B, Murphy WG, Ouwehand W, Waters AH. Guidelines for platelet transfusions. Transf Med 1992;2:311-18.

THE CLINICAL RELEVANCE AND BIOLOGICAL EFFECTS OF LEUKOCYTES PRESENT IN CELLULAR BLOOD COMPONENTS

M. A. Blajchman

The transfusion of allogeneic cellular blood components (platelets and red blood cells) is frequently associated with diverse biologic effects in the recipient. These occur despite careful blood donor selection and the pretransfusion testing of the blood collected. Recipient transfusion reactions (summarized in Table 1) include both positive and negative effects. Some of the negative effects include febrile non-haemolytic transfusion reactions (FNHTR), graft-versus-host disease, immunomodulation and the transmission of infectious agents. Over the past decade much relevant evidence has been reported indicating that many of these biological effects are related to allogeneic leukocytes present in the donor blood, or their products which are released during storage [1]. A review article detailing the biological effects of transfused leukocytes has been published previously [1] and therefore in this chapter, only some of these biological phenomena will be discussed.

Table 1. Positive and negative biologic effects experienced by recipients of allogeneic blood products.

Positive	a*	Improved renal allograft survival
	b	Reduced relapse rate in patients with Crohn's disease
	c*	Reduced rate of spontaneous recurrent abortions
Negative	d	Haemolytic transfusion reactions
	e*	Non-haemolytic transfusion reactions
	f*	Alloimmunization
	g	Transmission of infections
	h*	Immunosuppression causing increased susceptibility to infection
	i*	Immunosuppression associated with enhanced malignant cell growth
	j*	Graft-versus-host disease

* Associated with allogeneic leukocytes or their cell products.

Febrile non-haemolytic transfusion reactions (FNHTR)

An FNHTR is usually defined as a 1°C rise in temperature associated with an allogeneic blood transfusion. FNHTRs have been estimated to occur in association with approximately 1% of allogeneic red blood cell and approximately 30% of allogeneic platelet concentrate transfusions [2,3]. Until relatively recently, most FNHTRs were attributed to the presence of alloantibodies reactive with HLA or other alloantigens present on the surface of donor leukocytes, or the platelets, present in the recipient's plasma. Although a reduction in number of allogeneic leukocytes present in a cellular blood component has been shown to reduce the FNHTR rate, the clinical use of leukodepleted products has not been totally effective in preventing such reactions, particularly when the leukocytes are removed only prior to infusion to a patient (this type of leukodepletion is known as bedside or post-storage leukodepletion [1, 4-6]. Moreover, FNHTRs have been reported to occur in patients transfused with only the supernatant plasma from platelet concentrates, which contain very low numbers of platelets and leukocytes [5,7]. Moreover, FNHTR rates have been shown to correlate positively with increasing storage age for both red cell and platelet concentrates [5].

Following the infusion of platelet concentrates, a correlation has been noted between the levels of tumor necrosis factor (TNF), as well as other cytokines, and the frequency of FNHTRs [7,8]. Such data indicate that most FNHTRs may not be the result of antigen-antibody interactions but result from the infusion of various soluble biologically active agents (e.g. interleukins) that are actively synthesized during cellular blood product storage by the leukocytes present in such cellular components. These biologically active substances have been shown to accumulate during blood product storage and leukocyte removal shortly after blood collection (pre-storage leukodepletion) may be able to reduce the incidence of such reactions better than post-storage leukodepletion [9]. Direct evidence showing the clinical benefit of pre-storage leukodepletion has, however, not yet been provided. Relevantly, it has been reported by several groups of investigators that the pre-storage leukodepletion of platelet concentrates significantly reduces the level of accumulated cytokines in the supernatant plasma of stored platelet and red cell concentrates, compared to that seen in non-leukodepleted concentrates [9,10].

Platelet refractoriness and alloimmunization

Approximately 50% of transfused patients who receive non-leukodepleted allogeneic blood transfusions become refractory to pooled random donor platelet concentrates (Table 2). While most investigators suggest that most refractory episodes are due to alloimmunization to HLA antigens, it has been shown that HLA alloantibodies can be detected in only 50 percent of refractory patients receiving multiple random donor platelet concentrates.

Various methods have been advocated to try to prevent or to reduce the frequency of platelet alloimmunization. These include the use of single donor platelets, cross-match compatible platelets, single donor HLA-matched platelets, UVB irradiated platelets, and leukodepleted allogeneic cellular blood components. The latter recommendation is based on observations in patients who had received leukodepleted random donor cellular blood products who have a lower risk for

Table 2. Summary of 11 studies evaluating rate of platelet alloimmunization in recipients of either leukodepleted or non-leukodepleted allogeneic blood products.

First author (year published)	Non-leukodepleted		Leukodepleted	
	n	% alloimmunized	n	% alloimmunized
Eernisse (1981)	28	93	68	24
Schiffer (1983)	12	33	15	27
Fisher (1985)	-	NR	24	21
Murphy (1986)	31	48	19	16
Sniecinski (1988)	20	50	20	15
Andreu (1988)	35	31	34	12
Saarinen (1990)	17	71	18	0
van Marwijk Kooy (1991)	26	46	27	11
Oksanen (1991)	15	7	16	0
Handa (1993)	21	38	32	6
Sintnicolaas (1995)*	(21)	(43)	(25)	(44)
Total	205	48.3	273	14.7

NR = not reported.

* This study specifically evaluated patients with a history of prior allogeneic transfusions and/or pregnancies. The data from this study are not included therefore in the totals.

platelet refractoriness and HLA-alloimmunization than recipients of non-leukodepleted blood products. The result of 11 such studies are summarized in Table 2. Thus, the mean frequency of platelet alloimmunization in patients who had been transfused with non-leukodepleted blood components is considerably higher than that observed in patients who had received leukodepleted blood products. Recently two important studies have been published indicating that leukodepletion may be of limited efficacy, for the prevention of HLA-alloimmunization, in individuals with a history of prior pregnancy or prior transfusions [11,12]. These latter two studies indicate that the administration of leukodepleted cellular blood products to subjects who had been previously exposed to leukocytes will not prevent HLA-alloimmunization in such recipients.

Many other unresolved issues remain with regard to assessing the clinical impact of leukodepletion to prevent platelet refractoriness. These include establishing the extent and the optimal timing of the leukodepletion; establishing criteria to evaluate the correlation between alloimmunization and refractoriness; ascertaining the clinical risk of morbidity due to bleeding; and evaluating the cost-effectiveness of an intervention as costly as leukodepletion [13].

The issue of platelet refractoriness and alloimmunization has been studied also in two experimental animal models. In a mouse model, 50% of mice receiving platelet transfusions, containing very low numbers of residual leukocytes, became alloimmunized [14]. In a rabbit model, 3 $\log_{10}$ leukocyte reduction provided no significant advantage over 2 $\log_{10}$ leukocyte removal [15]. Thus both 2 $\log_{10}$ or 3 $\log_{10}$ pre-storage leukocyte removal resulted in approximately 30% of rabbits becoming refractory to allogeneic platelets compared to approximately 90% of rabbits that received non-leukodepleted blood products [16]. Interestingly, in this latter study, the extent of platelet refractoriness could be markedly reduced by combining plasma removal with pre-storage leukodepletion. An additional observation made in these studies was that pre-storage leukodepletion was associated with a markedly reduced frequency of platelet refractoriness, and therefore higher in vivo platelet survival, compared to that seen in animals that had received post-storage leukodepleted allogeneic blood.

Such data suggest that platelet refractoriness may be related not only to the number of white blood cells present in an allogeneic cellular blood component, but also to the presence of MHC or other antigens in a cellular blood component, either in a soluble form or as microparticles, that may escape leukocyte filtration. The increase in white cell fragment number with storage has recently been reported [17]. These studies also show poor retention of these white cell fragments by standard leukocyte filters. Such data indicate that the timing of the leukodepletion of a cellular blood component may be an important factor in the elimination of platelet refractoriness

Allogeneic blood transfusion and immunomodulation

Allogeneic blood transfusions have been shown to cause immunologic functional alterations in recipients. These effects are discussed in detail in reference 1 and summarized in Table 3. These alterations include: decreased helper to suppressor T-lymphocyte ratio; decreased NK cell function; defective antigen presentation; and reduction in cell-mediated immunity. The first evidence for an immunomodulatory effect of allogeneic blood transfusion was reported in renal allograft transplant recipients more than 20 years ago, when a highly significant correlation between pre-transplant blood transfusions and improved renal allograft survival was reported. These results have been replicated in studies in experimental animals and confirmed from many clinical renal transplant centres. The available information indicates that patients transfused with allogeneic blood have a significantly better survival of their renal allografts than do untransfused patients, regardless of the number of HLA mismatches. Even with HLA-identical siblings, it has been reported that 75% of untransfused recipients experience one or more episodes of graft rejection, while 33% of similar allogeneically transfused patients experience such episodes [18].

Although it is widely accepted that allogeneic blood transfusions can improve renal allograft survival, this therapeutic modality is not widely used clinically. There are three reasons that this effective therapeutic modality is not widely used: the advent of very effective immunosuppressive agents, improved patient management, and concern about the possible transmission of transfusion-associated infections. Nonetheless, a recent multicentre study reporting on over 58, 036 renal transplants from cadaver donors, transplanted since the advent of the use of cyclosporin, indicates that patients receiving allogeneic blood transfusion are still

Table 3. Reported alterations in immune function associated with allogeneic blood transfusions.

- Decreased natural killer (NK) cell function
- Altered delayed-type hypersensitivity
- Decreased helper T cell (CD4) count
- Altered CD4:CD8 T cell ratio
- Decreased lymphocyte mitogenic responses
- Suppression of lymphocyte blastogenesis
- Decreased phagocytic function
- Decreased cytokine production by lymphocytes (i.e. IL-2)

more likely to have a successful renal allograft than those who do not. This study reported that the one-year renal allograft survival rate was 3-5% better than in patients who did not receive such transfusions [19].

Blood transfusion and tumor growth

The possibility that an allogeneic blood transfusion might adversely affect patients with a malignancy was raised a number of years ago. In this author's opinion, no definitive clinical data either proving or disproving this effect of allogeneic blood transfusions have been published. The available clinical data are mainly from non-randomized, retrospective clinical studies. These have been summarized in detail elsewhere [1]. The available data show that approximately 50% of the reported studies indicate that allogeneic blood transfusions have an adverse effect on tumor growth in recipients; however, the remaining studies report no such effect.

There have been 7 prospective studies reporting on clinical outcome following perioperative allogeneic blood transfusion in patients with a malignancy. These are summarized in Table 4. Six studies involve patients with colorectal cancer and one is from prostate cancer patients. Four of these seven studies have been randomized prospective studies, and in 3 of them no adverse effect of allogeneic blood transfusions could be demonstrated. Overall in the 7 prospective studies, 5 indicate no adverse effect of allogeneic blood transfusions while 2 indicate an

Table 4. Summary of the results of four randomized and three non-randomized prospective studies reporting clinical outcome following perioperative allogeneic blood transfusions in patients with a malginancy.

Tumor site	No adverse effect reported		Adverse effect reported	
	Randomized	Non-randomized	Randomized	Non-randomized
Colorectal	2	2	1	1
Prostate	1	0	0	0
Total	3	2	1	1

adverse effect in recipients. Thus, in this author's opinion, the issue as to whether allogeneic blood transfusions can affect tumor growth in man is still an open issue.

The tumor growth-promoting effect of allogeneic blood transfusion has been studied also in experimental animals [20-24]. Data from both inbred and outbred animal models indicate that the tumor growth-promoting effect of allogeneic blood transfusions is a real biological phenomenon and that this effect is mediated immunologically. These studies also indicate that the allogeneic blood transfusion effect on promoting tumor growth is related to the presence of donor allogeneic leukocytes and that this allogeneic leukocyte effect can be ameliorated by the pre-storage leukodepletion of the allogeneic blood, but not by post-storage leukodepletion. Although results from experimental animals cannot necessarily be extrapolated to the clinical situation, the available data indicate that the post-storage leukodepletion of allogeneic blood products may not be effective in preventing the tumor growth-promoting effect of allogeneic blood transfusion.

Allogeneic blood transfusions and risk of bacterial infection

The association between perioperative allogeneic blood transfusions and increased risk of bacterial infection following surgery has been examined in both clinical and experimental animal studies [1]. The available studies indicate that allogeneic blood transfusions predispose recipients to bacterial infection. Six prospective clinical studies have reported the increased risk of postoperative infection following allogeneic blood transfusions. These are summarized in Table 5. Three of these studies have been randomized prospective studies while three were not. As outlined in Table 5, susceptibility to post-operative bacterial infection appears to be associated with the transfusion of non-leukodepleted allogeneic blood products and that the removal of the leukocytes from such allogeneic blood might mitigate the risk of bacterial infection.

Table 5. Summary of the six prospective studies reporting on the incidence of postoperative infections following allogeneic blood transfusions.

First author (year published)	**Randomized**	**Type of surgery**	**n**	**Infection rate**	
				Allogeneic recipients	**Controls**
NORGAS (1988)	No	Abdominal	1,537	22/357 (6%)	16/1,180 (1%)1)
Tartter (1988)	No	Abdominal	343	33/134 (25%)	9/ 209 (4%)1)
Jensen (1990)	No	Abdonimal	311	57/202 (28%)	2/ 109 (2%)1)
Triulzi (1992)	Yes	Orhtopaedic	84	5/ 24 (21%)	2/ 60 (3%)2)
Jensen (1992)	Yes	Abdominal	104	13/ 56 (23%)	1/ 48 (2%)3)
Heiss (1993)	Yes	Abdominal	120	17/ 62 (27%)	7/ 58 (12%)2)
Total			2,499	147/835 (17.6%)	37/1,664 (2.2%)

1) The control group of patients in this study did not receive any blood products.
2) The control group received autologous blood only.
3) The control group received leukodepleted allogeneic blood products only.

Leukocytes as the vector for transfusion-associated infections

Allogeneic blood transfusions are administered regularly to patients who are at increased risk for infections. Not only do allogeneic cellular blood transfusions cause immunomodulation, they also may be the source for a transfusion-transmitted infection [1]. In some of these instances the donor leukocytes may bet the vector for such transfusion-transmitted diseases. Such instances are summarized in Table 6.

Table 6. Transfusion-transmitted infections for which allogeneic leukocytes have been reported to be a vector for the transmission of the infectious agent.

- Cytomegalovirus (CMV)
- HIV-1/2
- HTLV-I/II
- Epstein-Barr virus (EBV)
- Hepatitis C virus (HCV)

Cytomegalovirus (CMV) infections

Transfusion associated CMV infections have been recognized as a significant pathogenic cause of morbidity and mortality in cellular blood product recipients. CMV is a virus that is associated almost invariably with leukocytes. It has thus been suggested that the removal of leukocytes from allogeneic donor blood may prevent much transfusion-associated CMV. In a multicentre study controlled trial, 20% of newborn infants transfused with unfiltered blood products were reported to have developed CMV infection, whereas no CMV infection was observed in a similar group of neonates transfused with leukodepleted blood products [25]. Data from a prospective randomized study involving 487 patients undergoing bone marrow transplantation have recently been reported [26]. The results from this study indicate that the use of leukodepleted blood products is approximately equivalent to the use of CMV serologically-negative blood products in preventing transfusion-associated CMV infections.

Other transfusion-associated infections

Leukocytes, particularly B and T lymphocytes, are the reservoir of many infectious agents that can be transmitted through the transfusion of cellular blood products (summarized in Table 6). While it is widely accepted that many viral infections can be transmitted by blood products, the role of leukocytes in such transmission has bot been fully established. For example, the minimum number of leukocytes capable of transmitting viral infections has not yet been determined. While leukocyte filtration can remove cells containing infectious agents, it is unlikely in most situations that the leukodepletion of cellular blood products will be sufficient to prevent such infections (except CMV, perhaps).

Allogeneic peripheral blood mononuclear cells have been shown recently to induce activation of cells containing HIV-1 and the subsequent dissemination of

HIV-1 to uninfected cells [27]. This in vitro effect was not observed with leukodepleted allogeneic blood. This aspect of the role of allogeneic leukocytes in transfusion-transmitted infections remains to be elucidated.

Bacterial contamination of blood products remains a significant problem in transfusion medicine [28]. Recently we have reported that approximately 1 in 1,000 units of random donor platelet concentrates contain detectable levels of bacteria, as contaminants [29]. One manoeuvre that has been shown to be able to reduce the level of bacterial contamination has been the use of leukodepletion. It appears that the removal of leukocytes from blood products causes the removal of those leukocytes which contain bacteria which have undergone phagocytosis. The removal of such phagocytic cells appears to lower the risk of transfusion-associated septic reactions. Thus, the removal of leukocytes from cellular blood products should be performed only after an appropriate incubation period (3-8 hours) to enable phagocytosis of the bacteria present to take place.

The leukocyte depletion of blood products

The leukodepletion of cellular blood products can be performed shortly after collection from the donor (pre-storage leukodepletion) or after storage, just before transfusion (post-storage leukodepletion) and at the bedside during transfusion. The latter is also known as bedside leukodepletion. Pre-storage leukodepletion of blood products has been shown to prevent some of the adverse effects caused by the metabolites that are released from leukocytes during blood product storage. Moreover, the pre-storage leukodepletion of blood products has been shown to be more effective than post-storage leukodepletion in preventing platelet alloimmunization as well as the tumor growth-promoting effect associated with allogeneic blood transfusions. As outlined above, most of the latter observations are from experimental animals and need to be confirmed for humans with properly designed clinical trials.

Conclusions

The clinical indications for the leukodepletion of cellular blood products include the prevention of: FNHTRs; the transmission of disease; platelet refractoriness; and immunomodulation. However, for most of these indications the effectiveness clinically of leukodepletion remains unproven. Moreover, the exact degree of leukodepletion required for the various proposed indications remains to be defined. Thus many of the results obtained with the use of leukocyte depletion filters are tantalizing but the actual clinical benefit of leukodepletion has not been established in many instances, as much of the available data are from retrospective or from uncontrolled clinical trials. Moreover, issues of cost-effectiveness and quality control have not been adequately considered. Properly designed prospective clinical trials are urgently required to provide data with which to answer such questions and also to define optimal conditions for the preparation of blood components.

References

1. Bordin JO, Heddle NM, Blajchman MA. The biologic effects of leukocytes present in transfused cellular blood products. Blood 1994;84:1703-21.
2. Menitove JE, McElligott MC, Aster RH. Febrile transfusion reaction: What blood component should be given next? Vox Sang 1982;42:318-21.
3. Chambers LA, Kruskall MS, Pacini DG, Donovan LM. Febrile reactions after platelet transfusion: The effect of single versus multiple donors. Transfusion 1990;30:219-21.
4. Mangano MD, Chambers LA, Kruskall MS. Limited efficacy of leukopoor platelets for prevention of febrile transfusion reactions. Am J Clin Pathol 1991;95:733-38.
5. Heddle NM, Klama LN, Griffith L, Roberts R, Shukla G, Kelton JG. A prospective study to identify the risk factors associated with acute reactions to platelet and red cell transfusions. Transfusion 1993;33:794-97.
6. Goodnough LT, Riddell J IV, Lazarus H, et al. Prevalence of platelet transfusion reactions before and after implementation of leukocyte-depleted platelet concentrates by filtration. Vox Sang 1993;65:103-7.
7. Heddle NM, Klama LN, Singer J, et al. The role of the plasma from platelet concentrates in transfusion reactions. N Engl J Med 1994;331:625-28.
8. Muylle L, Joos M, Wouters E, de Bock R, Peetermans ME. Increased tumor necrosis factor α (TNFα), interleukin 1, and interleukin 6 (Il-6) levels in the plasma of stored platelet concentrates: Relationship between TNFα and IL-6 levels and febrile transfusion reactions. Transfusion 1993;33:195-99.
9. Aye MT, Palmer DS, Giulivi A, Hashemi S. Effect of filtration of platelet concentrates on the accumulation of cytokines and platelet release factors during storage. Transfusion 1995;35:117-24.
10. Stack G, Baril L, Napychank P, Snyder E. Cytokine generation in stored, white cell-reduced, and bacterially contaminated units of red cells. Transfusion 1995;35:199-203.
11. Sintnicolaas K, van Marwijk Kooij M, van Prooijen HC, et al. Leukocyte depletion of random single-donor platelet transfusions does not prevent secondary human leukocyte antigen-alloimmunization and refractoriness: A randomized prospective study. Blood 1995;85:824-28.
12. Novotny VMJ, van Doorn R, Witvliet MD, Claas FHJ, Brand A. Occurrence of allogeneic HLA and non-HLA antibodies after transfusion of prestorage filtered platelets and red blood cells: A prospective study. Blood 1995;85:1736-41.
13. Heddle NM, Blajchman MA. Editorial: The leukodepletion of cellular blood products in the prevention of HLA alloimmunization and refractoriness to allogeneic platelet transfusions. Blood 1995;85:603-5.
14. Kao KJ. Effects of leukocyte depletion and UVB irradiation on alloimmunogenicity of major histocompatibility complex antigens in platelet concentrates. Blood 1992; 80:2931-27.
15. Bordin JO, Bardossy L, Blajchman MA. Experimental animal model of donor platelet refractoriness: The effect of plasma removal and the extent of leukodepletion on allogeneic alloimmunization. Transfusion 1993;33:798-801.
16. Blajchman MA, Bardossy L, Carmen RA, Goldman M, Heddle NM, Singal DP. An animal model of allogeneic donor platelet refractoriness: The effect of the time of leukodepletion. Blood 1992;79:1371-75.
17. Ramos RR, Curtis BR, Duffy BF, Chaplin H. Low retention of white cell fragments by polyester fiber white cell-reduction platelet filters. Transfusion 1994;34:31-34.

18. Blajchman MA, Singal DP. Renal transplantation: The role of red blood cell antigens, histocompatibility antigens and blood transfusions on renal allograft survival. Transf Med Rev 1989;3:171-79.
19. Opelz G. The role of HLA matching and blood transfusions in the cyclosporine era. Transplant Proc 1989;21:609-12.
20. Shirwadkar S, Blajchman MA, Frame B, Orr RW, Singal DP. Effect of blood transfusions on experimental pulmonary metastases in mice. Transfusion 1990;30:188-90.
21. Shirwadkar S, Blajchman MA, Frame B, Singal DP. Effect of allogeneic blood transfusion on solid tumor growth and pulmonary metastases in mice. J Cancer Res Clin Onc 1992;118:176-80.
22. Blajchman MA, Bardossy L, Carmen R, Sastry A, Singal DP. Allogeneic blood transfusion-induced enhancement of tumor growth: Two animal models showing amelioration by leukodepletion and passive transfer using spleen cells. Blood 1993;81:1880-82.
23. Bordin JO, Bardossy L, Blajchman MA. Growth enhancement of established tumors by allogeneic blood transfusion in experimental animals and its amelioration by leukodepletion: The importance of the timing of the leukodepletion. Blood 1994; 84:344-48.
24. Blajchman MA, Bordin JO. Tumor growth-promoting effect of allogeneic blood transfusion. Immunol Invest 1995;24:311-17.
25. Gilbert GL, Hayes K, Hudson IL, James J. Prevention of transfusion-acquired cytomegalovirus infection in infants by blood filtration to remove leukocytes. Lancet 1989;i:1228-31.
26. Bowden RA, Cays M, Schoch G, et al. Comparison of filtered blood (FB) to seronegative blood products (SB) for prevention of cytomegalovirus (CMV) infection after marrow transplant. Blood 1993;82(Suppl 1):204a.
27. Busch MP, Lee TH, Heitman J. Allogeneic leukocytes but not therapeutic blood elements induce reactivation and dissemination of latent human immunodeficiency virus type 1 infection: Implications for transfusion support of infected patients. Blood 1992;80:2128-35.
28. Blajchman MA. Editorial: Transfusion-associated bacterial sepsis: The phoenix rises yet again. Transfusion 1994;34:940-42.
29. Blajchman MA, Ali A, Lyn P, Klama L, Richardson H. A prospective study to determine the frequency of bacterial contamination in random donor platelet concentrates. Blood 1994;84(Suppl 1):529a.

PLATELETS: WHAT QUALITIES AND CHARACTERISTICS DO JUSTIFY THE NEED FOR TRANSFUSION?

S. Murphy

In the United States, the use of platelet transfusions increased progressively during the 1980's [1]. However, in many centres including our own at the Penn-Jersey Region of the American Red Cross, this use has maintained a plateau during the first half of the 1990's. Part of the explanation for this change may be the gradual adoption of a more stringent trigger for prophylactic platelet transfusion. The purpose of this paper is to review what is known about the pathophysiology of severe thrombocytopenia and the clinical data relevant to its management.

Among the first platelet transfusions given were those by Hirsch and Gardner [2] who transferred native blood (without anticoagulant) is siliconized syringes from thrombocytotic patients with myeloproliferative disease to patients with sever thrombocytopenia. They observed elevation of the platelet count, shortening of the bleeding time, cessation of clinical bleeding, and the development of the refractory state after repeated transfusion from the same donor. In addition, they made the first measurement of platelet survival time as they observed the decline in the platelet count during the week after infusion. They concluded that platelet survival time is approximately 6-7 days.

More recent studies using radioisotopic labelling have suggested that platelet survival time is closer to ten days in normal individuals [3]. However, platelet survival time is shorter in thrombocytopenic patients even when the mechanism of thrombocytopenia is failure of platelet production as in aplastic anaemia [4]. The best explanation for this observation is that a fixed number of platelets per unit time leave the circulation because they are required to maintain vascular integrity. Thus, with increasing severity of thrombocytopenia, an increasing fraction of the platelet mass is utilized for this function leading to a reduction in mean survival time which is proportional to the degree of thrombocytopenia. This explains the shorter survival time observed by Hirsch and Gardner.

Unfortunately, little is known about the nature of this function and how many platelets per unit time are required to perform it. In experimental animal models, thrombocytopenia has been produced by total body irradiation. The number of red cells appearing in lymph has been used as a reflection of the breakdown of vascular integrity produced by thrombocytopenia [5, 6]. Such breakdown is observed only with severe thrombocytopenia, at levels far below those required

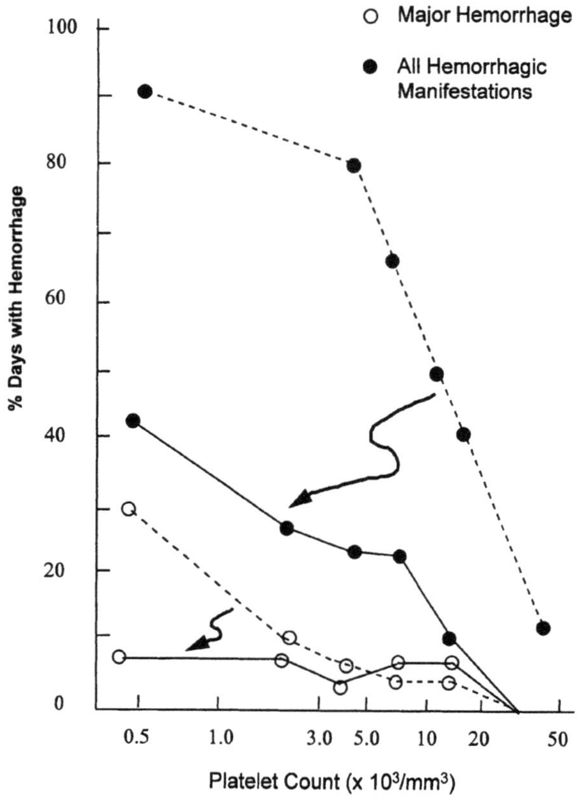

Figure 1. Percentage of days with haemorrage versus platelet count in patients with acute leukemia. The interrupted lines provide data from a period before platelet transfusion was available while the solid lines provide data during a period when prophylactic platelet transfsuion was routinely administered for a platelet count beloow 20,000/μl. Major haemorrhage was seen when the platelet count was below 20,000/μl but prophylactic transfusion only had a major impact when the platelet count was below 5,000/μl. Data taken from references 7 and 8. Figure redrawn from reference 13.

to prolong the skin bleeding time. Slichter used the appearance of radiolabelled red cells in the stool of humans with aplastic anaemia to detect such spontaneous bleeding and concluded that it appeared at approximately 5,000/μl [3].

Presumably, clinicians give prophylactic platelet transfusions to prevent such spontaneous bleeding. In the United States, the traditional transfusion trigger, 20,000/μl, appears to have had its origin in the work of Gaydos et al [7, 8] which is summarized in Figure 1. Thrombocytopenic children with leukemia were observed during a time period before platelet transfusion was available and correlations were made between the platelet count and clinical evidence of haemorrhage, both minor and major. Minor skin and mucous membrane haemorrhage began when the platelet count fell below 50,000/μl and was universal when the

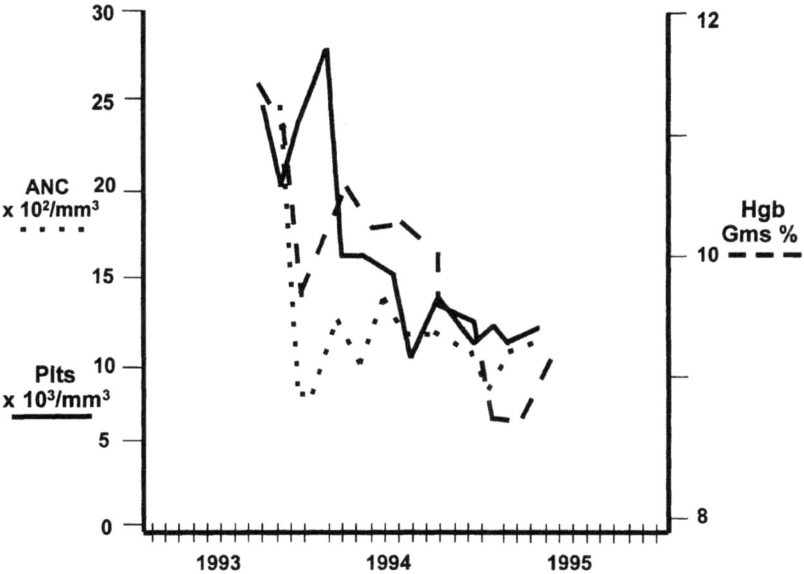

Figure 2. Clinical course of a 73 year old woman who presented with amegakaryocytic thrombocytopenia in 1993. Modest anaemia and neutropenia have developed after presentation. Over the past 18 months, the platelet count (plts) has been in the range, 10,000-15,000/μl. No therapy or platelet transfusions have been given and there have been no major haemorrhagic manifestations. ANC = absolute neutrophil count, Hgb = haemoglobin concentration.

platelet count reached very low levels of 5,000/μl and below. On the other hand, major, life-threatening haemorrhage did not appear until the platelet count was below 20,000/μl. Such severe haemorrhage was observed at a relatively low frequency in the range, 5,000-20,000/μl, but became very frequent in the range, 0-5,000/μl.

This group chose 20,000/μl as their transfusion trigger when they began a program of prophylactic platelet transfusion in a subsequent group of patients. Their experience with this group is also shown in Figure 1. The incidence of minor haemorrhage was certainly reduced. However, major haemorrhage was not eliminated and continued at the same rate as had been observed in the prior period in the range, 5,000-20,000/μl. However, a substantial difference was seen in the range, 0-5,000/μl, where major haemorrhage was clearly reduced by prophylactic transfusion. The data from the initial study [7] appears to have been responsible for the 20,000/μl trigger for prophylactic platelet transfusion that was used for many years in the United States. However, it is clear from Figure 1 that the data could just as easily have been used to suggest a trigger at 5,000/μl.

More recently, the 20,000/μl trigger has been questioned [9, 10]. Gmur et al have recently described their experience with a more stringent use of prophylactic

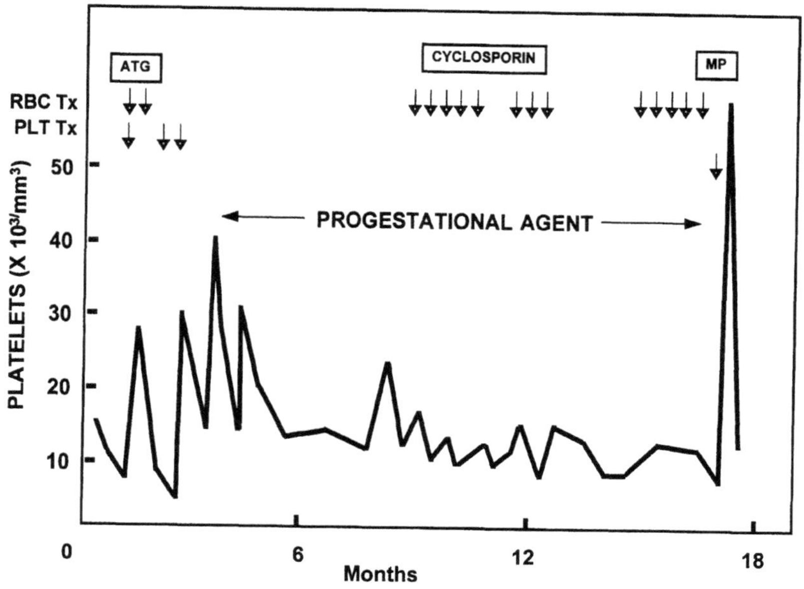

Figure 3. Clinical course of a 23 year old woman with aplastic anaemia. The patient presented with menorrhagia which responded to platelet transfusion. Subsequently, menses have been controlled with a progestational agent. Although the aplastic anaemia has not responded to antithymocyte globulin (ATG), cyclosporin, or high doses methylprednisolone (MP), the patient has had no serious haemorrage symptoms with a platelet count in the range, 10,000-15,000μl. Platelet transfusions were not given during a period of more than a year.

platelet transfusion during the treatment of patients with acute leukemia [10]. Prophylactic transfusion was administered to patients who were clinically uncomplicated only if the platelet count was less than 5,000/μl. These authors introduced a new level of complexity into decision making in that they transfused patients with platelet counts in the range, 6,000-10,000/μl, if there were fresh, minor haemorrhagic manifestations or if the body temperature was greater than 38° C. The authors were implicitly suggesting that spontaneous, severe haemorrhage was more likely if there was fever and presumably coexistent infection. Above 10,000/μl, transfusions were given only if there was a concurrent coagulation disorder or in anticipation of an invasive procedure.

In accordance with this protocol, platelet transfusion was withheld on 1,471 of 2,134 (69%) days in which the platelet count was in the range, 6,000-20,000/μl. There were only three haemorrhagic deaths, and two of these occurred at platelet counts greater than 50,000/μl. The third patient who died of haemorrhage was highly alloimmunized and completely refractory to platelet transfusions. No philosophy of platelet transfusion would have prevented these deaths. There were 25 other major but nonlethal bleeding episodes which responded to therapeutic platelet transfusions. In many of these, there were additional risk factors for haemorrhage such as extensive mucous membrane lesions. 78% of the patients were discharged in complete or partial remission. Thus, it is clear that this more restrictive policy did not endanger the welfare of the patients.

The author's own clinical experience has been in accord with that of Gmur et al. Figures 2-5 provide illustrative examples. Figure 2 shows the course of a 73 year old woman who presented with amegakaryocytic thrombocytopenia in July, 1993. Over the ensuing two years, she has developed a full pancytopenia, presumably related to aplastic anaemia or a dysmyelopoeitic syndrome. For the past 18 months, her platelet count has been stable in the range, 10,000-15,000/μl, without therapeutic intervention. She has had persistent petechiae of her lower extremities but no other haemorrhage complications. Figure 3 describes the course of a 23 year old woman with aplastic anaemia who presented with anaemia due to menorrhagia which responded to platelet transfusion. The underlying illness has been refractoriness to therapy with antithymocyte globulin, cyclosporin and high-dose methylprednisolone. However, menorrhagia was controlled with a progestational agent, and there were no significant haemorrhagic symptoms without platelet transfusion although the platelet count was in the range, 10,000-15,000/μl.

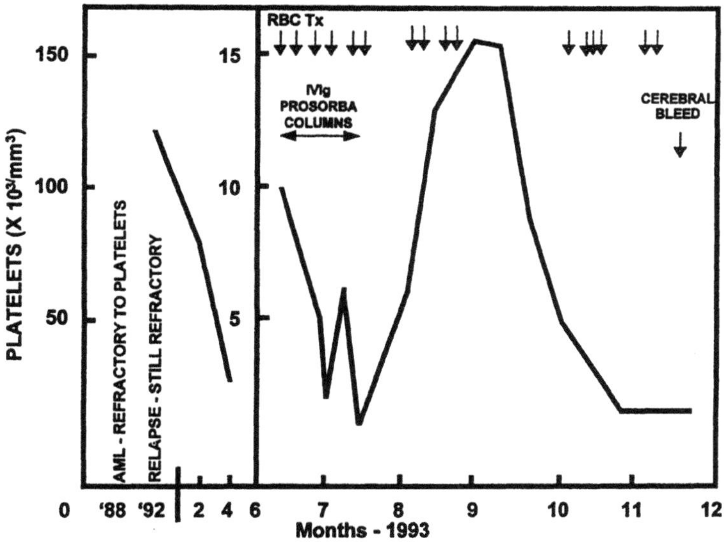

Figure 4. Clinical course of a 63 year old woman with acute leukemia. The patient was highly alloimmunized and never responded to platelet transfusion. After an initial four-year remission, the patient relapsed with severe thrombocytopenia. Attempts to reverse alloimmunization with intravenous gammaglobulin (IVIg) and Prosorba column apheresis were unusccessful. However, the patient's platelet count rose to approximately 15,000/μl for 1-2 months. Thereafter, it fell to a persistent level below 5,000/μl and a spontaneous cerebral haemorrhage occurred.

Figure 4 and 5 present cases with more severe thrombocytopenia who did poorly. In Figure 4, a woman with acute leukemia presented already highly alloimmunized by pregnancy and previous transfusions. Nonetheless, chemotherapy produced a complete remission which lasted for four years. At relapse, the platelet count ultimately fell to a level persistently below 5,000/μl. Therapy with IVIg and Prosorba column apheresis was administered in an unsuccessful attempt to reverse alloimmunization. However, the platelet count rose to 10,000-15,000/μl for 1-2 months. When the platelet count fell to a persistent level below 5,000/μl,

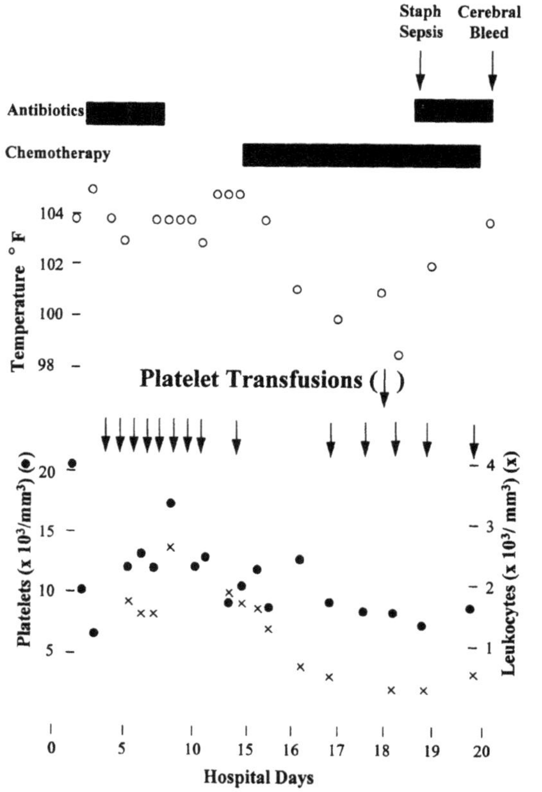

Figure 5. Clinical course of a 56 year old woman with smoldering acute leukemia. High fever did not respond to antibiotics and thrombocytopenia did not improve in response to platelet transfusions due to profound alloimmunization (100% PRA) and the patient's rare HLA (32,--/18, 44). Chemotherapy for acute leukemia lead to reduction of the fever and the leukocyte count. Fever recurred with an episode of staphylococcal bacteraemia which required readministration of antibiotics including a penicillin derivative which interferes with platelet function. A cerebral haemorrhage occurred on the twentieth hospital day when the platelet count was 8,000μl. It is believed that this spontaneous haemorrhage occurred because of the combination of thrombocytopenia, fever, bacteraemia, and the antiplatelet effect of a semisynthetic penicillin derivative.

a spontaneous intracerebral haemorrhage eventually occurred. In Figure 5, a 56 year old woman with smouldering acute leukemia is shown. She was admitted with high fever and pancytopenia. She was highly alloimmunized (100% PRA), had a rare HLA type, and did not respond to repeated platelet transfusions. Nonetheless, there were no major haemorrhagic signs when the platelet count was in the range, 6,000-12,000/μl. It was decided to give her chemotherapy which lowered her temperature and her leukocyte count. She developed staphylococcal bacteraemia on the nineteenth hospital day which necessitated the use of antibiotics including those in the penicillin family which interfere with platelet function. She died from a cerebral haemorrhage on the twentieth hospital day while she was receiving a platelet transfusion for a platelet count of 8,000/μl. We presume that bacteraemia and the use of drugs inhibiting platelet function predisposed to haemorrhage at this point.

Of course, these anecdotal experiences prove nothing. However, they are in line with the philosophy of Gmur et al. I believe that platelet transfusion can be omitted in the stable patient with a platelet count greater than 10,000/μl. On the other hand, major haemorrhage is to be expected if the platelet count remains persistently below 5,000/μl over an extended period of time. The range, 5,000-10,000/μl, is a grey area for all patients. It is wise to raise the platelet count by transfusion if there is coexisting fever, infection, coagulation factor deficiency, use of a drug that interferes with platelet function, or an anatomic lesion which predisposes to haemorrhage. It is likely that extreme leukocytosis also predisposes to intracerebral haemorrhage. One could not argue with a somewhat less stringent philosophy which calls for transfusion of all patients with platelet counts below 10,000/μl and platelet counts in the range 10,000-15,000/μl if accompanied by the coexistent, complicating clinical factors listed above.

Prophylactic platelet transfusion may also be considered in anticipation of an invasive, surgical procedure. What literature there is [11, 12] suggests that there will be increased bleeding if the platelet count is below 50,000/μl particularly if the procedure is "blind" in that the surgeon cannot achieve haemostasis mechanically. On the other hand, splenectomy can be done safely for idiopathic thrombocytopenic purpura (ITP) without platelet transfusion at extremely low platelet counts, often below 10,000/μl. Important considerations here are that the surgeon can achieve haemostasis mechanically, the surgical field is not highly vascular, and a small bleed would not be disastrous as it might be in the central nervous system. Thus, platelet transfusion is recommended to raise the platelet count to greater than 50,000/μl if mechanical haemostasis would be difficult or impossible to achieve, if the surgical field is highly vascular due, for example, to infection or portal hypertension, or if the surgery is in a critical area such as the eye or central nervous system.

References

1. Surgenor DM, Wallace EL, Hao SH, Chapman RH. Collection and transfusion of blood in the United States, 1982-1988. N Engl J Med 1990;322:1646-51.

2. Hirsch Gardner FH. The transfusion of human blood platelets: With a note on the transfusion of granulocytes. J Lab Clin Med 1952;39:556-59.
3. Slichter SJ. Controversies in platelet transfusion therapy. Ann Rev Med 1980;31:509-50.
4. Hanson SR, Slichter SJ. Platelet kinetics in patients with bone marrow hypoplasia: Evidence for fixed platelet requirement. Blood 1985;56:1105-9.
5. Aursnes I. Blood platelet production and red cell leakage to lymph during thrombocytopenia. Scand J Haematol 1974;13:184-95.
6. Roy AJ, Djerassi I. Effects of platelet transfusions: Plug formation and maintenance of vascular integrity. Proc Soc Exp Bio and Med 1972;139:137-42.
7. Gaydos LA, Freireich EJ, Mantel N. The quantitative relation between platelet count and hemorrhage in patients with acute leukemia. N Engl J Med 1962;266:905-9.
8. Freireich EJ, Kliman A, Gaydos LA, et al. Response to repeated platelet transfusion from the same donor. Ann Intern Med 1963;59:277-87.
9. Beutler E. Platelet transfusions: The 20000/μl trigger. Blood 1993;81:1411-13.
10. Gmur J, Burger J, Schanz U, et al. Safety of stringent prophylactic platelet transfusion policy for patients with acute leukemia. Lancet 1991;338:1223-26.
11. McVay PA, Toy PTCY. Lack of increased bleeding after liver biopsy in patients with mild hemostatic abnormalities. Amer J Clin Path 1990;94:747-53.
12. McVay PA, Toy PTCY. Lack of increased bleeding after paracentesis and thoracentesis in patients with mild coagulation abnormalities. Transfusion 1991;31:164-71.
13. Murphy S. Platelet transfusion. Prog Haemostasis and Thrombosis 1976;3:289-310.

CLINICAL RELEVANCE OF CLOTTING FACTOR CHARACTERISTICS

Ch.A. Ludlam

The availability of coagulation factor concentrates has transformed the lives of those with haemophilia both by improving its quality and duration. The indisputable benefits have, as is well know, been attained at some considerable cost to those who have used Factor VIII and Factor IX containing products. All concentrates whether derived from plasma, or by recombinant DNA technology, can potentially lead to untoward side effects. This review will highlight those characteristics of concentrates that are clinically relevant in deciding upon the most appropriate treatment for patients (Table 1).

*Table 1.*Clinically important features of coagulation factor concentrates.

The concentrate should have the following features:
– It should be free of viruses
– The coagulant protein should be "native"
– The concentrate should contain only the factor required by the recipient
– It should be of high purity and potency
– The potency on the label should be correct
– Stability, when reconstituted, should be prolonged
– Absence of adverse undesirable haematological effects following administration, e.g. thrombocytopenia or activation of the haemostatic system
– Allergic reactions following transfusion should be rare

As with all patients it is necessary to be certain that a concentrate is actually required and that a particular bleed, or surgical procedure, could not be adequately managed without exposing the individual to a Factor VIII containing product. Haemostasis might be achieved by the use of desmopressin, for example, in an individual with mild haemophilia or vWD. Menorrhagia may be controlled with desmopressin (via the intra nasal route) or by hormone therapy. The topical application of fibrin glue may be preferable to giving a factor concentrate intravenously [1]. Only when local measures or other therapeutic options are insufficient should patients be considered for concentrates containing coagulation factors.

The reason for such caution in the use of these products is because of their potential to cause serious and permanent harm to the recipients.

It is the safety of all coagulation factor concentrates that should be of prime concern to prescribing physicians. The principal complications reported following their use are given in Table 2.

Table 2. Complications of coagulation factor use.

- Virus transmission
- Anti-Factor VIII antibodies
- Immune modulation in recipients
- Thromboembolism
- Thrombocytopenia
- Allergic reactions

Viral safety

Despite careful donor selection and the screening of individual donations for HBsAg, anti-HCV and anti-HIV 1 and 2, along with virucidal treatment during manufacture, there are still reports of transmission of these viruses (Table 3). Some other viruses, particularly of the herpes virus group, are not transmitted by freeze dried concentrates because they are only transmissible as intracellular pathogens. Coagulation factor concentrates, therefore, do not transmit EBV or CMV or other intracellular viruses. This may explain why haemophiliacs do not get Kaposi's sarcoma if it is, as seems increasingly likely, due to a Kaposi sarcoma associated herpes virus, unlike individuals who become infected with HIV sexually where there is the possibility of transmission of viable leukocytes [2].

Table 3. Recent reports of seroconversions in haemophiliacs.

	References
– Hepatitis A	[5, 53–58]
– Hepatitis B	[59, 60]
– Hepatitis C	[9, 10, 11]
– HIV	[61, 62]
– Parvovirus	[6, 63–66]

Why are virus that should be eliminated by screening of individual donations still being transmitted? Some of the possible mechanisms are given in Table 4. For some the reason is straightforward, for example parvovirus is neither screened for, nor do any of the current viral inactivation methods result in its elimination because it is neither heat labile nor is it sensitive to solvent detergent techniques as it lacks a lipid envelope [3]. Other viruses may be transmitted because the detection method is insufficiently sensitive to identify all infectious donations, e.g. hepatitis B virus [4]. A change in the manufacturing method may result in products previously considered safe becoming infectious. An example of this in an allied area of therapy is the transmission of HCV by intravenous immunoglobulin after the introduction of anti-HCV screening.

Table 4. Why are viruses still being transmitted by coagulation factor concentrates?

- Donor in viraemic "window" period
- Absence of screening for virus or specific antibody
- Not sensitive to virucidal process
- Change in epidemiology of virus prevalence in donors and/or recipients
- Change in method of manufacture
- Recipients not appropriately vaccinated

It is also disturbing that viruses previously hardly ever recorded as causing infection in recipients have recently caused concern. Prior to 1990 there were only occasional reports of hepatitis A being transmitted by transfusion of single donor products but recently four separate outbreaks have been reported in Europe (Table 3). These were all due to an ion-exchange Factor VIII concentrate treated by a solvent detergent process and manufactured by a very similar processes. That HAV was undoubtedly transmitted by the concentrate was considered by some to be specific to a particular licensed manufacturing process rather than a generic problem with all ion-exchange purified concentrates. The recent report of HAV transmission by an intermediate purity concentrate has reopened the debate as to the reason for the European outbreaks [5]. One possible explanation is that more haemophiliacs are now at risk because the mean age for acquiring HAV from the community has risen from childhood to young adults and this has resulted in more adult donors being viraemic and haemophilic recipients susceptible. Formerly when haemophiliacs were treated with intermediate purity concentrate they also received donor immunoglobulin as an "impurity" which may have provided a degree of passive immunity.

These reports of hepatitis A infection have been disturbing for two reasons. Firstly because a virus that was not previously considered transmissible has infected five groups of haemophiliacs and secondly because infection has in many individuals resulted in clinical illness. In children acute HAV infection is often asymptomatic but in adults it is more like to result in symptomatic jaundice. The situation in HCV infected haemophiliacs is more serious because the acute HAV infection further damages an already compromised liver.

In a similar way parvovirus infection is either asymptomatic or results in the mild illness of erythema infectiosum or fifth disease. In adults, however, the situation can be very different when parvovirus can result in serious clinical sequelae including chronic arthralgia [6], spontaneous abortion, hydrops fetalis and red cell aplasia [7]. Infection in an adult haemophiliac can cause pancytopenia and severe systemic malaise [8].

The hepatitis C virus (HCV), because of its lipid envelope, is sensitive to solvent detergent virucidal treatment and to heating both at 60 degrees during Pasteurization and to dry heat at 80 degrees. Lower temperatures in the lyophilised state may be ineffective at preventing transmission. The risk, therefore, of transmission by currently available concentrates is exceedingly small. There are still, however, reports appearing of servoconversions to HCV being observed in haemophiliacs but these are difficult to evaluate because the data is often incomplete and because these sporadic events are discovered long after the seroconversion has occurred [9-11]. To try and help in the evaluation of the reports the National Haemophilia Foundation has drawn up some criteria which should be fulfilled before it is reasonable to conclude that a seroconversion is highly likely to be due to a particular concentrate.

What is very clear is that it is imperative that strenuous efforts are made to prevent transmission of HCV because there is now very strong evidence that it is the cause of serious and progressive liver disease in haemophiliacs [12,13]. Virtually all patients treated with non-virally inactivated concentrates prior to the introduction of effective virucidal processes in the mid to late 1980s became infected by HCV [14,15]. During the past 10 years it has become clear that the resultant liver disease is progressive in many individuals although in the small percentage who become PCR negative and have normal ALTs they may have minimal damage. HCV is composed of at least 6 major genotypes and recent studies demonstrate that the spectrum of genotype distribution in haemophiliacs reflects that in the donor plasma from which concentrates were derived [16]. In HIV negative recipients the same predominant genotype tends to be found in the serum over prolonged periods of time whereas in those who are HIV positive there is more likely to be a change in the circulating genotype. Furthermore there is accumulating evidence that the rate of progression of liver disease is much more rapid in those patient co-infected with HIV [17]. In the UK liver disease is now the second commonest cause of death in haemophiliacs after AIDS. There is controversy as to whether a particular genotype is more likely to lead more rapidly to serious liver disease. Initial studies suggested that genotype Ib was associated with more rapid progression but this genotype is also associated with higher serum concentrations of virus which may in turn reflect infection of longer duration. When viral load is taken into account it now seems likely that genotype does not affect progression. The difficulty in relating genotype to severity of liver disease in haemophiliacs is that the studies that have been published are too small to give a reliable guide.

Hepatocellular carcinoma (HCC) is now established as a sequelae to HCV infection and it occurs in haemophiliacs at a rate 30 times that in the general population [18]. Whereas the majority of cases arise in those who have progressed to cirrhosis it can arise secondary to chronic non-cirrhotic hepatitis. There is some evidence that genotype Ib infection may be more likely to lead to HCC but this may merely be a consequence of this genotype having been in the population for a longer period of time. As HCC is potentially curable if diagnosed early, either by excision or liver transplantation, it is now recommended policy in the UK that all patients likely to have cirrhosis should be screened for the development of HCC by ultrasound every four months [19].

The only licensed treatment of HCV is α-interferon. In non-haemophiliacs this will produce a response in about 50-70% of patients after the initiation of treatment and of these about half will remain in remission after therapy is discontinued. Unfortunately it has recently become clear that in haemophiliacs the response is less good despite initial studies suggesting that it would be as good as in non-haemophiliacs [20]24]. Furthermore even those patients who obtained a remission with α-interferon relapsed when therapy was discontinued. The reasons why α-interferon has been disappointing are difficult to discern at present but may relate to the fact that infection has in many individuals been lifelong and that many have advanced liver disease which is known to be associated with a less favourable outcome. As in non-haemophiliacs, those with genotypes 2 and 3 have a better response than those with type 1. Most of the published studies in haemophiliacs have given 3MU α-interferon 3 times weekly for 6 months but there is now increasing evidence that therapy for a longer duration may be more effective is maintaining remission [25]. Although initial studies suggested that the response to α-interferon may be independent of HIV, recent evidence suggests that those with HIV fare less well. The reason for the difference between the results of earlier studies and the later ones may be due to the advance of HIV such that immune function has deteriorated to such an extent that α-interferon is now unable to achieve an appropriate immune response.

Thus there is very substantial evidence that HCV results in considerable morbidity and mortality in haemophiliacs and it is essential to ensure that concentrates do not transmit this virus in future.

The situation in haemophiliacs may be more complicated than originally envisaged so far as hepato-tropic viruses are concerned as evidence is starting to emerge that there may be other viruses such as hepatitis G virus and GBV-C which may be transmitted by concentrates.

Anti-Factor VIII antibodies

It is currently unclear what determines whether, or when, an individual may develop an antibody to transfused Factor VIII. What has been of concern recently is whether patients are more likely to develop an antibody after use of recombinant Factor VIII than following the use of plasma derived concentrate. It has, however, become apparent that transient low titre inhibitors in children are probably more common than previously considered. If patients are tested more frequently for the presence of an antibody, as has happened in the PUP studies of rVIII, then these low level, and often short lived, antibodies will be detected in vitro although the patients will apparently still respond clinically to standard doses of concentrate given on demand to treat a bleeding episode [26,27].

Of those with severe haemophilia in receipt of plasma derived concentrate up to 54% may at one time or another develop an antibody. Other estimates are as low as 5% of recipients of plasma derived concentrates being at risk although one intermediate purity product did not apparently result in the development of any anti-Factor VIII antibodies when given to 34 individuals [28]. What is now clear is that when patients are treated with rVIII and tested every three months for the presence of an inhibitor about 28% will develop one within two years. This is irrespective of which of the current two rVIII concentrates they receive despite there being minor differences in the degree of glycosylation of the two different products. This observed rate of antibody development cannot be distinguished from the rate of inhibitor appearance in recipients of plasma derived concentrate [29,30].

Many would now concede that because the rate of inhibitor development is probably similar in recipients of plasma derived and recombinant concentrate, it is likely that the antigenicity of rVIII is similar to native plasma derived Factor VIII. What has become a major concern, however, is that plasma derived Factor VIII may become denatured following fractionation during its virucidal treatment. Ever since the introduction of viral inactivation steps, particularly heat treatment, there has been anxiety that the Factor VIII molecule might become altered in such a way that neoantigens will be produced which will provoke recipients to develop inhibitors. Despite heating of concentrates up to 60 degrees by Pasteurization and up to 100 degrees when lyophilised these particular processes do not appear to alter the antigenicity of Factor VIII.

What has become clear, however, is that subtle changes in the molecular configuration may result from use of apparently well established and apparently safe viral inactivation procedures. This has been well exemplified by the appearance of anti-Factor VIII antibodies in previously treated adult severe haemophiliacs following the introduction of a new intermediate purity concentrate which was virucidally treated by Pasteurization. Two clusters of patients were identified in The Netherlands and Belgium shortly after its introduction [31,32]. That this concentrate had neoantigens rapidly became apparent because the inhibitors appeared in multiply the incidence of such new antibodies in adult severe haemophiliacs is exceedingly low. Of interest was the observation that the kinetics of the Factor VIII inhibitory activity was different from that observed with the more usual alloantibodies that appear typically in children. A further unusual feature of these two small epidemics was that when the patients were switched to being treated with another Factor VIII concentrate the alloantibodies disappeared. What has been unsettling about this episode is that, despite testing with monoclonal antibodies in vitro to a range of epitopes on Factor VIII, it has not been possible to identify clearly that this concentrate has neoantigens, unfortunately therefore this technique may be of limited value in screening new Factor VIII concentrates for neoantigenicity.

Do Factor VIII concentrates cause immune modulation?

Shortly after the appearance of the clinical syndrome of AIDS in the US it became clear that in many haemophiliacs it was possible to demonstrate a range of immune disturbances. While in those in whom it was subsequently found were infected with HIV, immune modulation was to be expected, what was unexpected was the finding of immune changes in those that were not infected with HIV [33, 34]. These range from a reduction in delayed hypersensitivity responses to common antigens, to an increase in the serum immunoglobulin levels and altered function of lymphocytes and monocytes. What was not clear was whether these changes were due to "contaminants" in the concentrates or whether they were the result of other putative viruses, e.g. the non-A non-B hepatitis agent. The importance of these observations was whether immunomodulatory components of Factor VIII concentrates might reduce the ability of the patients to maintain their immune status in the presence of HIV. This led to studies which attempted to identify components which had immunomodulatory activities. Various in vitro systems were used to assess the concentrates, but the ones most widely used were to assess modification of the response to lymphocyte mitogens, e.g. PHA, IL2 secretion or receptor expression. Whereas many concentrates reduced the response to mitogens some resulted in an enhancement. In general the higher purity concentrates particularly those prepared using monoclonal antibodies had less ability to modulate in vitro immune reactions. Attempts to identify the component(s) which may be responsible for the in vitro effects have demonstrated several inhibitory fractions. The identity of the factor(s), however, remains obscure. It has been proposed that TGF B may be an important immunomodulatory constituent but other studies, although having confirmed that it is present in concentrates, question its importance to the observed effects in vitro, or in vivo [35,36].

In an attempt to ascertain whether concentrate purity might influence the clinical rate of HIV progression several prospective studies were established. These compared intermediate purity with high purity, either ion exchange chromatographically purified, or monoclonally prepared, concentrates on the rate of change of CD4 cell counts over time, this being used as a surrogate marker for HIV progression. The difficulty with all the studies is that the number of patients included has been small and in some there have been significant numbers of patient withdrawals. Two studies report stabilization or CD4 cell numbers with monoclonally prepared concentrates [37,39] whereas no difference could be distinguished between recipients of ion exchange, compared to intermediate purity concentrate [39]. A further study reports that monoclonally prepared concentrate is beneficial when compared to an ion exchange manufactured one but the patient groups in this study had markedly different initial CD4 counts [40]. None of these studies has demonstrated a reduction in the clinical progression to AIDS defining illnesses with high purity concentrates.

The importance, or otherwise, of concentrate purity in the determination of HIV progression has been studied epidemiologically. What has become clear from these studies is that the rate of development of AIDS and death after HIV infection is independent of the severity of the haemophilia and the annual Factor VIII usage [41]. Furthermore a recent large UK study has revealed that mortality of HIV infected subjects is independent of severity of haemophilia and therefore by presumption independent of Factor VIII use; this argues against concentrates having a significant effect on HIV progression and that non-Factor VIII proteins, or other constituents, do not have an important detrimental effect in vivo following infusion [42].

As a result of improvements in the manufacturing processes for Factor VIII concentrates the majority of products now available are of high purity. Whether there is any difference in the rate of HIV progression between patients treated with monoclonally, compared to ion exchange, prepared concentrates must await the outcome of a current large study in the UK.

A useful development that has become possible with the ready availability of high purity concentrates has been the ability to give a continuous intravenous infusion of Factor VIII. This has been particularly useful in the postoperative period where it has led to the reduction in the total amount of concentrate used to about half that needed when given by bolus infusions [43].

Factor IX concentrates

Until recently those with haemophilia B were treated with prothrombin complex concentrates which contained in addition to Factor IX, Factors II and X, and in some cases also Factor VII. While these concentrates were effective in the treatment and prevention of bleeding their use was associated with the development of a hypercoagulable state as evidenced by the appearance of DIC, venous thromboembolism, stroke and myocardial infarction. The mechanism by which these concentrates predispose to thrombosis is not entirely clear but is probably related to their possession of activated coagulation factor(s). Recent studies indicate that Factor IXa may be responsible although previously it has been suggested that it might be Xa [44,-46].

The more recently developed high purity single Factor IX containing products result in much less activation of the haemostatic system following infusion, as evidenced by an absence of a rise in prothrombin fragment 1.2 [46-49]. Furthermore their clinical use in situations likely to lead to thrombosis has been reassuring in that venous thromboembolism has not been observed [50].

For the treatment of patients with anti-Factor VIII antibodies FEIBA (which is an activated prothrombin complex concentrate) has been used for many years despite its record of being associated with thrombotic episodes. Factor VIIa is still under assessment and may be effective treatment without predisposing to thromboembolic complications.

Porcine Factor VIII also has an established place in the treatment of individuals with allo and auto anti-Factor VIII antibodies [51,52]. Apart from thrombocytopenia, which is normally mild and dose dependent, and occasional systemic reactions, it has a high safety record. It is the only plasma derived concentrate, however, now available that does not include a virucidal step in its manufacture.

Conclusion

Over the last ten years plasma derived coagulation factor concentrates have become much safer both from virus transmission and thromboembolism. There is still considerable concern about viruses that are resistant to the current viral inactivation procedures, e.g. hepatitis A and parvovirus, not only for the risk that these known viruses pose to patients who are not immune, but more particularly because they illustrate very clearly the shortcomings of the current virucidal processes. Recombinant Factor VIII is now available, appears safe and probably no more antigenic than that derived from plasma. Studies are at an advanced stage in the assessment of a novel B domainless recombinant Factor VIII concentrate. Recombinant Factor VIIa is now widely used for the treatment of individuals with anti-factor antibodies and appears to have a high degree of safety. Recombinant IX is currently under active clinical evaluation.

References

1. Martinowitz U, Schulman S. Fibrin sealant in surgery of patients with a haemorrhagic diathesis. Thromb Haemost 1995;74:486-92.
2. Whitby D, Howard MR, TenantFlowers M, et al. Detection of Kaposi sarcoma associated herpesvirus in peripheral blood of HIV -infected individuals and progression to Kaposi's sarcoma. Lancet 1995;347:799-802.
3. Prowse CV, Ludlam CA, Yap PL. Human parvovirus B19 and blood products. Vox Sang 1996;(in press).
4. Stirling ML, Murray JA, Mackay P, Black SH, Peutherer JF, Ludlam CA. Incidence of infection with hepatitis B virus in 56 patients with haemophilia A 1971-1979. J Clin Pathol 1983;36:577-80.
5. Cohn RJ, Schwyzer R, Field SP, FemandesCosta F, Armstrong D. Acute hepatitis A in haemophiliacs (4). Thromb Haemost 1994;72:785-86.
6. Lyon DJ, Chapman CS, Martin C, et al. Symptomatic parvovirus B19 infection and heattreated factor IX concentrate (letter). Lancet 1989;1:1085.
7. Brown KE, Green SW, De M, et al. Congenital anaemia after transplacental B19 parvovirus infection. Lancet 1994;343:895-96.
8. Yee TT, Lee CA, Pasi KJ. Life-threatening human parvovirus B29 infection in immunocompetent haemophilia (9). Lancet 1995;345:794-95.
9. Schulman S, Lindgren AC, Petrini P, Allander T. Transmission of hepatitis C with pasteurised factor VIII. Lancet 1992;340:305-6.
10. Gerritzen A, Scholt B, Kaiser R, Schneweis KE, Brackmann HH, Oldenburg J. Acute hepatitis C in haemophiliacs due to "virus-inactivated" clotting factor concentrates. Thromb Haemost 1992;68:781.
11. Koehler-Vajta K, Guertier L, Schaetzl H. Frequency of HCV-RNA in anti-HCV positive hemophilic children and young adults. Thromb Haemost 1993;69:853(abstract 1115).
12. Hay CR, Preston FE, Triger DR, Underwood JC. Progressive liver disease in haemophilia: An understated problem? Lancet 1985;1:1495-98.
13. Hanley JP, Jarvis LM, Andrews J, et al. Investigation of chronic hepatitis C infection in individuals with haemophilia: Assessment of invasive and non-invasive methods. Brit J Haematol 1996;(in press).

14. Fletcher ML, Trowell JM, Craske J, Parvier K, Rizza CR. Non-A non-B hepatitis after transfusion of factor VIII in frequently treated patients. Brit Med J [Clin Res] 1983; 287:1754-57.
15. Kernoff PB, Lee CA, Karayiannis P, Thomas HC. High risk of non-A non-B hepatitis after a first exposure to volunteer or commercial clotting factor concentrates: Effects of prophylactic immune serum globulin. Brit J Haematol 1985;60:469-79.
16. Jarvis LM, Watson HG, McOmish F, Peutherer JF, Ludlam CA, Simmonds P. Frequent reinfection and reactivation of hepatitis c virus genotypes in multitransfused hemophiliacs. J Inf Dis 1994;170:1018-22.
17. Eyster ME, Diamondstone LS, Lien JM, Ehmann WC, Quan S, Goedert JJ. Natural history of hepatitis C virus infection in multitransfused hemophiliacs: Effect of co-infection with human immunodeficiency virus. J Acquir Immune Defic Syndr 1993; 6:602-10.
18. Preston FE, Dusheiko G, Giangrande PLF, et al. Hepatocellular carcinoma in UK haemophiliacs. Brit J Haematol 1995;89:9[Abstract].
19. Preston FE, Dusheiko G, Lee CA, Ludlam CA, Giangrande PLF. Guidelines on the diagnosis and management of chronic liver disease in haemophilia. Haemophilia 1995;1:41-42.
20. Makris M, Preston FE, Trigger DR, Underwood JCE, Westlake L, Adelman MI. A randomized controlled trial of recombinant interferon-α in chronic hepatitis C in hemophiliacs. Blood 1991;78:1672-77.
21. Reesink HW, Bresters D, Van DP, Cuypers HTM, Lelie PN. New developments in hepatitis C. Scand J Gastroenterol 1992;27(Suppl):82-86.
22. Peerlinck K, Willems M, Sheng L, et al. Rapid clearance of hepatitis C virus RNA in peripheral blood mononuclear cells of patients with clotting disorders and chronic hepatitis c treated with alpha-2b interferon is not a predictor for sustained response to treatment. Brit J Haematol 1994;86:816-19.
23. Telfer P, Devereux H, Colvin B, Hayden S, Dusheiko G, Lee C. Alpha interferon for hepatitis C virus infection in haemophilic patients. Haemophilia 1995;1:54-58.
24. Hanley JP, Jarvis LM, Andrews J, et al. Interferon treatment for chronic hepatitis C infection in haemophiliacs: Influence of virus load, genotype and liver pathology on response. Blood 1996;87:1704-09.
25. Reichard O, Foberg U, Fryden A, et al. High sustained response rate and clearance of viremia in chronic hepatitis C after treatment with interferon alpha2B for 60 weeks. Hepatology 1994;19:280-85.
26. Lusher JM, Arkin S, Abildgaard CF, et al. Recombinant factor VIII for the treatment of previously untreated patients with hemophilia A - A safety, efficacy, and development of inhibitors. N Engl J Med 1993;328:453-59.
27. Bray GL, Gomperts ED, Courter S, et al. A multicenter study of recombinant factor VIII (recombinate): Safety, efficacy, and inhibitor risk in previously untreated patients with hemophilia A. Blood 1994;83:2428-35.
28. Pasi KJ, Hamon MD, Perry DJ, Hill FG. Factor VIII and IX inhibitors after exposure to heat-treated concentrates. Lancet 1987;1:689(letter).
29. Briet E, Rosendaal FR. Inhibitors in hemophilia A: Are some products safer? Sem Hematol 1994;31:11-15.
30. Briet E, Rosendaal FR, Kreuz W, et al. High titer inhibitors in severe haemophilia A, a meta-analysis based on eight long-term follow-up studies concerning inhibitors associated with crude or intermediate purity factor VIII products (4). Thromb Haemost 1994;72:162-64.

31. Rosendaal FR, Nieuwenhuis HK, Van B, et al. A sudden increase in factor VIII inhibitor development in multitransfused hemophilia A patients in the Netherlands. Blood 1993;81:2180-86.
32. Peerlinck K, Arnout J, Gillies JG, Saint-Remy JM, Vermylen J. A higher than expected incidence of factor VIII inhibitors in multitransfused haemophilia A patients treated with an intermediate purity pasteurized factor VIII concentrate. Thromb Haemost 1993;69:115-18.
33. Carr R, Veitch SE, Edmond E, et al. Abnormalities of circulating lymphocyte subsets in haemophiliacs in an AIDS-free population. Lancet 1984;1:1431-34.
34. Watson HG, Ludlam CA. Immunological abnormalities in haemophiliacs. Blood Rev 1992;6:26-33.
35. Wadhwa M, Dilger P, Tubbs J, MireSluis A, Barrowcliffe T, Thorpe R. Identification of transforming growth factor-beta as a contaminant in factor VIII concentrates: A possible link with immunosuppressive effects in hemophiliacs. Blood 1994;84:2021-30.
36. Spiers HJL, Stirling D, Ludlam CA. TGF-Beta 1 is only a minor immunosuppressive contaminant of factor VIII concentrates. Tromb Haemost 1995;73:525[Abstract].
37. Seremetis SV, Aledort LM, Bergman GE, et al. Three-year randomised study of high-purity or intermediate-purity factor VIII concentrates in symptom-free HIV-seropositive haemophiliacs: Effects on immune status. Lancet 1993;342:700-3.
38. de Biasi R, Rocino A, Miraglia E, Mastrullo L, Quirino AA. The impact of a very high purity factor VIII concentrate on the immune system of human immunodeficiency virus-infected hemophiliacs: A randomized, prospective, two-year comparison with an intermediate purity concentrate. Blood 1991;78:1919-22.
39. Mannucci PM, Gringeri A, Debiasi R. Immune status of HIV-positive haemophiliacs: A randomised prospective comparison of treatment with a high-purity or an intermediate-purity factor VIII concentrate. Thromb Haemost 1991;65:824[Abstract].
40. Varon D, Schulman S, Dardik R, Barzilai A, Bashari D, Martinowitz U. High versus ultra high purity factor VIII concentrate therapy: Prospective evaluation of immunological and clinical parameters in HIV seronegative and seropositive hemophiliacs. Thromb Haemost 1994;72:359-62.
41. Goedert JJ, Kessler CM, Aledort LM, et al. A prospective study of human immunodeficiency virus type 1 infection and the development of AIDS in subjects with hemophilia. N Engl J Med 1989;321:1141-48.
42. Darby SC, Ewart DW, Giangrande PLF, et al. Mortality before and after HIV infection in the complete UK population of haemophiliacs. Nature 1995;377:79-82.
43. Martinowitz U, Schulman S, Gitel S, Horozowski H, Heim M, Varon D. Adjusted dose continuous infusion of factor VIII in patients with haemophilia A. Brit J Haematol 1992;82:729-34.
44. Gray E, Tubbs J, Thomas S, et al. Measurement of activated factor IX in factor IX concentrates: Correlation with in vivo thrombogenicity. Thromb Haemost 1992;73:675-79.
45. Limentani SA, Gowell KP, Deitcher SR. In vitro characterization of high purity factor IX concentrate for the treatment of hemophilia B. Thromb Haemost 1995;73:584-91.
46. Philippou H, Adami A, Lane D, et al. High purity factor IX and prothrombin complex concentrate (PCC): Pharmacokinetics and evidence that factor IXa is the thrombogenic trigger in PCC. Tromb Haemost 1996;(in press).
47. Mannucci PM, Bauer KA, Gringeri A, et al. Thrombin generation is not increased in the blood of hemophilia B patients after the infusion of a purified factor IX concentrate. Blood 1990;76:2540-45.

48. Kim HC, Matts L, Eisele J, Czachur M, Saidi P. Monoclonal antibody-purified factor IX: Comparative thrombogenicity to prothrombin complex concentrate. Sem Hematol 1991;28:15-19.
49. Mannucci PM, Bauer KA, Gringeri A, et al. No activation of the common pathway of the coagulation cascade after a highly purified factor IX concentrate. Brit J Haematol 1991;79:606-11.
50. Thomas DP, Lee CA, Colvin BT, et al. Clinical experience with a highly purified factor IX concentrate in patients undergoing surgical operations. Haemophilia 1995; 1:17-23.
51. Donohue SM, Wonke B, Hoffbrand AV, et al. Alpha interferon in the treatment of chronic hepatitis C infection in thalassaemia major. Brit J Haematol 1993;83:491-97.
52. Hay CRM, Lozier JN, Lee CA, et al. Porcine factor VIII therapy in patients with congenital hemophila and inhibitors: Efficacy, patient selection, and side effects. Sem Hematol 1994;31:20-25.
53. Mannucci PM. Outbreak of hepatitis A among Italian patients with haemophilia. Lancet 1992;339:819.
54. Gerritzen A, Schneweis KE, Brackmann HH, et al. Acute hepatitis A in haemophiliacs. Lancet 1992;340:1231-32.
55. Peerlinck K, Vermylen J. Acute hepatitis A in patients with haemophilia A (10). Lancet 1993;341:179.
56. Temperley IJ, Cotter KP, Walsh TJ, Power J, Hillary IB. Clotting factors and hepatitis A. Lancet 1992;340:1466.
57. Mariani G, Di Paolantonio T, Baklaja R, Mannucci PM. Prospective hepatitis C safety evaluation of a high purity solvent detergent treated FVIII concentrate. Blood 1991;78(Suppl):55a.
58. Mannucci PM, Gdovin S, Gringeri A, et al. Transmission of hepatitis A to patients with hemophilia by factor VIII concentrates treated with organic solvent and detergent to inactivate viruses. Ann Int Med 1994;120:1-7.
59. Brackmann HH, Egli H. Acute hepatitis B infection after treatment with heat-inactivated factor VIII concentrate (letter). Lancet 1988;2:967.
60. Arzneimittelkommission. Information. Beriplex HS250 and 500. Pharm Ztg 1994;139: 2192-93.
61. Karcher H. German haemophilic patients infected with HIV [news]. Brit Med J 1991;303:1352-53.
62. Kleim JP, Bailly E, Schneweis KE, et al. Acute HIV-1 infection in patients with hemophilia B treated with beta-propiolactone-UV-inactivated clotting factor. Thromb Haemost 1990;64:336-37.
63. Williams MD, Cohen BJ, Beddall AC, Pasi KJ, Mortimer PP, Hill FG. Transmission of human parvovirus B19 by coagulation factor concentrates. Vox Sang 1990;58:177-81.
64. Girolami A, Sartori MT, Simioni P. An updated classification of factor XIII defect [letter; comment]. Brit J Haematol 1991;77:565-66.
65. Santagostino E, Mannucci PM, Gringeri A, Azzi A, Morfini M. Eliminating parvovirus B19 from blood products (17). Lancet 1994;343:798.
66. Bermejo E, Woods A, Pieroni G, Meschengieser S, Penalva L, Lazzari MA. Current status of DDAVP formulations and their use in haemostatic disorders DDAVP: Variaciones de la hemostasia producidas por su uso. Prensa Med Argent 1992;79: 376-80.

DISCUSSION

H.J.C. de Wit and P.V. Holland – moderators

R.S. Eisenstaedt (Philadelphia, PA, USA): Dr. Blajchman about the Busch study[1], you speculated that the equivalency of the allogeneic and autologous blood in cancer occurrence may be due to a kind of superior allogeneic product by virtue of the buffy coat being removed. What about the possibility that it was the autologous product that was kind of inferior by virtue of those white cells desintegrating or in the least the same cytokines that might have been seen in an allogeneic unit.

M. Blajchman (Hamilton, C): In fact we have been looking recently at this very issue in our animal models, carefully as a result of the Busch study. It would appear from our animal data that autologous blood that is stored for a week also has a tumour growth-promoting effect. This appears to be due to at least two distinct phenomena occurring: one is allogeneic related and the second is independent of the allogeneic phenomenon, that also occurs with stored autologous blood. If this turns out to be the case we may have to do prestorage leukodepletion of autologous blood. That is to prevent the potential immunomodulatory effect of some of the cytokines that are released by the leukocytes in autologous blood, during storage. So, we have some preliminary evidence that non-leukodepleted autologous blood may be immunomodulatory.

R.S. Eisenstaedt: In a somewhat different direction but from the same study we have heard a number of speakers lamenting the lack of controlled clinical investigation and transfusion. These people made good effort to try to randomise their study. You pointed out the ethical problems with randomising people to transfusion or no transfusion. What about the ethics of randomising people to autologous blood versus allogeneic blood?

M. Blajchman: On the basis of current knowledge I do not think there is an ethical issue with such a randomisation. I think most people would agree that autologous blood is probably the safest blood that you can give a patient. The other thing

1. Busch ORC, Hop WJC, van Papendrecht MAWH, Marguet RL, Jeekel J. Blood transfusions and prognosis in colorectal cancer. N Engl J Med 1993;328:1372-76.

that must be mentioned is that autologous blood also has risks. There have been four reports[1-4] in recipients of autologous blood of serious bacterial infectious complications. There are also reports that autologous blood has on occasion been given to the wrong individual; so autologous blood is not without risk. It is no doubt safer than allogeneic blood, but perhaps the absolute safety of autologous blood may have been overstated. But at this point in time the use of autologous blood is not an unethical practice in my opinion.

H.P. Olthuis (Nijmegen, NL): I think in many cases we have the problem to make a good study design with comparable study groups. We participated in the Rotterdam study[5] and one of the major disadvantages of this study was that the group who should not receive the autologous transfusion were not collected blood before the operation. That made the two groups completely different in handling and so on.

Dr. de Wolf mentioned a study which was done by Novotny about the reaction of platelet transfusion in Holland. This was not a study, this was an interview in preparation of a lecture where she interviewed by telephone about the incidence rate on platelet transfusion and because the questions were not addressed very strict, the reason that there was such a big difference between Amsterdam and Nijmegen can be explained.

J.Th.M. de Wolf (Groningen, NL): It was not meant to suggest that it was a study, it was to show you that there is reported an enormous difference in transfusion reactions caused by platelet transfusions in the literature ranging from 0-70%, also in the Netherlands. I wonder, when you start a study investigating transfusion reactions, if you know where to look at when reactions to platelet concentrates are concerned. It is remarkable that two centres using platelets from the same blood bank have reported reactions; one centre 0.3% and the other at least 30% of the cases.

M. Blajchman: I think that it is crucially important when doing such studies that the investigators define the criteria and make sure that appropriately trained per-

---

1. Richards C, Kolins J, Trindade CD. Autologous transfusion-transmitted *Yersinia enterocolitica* (letter). JAMA 1992;268:1541-42.
2. Sire JM, Michelet C, Mesnard R, et al. Septic shock due to *Yersinia enterocolitica* after autologous transfusion. Clin Infect Dis 1993;17:954-55.
3. Duncan KL, Ransley J, Elterman M. Transfusion-transmitted *Serratia liquefociens* from an autologous blood unit (letter). Transfusion 1994;34:738-39.
4. Haditsch M, Birder L, Gabriel C, et al. *Yersenia enterocolitica* septicemia in autologous blood transfusion. Transfusion 1994;34:907-9.
5. Hoynck van Papendrecht MAW, Hop W, Langenhorst BLAM, Kothe FC, Marquer RL, Jeekel J. Feasibility of a predeposit autologous blood donation program in colorectal cancer patients: Results from a randomized clinical study. Vox Sang 1992;62:102-07.

sonnel are available to make the observations. If you rely on the nurses or the patients to report reactions, they would be very underreported.

C.Th. Smit Sibinga (Groningen, NL): Dr. Blajchman, I fully agree on that; it actually boils down to the communication mechanisms between the bedside and the blood bank trying to unravel these phenomena.

A few questions to dr. Blajchman and dr. de Wolf. Is it not becoming more clear and apparent that with respect to the fashion so to speak to get to more pure cellular products and specifically the elimination of white cells, we are grossly overlooking the functional aspects and how these cells behave over ageing in the ex vivo situation; the focus so far is on the physical presence of these cells as elements. Because if you look at the studies now there is a tremendous amount of information not being provided at least not in writing. We do not know what the ages have been of units transfused in most of these studies and then try to compare the one study to the other. That is particularly true in the cancer studies, but also in a number of studies in relation to alloimmunization and the occurrence of refractoriness. Dr. de Wolf showed his study and that is only part of a series of studies we have done, because there is also a substantial amount of retrospective material, which brings quite a bit of pieces of your puzzle to the surface. It does not mean that we all solve that puzzle, we are left with the puzzle. I would like you both to comment.

M. Blajchman: Dr. William Murphy indicated that platelets on day 1 were different from platelets on day 5. In a study that we are currently doing, looking at the reaction rate following platelet transfusions at different centres, one centre which has a limit on platelet storage of 3 days has very few reports of transfusion reactions. In another centre where outdating is 5 days we are seeing a reaction rate of 20-30%. Certainly when you look at the literature very few investigators report the age of the related platelets to the reaction rate.

C.Th. Smit Sibinga: There is now emerging the controversy of two studies: a retrospective 90 patients well controlled and a prospective 63 patients well controlled. There have been transfusions when I understand correctly with platelets non-depleted, so full amount of white cells left and 3-5 days old platelets, but there were not that amount of reactions reported back through the study of dr. de Wolf, is that correct?

J.Th.M. de Wolf: These 63 acute leukaemia patients received about 1000 transfusions with 3-5 days stored platelets and there were something more than 2% reactions but no serious reactions.[1] In our retrospective study concerning 90 patients we filtered red blood cell concentrates after a storage time of three weeks

1. De Wolf JThM, Westerterp A, Smit Sibinga CTh, Halie MR. Prestorage leukocyte depletion is not necessarily required for the prevention of refractoriness to platelet transfusion. Blood 1995;86:3263.

resulting in the same percentage of reactions and an HLA immunisation percentage of about 3-4%. This is different from what dr. Blajchman showed in animal studies, in which leukocyte depletion of stored RBC caused clinically important HLA-immunization in animals. In our study it seems not to be the case.

H.J.C. de Wit (Leeuwarden, NL): I was very interested in dr. Blajchman's report, that one centre exclusively transfuses platelets that are less than 3 days old. You talked about side-effects. It is very interesting to know whether there is also a difference between that centre and the rest in terms of percentage of chronically transfused patients that become refractory for platelets, because that would add to the research that dr. de Wolf does.

M. Blajchman: Well, this is one of the things that will be looked at in our current studies.

W. Flegel (Ulm, D): We are actually dealing with two types of platelet components which are quite different in respect to the rates of febrile transfusion reactions associated with these preparations.[1,2] One type is the platelet-rich-plasma which usually has a high white blood cell contamination. This preparation may be associated with a high rate of febrile reactions particularly if stored for 5 days. The second type is the buffy coat derived platelet concentrate which has generally a low white blood cell contamination and no cytokine contamination even at the end of the storage time. My question for dr. de Wolf is: you wondered why one type of platelet component caused different rates of febrile transfusion reactions at two different locations. Could it be that there was a difference in the storage time before these blood products were transfused? The question to dr. Blajchman: you suggested that the filtration of platelet components may reduce the cytokine exposure of the patients. Do you have data showing that filtration is also recommended for buffy coat derived platelet concentrates or might it be that they do not need to be filtered?

J.Th.M. de Wolf: In Groningen we used platelet concentrates produced from platelet rich plasma, and stored 3-5 days. I showed you the figures in the Netherlands; the difference between the blood banks was not coming from a different product, it was buffy coat derived.

M. Blajchman: There is no doubt that the cytokine levels in buffy coat depleted platelets has been with prestorage leukodepleted platelets, but I cannot provide the data, at this time.

---

1. Flegel WA, Wiesmeth M, Stampe D, Koerner K. Low cytokine contamination in buffycoat derived platelet concentrates without filtration. Transfusion 1995;35:917-20.
2. Klüter H, Müller-Steinhardt M, Danzer S, Wilhelm D, Kirchner H. Cytokines in platelet concentrates prepared from pooled buffycoats. Vox Sang 1995;69:38-45.

H.J.C. de Wit: I think dr. Muylle[1] in Antwerp published about that but I cannot reproduce.

B. Justiça (Oporto, P): Dr. Ludlam, could you add some programme like lyophilization of the products.

C.A. Ludlam (Edinburgh , UK): Clearly the products have to be lyophilized and I know that fractionators spend a lot of time quality controlling the process. I think we never know what is going to happen next. I remember back in the end of 1984 having had very long discussions about heat-treatment of FVIII whether we should do it or whether we should not, how sensitive was HIV to heat-treatment and so on. We were all scared that heating FVIII would be a danger, it might create neo-antigens. If in that discussion someone had talked about heating FVIII at 80° C let alone a 100° C as people have done now in a dry or wet state, we would almost certainly have had very, very major reservations with the thought of dry-roasting.

E.L. Snyder (New Haven, CT, USA): Dr. Murphy, I have a question. We know how difficult it is to count cells when you get to low levels. I think people would agree that Coulter counters or Baker counters or whatever counters you are using for platelets have their limits. Some people seem to live or die based on whether someone is using 5,000/μl or 10,000/μl as a cut-off trigger if you are considering giving a platelet transfusion. I personally do not think a count of 5,000/μl on a patient one day and a count of 10,000/μl the next day is an increment. It is all sort of background noise to me. I know the platelet count is low. Do you think that someone should be so precise in distinguishing between a 5,000/μl and a 10,000/μl count that you could criticise someone's transfusion practices because they use a number that is a little higher or a little lower when you are talking about platelets at that level.

S. Murphy (Philadelphia, PA, USA): this is an extremely important point. Where I work, patients are between 10 and 15,000 as they come into the office, really do stay between 10 and 15,000 and the ones who are between 0-5,000 stay between 0-5,000. We do not see people bouncing from 1 to 15,000. There are substantial numbers of patients chronically in the 10-20,000 range who do not need transfusion. Some of my colleagues in the Philadelphia area routinely transfuse these patients week after week, but my own experience has been that in most of those patients, transfusion is not necessary. If you are working in a

---

1. Muylle L, Joos M, Wouters E, de Bock R, Peetermans ME. Increased tumor necrosis factor α (TNFα), interleukin 1 and interleukin 6 (IL-6) levels in plasma of stored platelet concentrates; relationship between TNFα and IL-6 levels and febrile transfusion reactions. Transfusion 1993;33:195-99.

setting where a clinically stable patient is bouncing between 2,000 and 15,000, you might have to have a much higher trigger for transfusion. This is certainly not the situation where I work.

M.K. Elias (Gronignen, NL): Dr. de Wolf, a consensus conference was held by the Royal College of Physicians of Edinburgh two years ago on leukocyte reduction[1] in which the prevention of alloimmunization to platelet transfusion was not a solid indication, but it was a possible one. I am waiting for further studies. In the mean time you have rounded your elegant study, the 'leukotol', in which you addressed a totally different mechanism for induction of tolerance other than removal of the MHC class II bearing leukocytes. In view of these results what would be the solid indications for the use of leukodepleted blood components.

J.Th.M. de Wolf: I think they have not changed neither in the light of my results. I like to do a good randomized clinical study before there is something more to say about solid indications.

P.V. Holland (Sacramento, CA, USA): Dr. Blajchman, there is another dr. Busch[2] in Australia who made an interesting observation about the survival of patients with cancer of the cervix, who had received radiation therapy in relation to their anaemia. Are you familiar with the study? Basically those patients who were anaemic and got radiation therapy had a much shorter survival with cancer recurrence than those who were not anaemic at the time they were receiving radiation therapy. It is known that radiation works better in the presence of oxygenated cells rather than non-oxygenated cells. So, he actually transfused a number of these patients, the anaemic ones, into the normal range to haemoglobins above twelve g/dl prior to radiation therapy. Not only did he not see the same poor survival, but he, in fact, corrected their survival to the same as those who were not anaemic. I believe in immunomodulation effects, certainly for a kidney transplant. I would have expected that either he would not have improved the survival or he would have made it even worse by transfusing his patients. But, in fact, he made the survival equivalent to those who were not anaemic by transfusing them. You have any comment?

M. Blajchman: I am not familiar with the study you quote, at least I do not remember it. There is no question that anaemia is a relevant factor for the efficacy of irradiation as you pointed out. Anaemia has other effects as well. We have

1. Consensus conference leukocyte depletion of blood and blood components. Royal College of Physicians of Edinburgh, 1993.
2. Bush RS, Jenkin RDT, Allt WEC, et al. Definitive evidence for hypoxic cells influencing cure in cancer therapy. Brit J Cancer 1978;37:302-6.

recently published[1] a paper indicating that anaemic animals bleed more than non-anaemic animals. So, one of the things you might do for a bleeding thrombocytopenic patient is to correct the anaemia and if you correct the anaemia you probably will partially correct the bleeding tendency.

It is possible therefore that other positive biological effects associated with anaemia may have been corrected neutralizing the possible immunosuppressive effects of the transfusions. This is, of course speculation on my part.

E.L. Snyder: I am concerned that every time I think I have seen another study on leukodepletion that gives me something solid to hang my hat on. Then someone comes along and says you cannot hang your hat on this, because that is not a good study for the following reasons. Everyone has some concern and our concern about 14 day red cells versus 42 day red cells I think is the way I look at leukodepletion. It is a wall that is being built and every time I hear dr. Blajchman talk I come away believing that yes we have more bricks in this wall but he always concludes we still need more data. I am beginning to think that we will never ever get a study that can be done reasonably in our life times that we all will say, yes now we have a good indication for anything regarding leukodepletion.

P.V. Holland: So briefly, what is your point dr. Snyder: is it possible yes or no? I mean we can spend hours on this to really devise a study that would say yes leukodepletion is indicated other than for like on a Wednesday when it is raining in Borneo. I mean is it possible to even do a study or are we just going to sit around and meet for the rest of our lives discussing how we need to study?

I take that as a rhetorical question; we have several people who want to respond. Dr. Murphy I will give you the first chance.

W. Murphy (Edinburgh, UK): I do not think that you need to do further studies to demonstrate efficacy. What we need to find out is whether we can afford it. I do not think that you have to show conclusively that it is much better; it is almost certainly better than non-leukodepletion. In some instances it may be a lot better. If we can afford to do it we should do it.

However, I should like to raise one point. We are now saying that there is no downside to leukodepletion. That was an original small study by Tucker et al.[2] that suggested there might be an antileukaemic effect from transfused leukocytes

1. Blajchman MA, Bordin JO, Bardossyl L, Heddle NM. The contribution of the haematocrit to thrombocytopenic bleeding in experimental animals. Brit J Haemat 1994;86:47-50.
2. Tucker J, Murphy MF, Gregory WM, et al. Apparent removal of graft versus leukaemia effect by the use of leucocyte poor blood components in patients with acute myeloblastic leukaemia. Brit J Haematol 1989;73:572-74.

and that this effect is removed by leukodepletion. Subsequent reports[1-3] of which only that of Marwijk Kooy et al.[1] was a prospective randomized trial, failed to confirm the initial findings. However, in at least two of these studies[1,2] the standard non-leukodepleted blood products were buffy coat removed red blood cells and buffy coat derived platelets, in contrast to the standard blood products used in the initial study. In addition to the studies not being strictly comparable in terms of treatment, they are also very small, and lack the statistical power to establish or refute the presence of an antileukaemic effect. If this issue is to be addressed, it will have to be in a large prospective trial; outside of such a trial there is no reason at present to support use of non-leukodepleted blood products to avoid leukaemic relapse.

M. Blajchman: Dr. Murphy, your point is very important because it illustrates the problem about the decision making process in healthcare. The point is that scientists want proof, it is not always possible to have proof and therefore the scientist should not be making the decisions. We have a vacuum in North America and I think also in Europe, about the decision making process for transfusion medicine. This is the basis of the jury system. The jury consists of non-experts, who listen to the evidence and come up with a decision. I think it should be the same way decisions in healthcare and for leukodepletion specifically. There are many pieces to the puzzle and they should be presented and a rational decision made on the basis of the evidence available. The scientist has nonetheless a very important part as do such people who are knowledgeable in healthcare policy and cost effectiveness. Concerning the latter, there are all sorts of decisions being made that are not very cost effective. For example, the FDA has made a decision about HIV-1 antigen testing in the face of the likelihood that preventing one case of HIV will cost 25-30 million dollars. In other healthcare situations that would be a cost that would be deemed unacceptable.

H.J.C. de Wit: I agree with you and in the discussion leukocyte depletion or not I would add that if you cannot find any scientific proof that the one is better than the other, perhaps non-scientific factors might add as cost effectiveness but also the concept of going back to pure component therapy. We stopped transfusing whole blood a few years ago. I think if you can let benefit more patients from one donation, you should go as far as you can to optimally use the blood that you have. A second thing, what dr. Blajchman did is add studies so I would not

1. Van Marwijk Kooy M, van Prooijen HC, Bosma-Stants I, et al. Use of leukocyte-depleted concentrates for the prevention of refractoriness and primary HLA alloimmunization: A prospective randomised trial. Blood 1991;77:201-5.
2. Oksanen K, Elonen E. Impact of leucocyte depleted blood components on the haematological recovery and prognosis of patients with acute myeloid leukaemia. Brit J Haematol 1993;84:639-47.
3. Rebulla P, Pappaletrera M, Barbui T, et al. Duration of first remission in leukaemia recipients of leucocyte poor blood components. Brit J Haematol 1990;75:157-57.

disencourage any scientist to do more studies but I would encourage some scientists to add all those studies to make the parts of proof that we have stronger.

III. TRANSFUSION POLICIES AND CLINICAL PRACTICE

FACTS, FEARS AND FORMULAS ABOUT BLOOD TRANSFUSIONS: ON THE ASSESSMENT, ACCEPTANCE AND CONTROL OF RISKS

C.A.J. Vlek

Introduction

Giving blood and receiving others' blood are intimate things that easily raise sensitivities. A patient in need must trust the doctor who hopes that the donor is a responsible person. When there is doubt, there is risk. And risk-taking demands a balancing of risks against expected benefits. For a small or an anonymous benefit, you don't take a large risk. When the benefits are visibly large, you may get daring. But a blood recipient has little control, and the donor is not in charge either. So: how much fear is reasonable, how much trust is required, and what should you know to decide what to do?

In the area of behavioural decision theory, risk perception, risk acceptance and safety management have been topics for research and scientific debate for about twenty years now [1-5]. Initially, psychologists aspired to explain why "subjective risk" so often deviates from "objective risk" as assessed by technical engineers, statistical biologists, or epidemiologists. Later on, several disciplinary perspectives were brought together in various attempts to more fully understand basic conceptions of risk as well as entire processes of risk management [6-8].

In the present paper a behavioural-science perspective is given on risk management as comprising risk assessment, decision-making and risk acceptance, and risk control. Also, the relevance of this perspective for dealing with risks in and around blood transfusions is systematically considered. The paper successively goes along: three basic questions about risks and safety; formal definitions and cognitive dimensions of risk; probability and uncertainty; the multi-stage process of risk generation and risk management; the multi-attribute characterisation of risky activities or situations; decision-making and risk acceptance; and risk communication as an overall "trust-building" activity. At the end of each section of the paper "conclusions on blood transfusions"[1] are drawn so as to bring forward the implications of general theory and methods for practical risk management.

1. Throughout the paper the term "blood transfusion" is mostly used in a broad sense, to indicate the entire business of blood collection, processing, storage, distribution and administration to patients.

Three basic questions

Research questions and policy issues about risks and risk-taking are revolving around risk assessment, risk acceptance, risk decision-making, and risk control. How individuals deal with personal risks is a topic for psychologists: risk assessment, acceptance and control are all "in one hand". How a larger community deals with public or collective risks is another matter. For this may involve expert analysis and assessment, socio-political evaluation and decision-making, and well-organized risk control. These three key activities may be conducted by different parties having differing basic knowledge, values, decision power and control abilities vis-à-vis the risks. The three key activities naturally follow from three essential questions that any theoretical framework and practical methodology for dealing with risks should be able to handle:

1. How risky is a given activity or situation? (or: how safe is it?)
2. Is it not too risky? (or: is it safe enough?)
3. How could its riskiness be reduced? (or: how could its safety be increased?)

Answering these questions requires a conceptualisation and a methodology for: 1) the analysis and assessment of risk; 2) the evaluation of, and decision-making about risk acceptance; and 3) effective risk control and general safety management.

Most often "risk" is not a static component of an activity or situation (or system of activities), which can be easily measured and decided about, such as in one-shot, well-defined gambles. Instead, in most real-life situations risk is a function of so many factors, technical-physical as well as cognitive-behavioural and social-organizational, that risk may well be seen as a *process* rather than some kind of "substance" which could be clearly pinpointed. Therefore, conceptual tools and methods for risk assessment, decision-making and risk control must be supplemented with useful procedures for applying these tools and methods in multi-stage, multi-party risk situations.

Conclusions on blood transfusion

The three basic questions above directly apply to blood transfusions. Their answering, however, very much depends upon the position of the person asking the questions, and particularly upon the information, the expertise, and the technical means available for underpinning the answers. Obviously, a blood donor, a nurse, a doctor and a patient all have different interests, presuppositions, and convictions. Knowing these and acknowledging their differences are vital for the quality of the overall process of risk-benefit communication and safety management.

Definitions and dimensions of risk

Twenty years ago, when social scientists started to get involved in acceptable-risk debates [1,9,10], there seemed to be a solid belief in the statistical and engineering community that "risk" was a one-dimensional concept whose size or seriousness could be quantitatively assessed. Fairly soon, however, this idea was strongly criticized. Following Kaplan and Garrick [11] risk cannot be properly expressed in terms of a single number or even a single curve. In their view the best formal definition of risk is a probability distribution of possible (future) frequencies of harmful consequences, which themselves may be multi-dimensional in nature. More complicating still was the gradual unfolding of a host of differing definitions of risk [3,12,13]. A recent survey [14] yielded about ten distinct formal risk definitions, as summarized in Table 1.

Table 1. Formal definitions of risk and riskiness [adapted from ref. 14].

1. Probability of undesired consequence
2. Seriousness of (maximum) possible undesired consequence
3. Multi-attribute weighted sum of components of possible undesired consequences
4. Probability x seriousness of undesired consequence ("expected loss")
5. Probability-weighted sum of all possible undesired consequences ("average expected loss")
6. Fitted function through graph of points relating probability to extent of undesired consequences
7. Semivariance of possible undesired consequences about their average
8. Variance of all possible consequences about mean expected consequence
9. Weighted sum of expected value and variance of all possible consequences
10. Weighted combination of various parameters of the probability distribution of all consequences (encompasses definitions 8 and 9)
11. Weight of possible undesired consequences ("loss") relative to comparable possible desired consequences ("gain")

This collection of risk definitions may be condensed by viewing risk as the characterisation of: a) a single possibility of accident, loss or disease (defs. 1-4); b) a collection of accident possibilities (defs. 5-7); and c) an *activity* having accident (and other) possibilities (defs 8-11). Table 1 does not contain various informal definitions of risk, such as "set of possible negative consequences" or "lack of perceived controllability". The variety of risk definitions reflects the difficulty of answering the basic question of any risk manager: "What should, and what should not be comprehended by a concept that could be meaningfully called 'risk'?"

In their own search for a valid answer to this question, social and behavioural scientists have discovered a variety of basic dimensions of perceived risk or riskiness. They found out that different groups of "risk perceivers" rated, or compared, the riskiness of heterogeneous sets of risky activities and situations as following various basic risk characteristics. Differing tasks have been presented to available respondents, such as, e.g., ratings of risky activities on a set of explicit risk variables, rank ordering of risky activities following their perceived riskiness and/or acceptability, and sorting a collection of risky activities in groups of similar items. Some relevant studies are: Fischhoff, Slovic, Lichtenstein, Read and Combs [15], Slovic et al. [2], Vlek and Stallen [17], Renn [18] Kuyper and Vlek [19], Kraus and Slovic [20], and Gardner and Gould [21].

Apart from this there have been theoretical analyses of activities and situations, which have yielded a number of characteristics that policy makers are recommended to take into account when approaching particular risky decision situations; see Vlek and Stallen [3], Otway and Von Winterfeldt [22], Hohenemser, Kates and Slovic [23], Hansson [24], and Jungermann [25].

From this empirical and theoretical work Vlek and Keren [25] have compiled the list of basic dimensions underlying the perceived riskiness of any activity or situation which is given in Table 2. Using this set of dimensions one may either diagnose the reasons why a particular activity or situation is (to be) perceived as "risky", or one may deliberately change a given activity or situation such that it appears to be riskier, or safer, than it originally was. One problem here is that various groups of respondents attach varying weights to such dimensions and hence also to judged riskiness; this is related to group attitudes towards the expected benefits of a risky activity [17, 19-21,27].

Table 2. Basic dimensions underlying perceived riskiness.

1. Potential degree of harm or fatality
2. Physical extent of damage (area affected)
3. Social extent of damage (number of people involved)
4. Time distribution of damage (immediate and/or delayed effects)
5. Probability of undesired consequence
6. Controllability (by self or trusted expert) of consequences
7. Experience with familiarity, imaginability of consequences
8. Voluntariness of exposure (freedom of choice)
9. Clarity, importance of expected benefits
10. Social distribution of risks and benefits
11. Harmful intentionality

The eleven risk dimensions in Table 2 may be seen as elaborations of, or as supplements to the formal risk definitions in Table 1. Dimensions 1-4 provide specifications for the terms "undesired consequence" and "components of undesired consequences" in Table 1. Dimensions 5-7 qualify the terms "probability" and "probability distribution" in Table 1, and they convey the message that these may be under partial control of the people involved. Control over possible consequences often correlates with decision control and freedom of choice, covered by dimension 8 in Table 2, which is absent in Table 1 because formal risk definitions stem from frameworks in which full autonomy of decision makers (i.e., complete voluntariness of exposure to risk) is presupposed. Dimension 9 in Table 2 may sound somewhat disturbing: the perceived riskiness of an activity varies with the clarity and importance of its benefits. This means that riskiness is perceived *relative* to expected benefits, which is in line with risk definition 11 in Table 1. Having emerged from *risk* perception research, dimension 9 badly needs closer investigation so that *its* underlying dimensions ("perceived beneficiality") may be differentiated.

Conclusions on blood transfusion

The "risk" of a blood transfusion is a multi-dimensional concept which is very hard to assess numerically. The observed relative frequency of transfusion deaths – e.g., 1 per 100,000 [28] or 2 per 10,000 recipients [29], or of transfusion-transmitted AIDS – e.g., 1 per 100,000 [30] or 1 in a million [31], constitutes only one dimension of risk. Other important dimensions have to do with the possible consequences – e.g., their controllability, and with the decision context – e.g., the subject's freedom of choice and the expected benefits of transfusion. Due to the multi-dimensional nature of most risks, risk comparisons across divergent activities or situations are not easy to justify. Particularly when freedom of choice (or voluntariness), subjective degree of control, and the importance of expected benefits co-vary with the possibility of adverse effects, differing activities or situations cannot be meaningfully compared with respect to their riskiness.

Probability and uncertainty

Given that one adopts a core definition of risk as a function of probability and seriousness (disutility) of undesired consequences (def. 4 in Table), the measurability of (accident) probabilities and (dis)utilities deserves special attention. Multi-attribute (dis)utility evaluation will be discussed in the next section. Regarding probability, there are variations and limitations in the information basis for probability assessment. There exist three interpretations of "probability": the frequentistic, logical and personalistic interpretations, respectively. High-quality statistical information to assess "frequentistic" probabilities is often not available. "Logical" probabilities can only be deduced if one has sufficient information about the properties of a stochastic apparatus or process (such as a roulette wheel, or genetic inheritance). And "personal" probabilities of uncertain outcomes can only be validly assessed via somewhat artificial and laborious betting methods [32]. In empirical research on risk judgement it appeared that frequency information and scenario information on past and possible accidents are both relevant, depending upon their availability and (but not always) their quality [33].

Even more important perhaps is the distinction between controllable and uncontrollable risks: in some cases the probability of an accident may be influenced by the decision maker's effort (through safety precautions, safe behaviour etc.). In other cases the accident probability is fixed a priori and the situation amounts to gambling. Following up on Howell and Burnett [34] and Kahneman and Tversky [35], Hendrickx et al. [33] have proposed a simple taxonomy of uncertainty, related to four different kinds of (risk) information. These are, respectively: frequency information on external (pure chance) events such as a lightning stroke; frequency information on "internal" (i.e., human-controllable) events such as in repeated dart throwing; scenario information on external events (a description of "how this might occur to you"); and scenario information about "internal", human-controllable events (a description of "how you might make this happen or prevent this from happening"). The idea of this taxonomy is that uncertainty and probability mean different things across these four combinations, and hence "risk" – as dependent on probability – also varies in nature.

Conclusions on blood transfusion

Obviously, the information basis for probability assessment in blood transfusion varies across different cases (patients, institutions and circumstances). Sometimes high-quality relative frequencies are available concerning accidents in similar transfusion cases from the past. Sometimes one just does not know enough and one has to go by expectations and presuppositions about what might happen in a particular case and how this could be managed. External probabilities (concerning "acts of god") may be more reliable (if you trust "god") than internal probabilities which depend on unreliable human factors. So: be explicit about your sources of uncertainty and about the evidence and/or the arguments you can bring to bear upon your probability estimates in the context of risk assessment.

Risk generation and management as a process

A golden rule for any kind of problem-solving is: first diagnose, then decide, and finally intervene (and evaluate). For risk management this would involve that the origins and causes of risk are clearly charted, before any decision on risk acceptance is made and risk control is being conducted. Or, if conceived dynamically, there should be a continuous interaction between risk assessment as diagnosis (and evaluation), decision-making on risk acceptance, and risk control as intervention. Such diagnosis and planned intervention for risk control may be done explicitly, with the aid of human cognitive, social and/or technical facilities. In everyday life, however, diagnosis and intervention for risk control often proceed "automatically", on the basis of some well-established habitual behaviour (such as, e.g., in city bicycling or during medical surgery – by the doctor).

Stage-models of risk generation, decision-making and risk control have been proposed by several authors. Table 3 summarises three different views, as developed by Hohenemser et al. [23], Merkhofer [36] and Vlek and Keren [26], respectively. An intriguing question, of course, is whether such models as in Table 3 can be extended so as to *both* cover the phases of risk assessment, decision-making and risk control, *and* accommodate the basic dimensions of risk as summarized in Table 2.

Table 3. Multi-stage models of risk generation and management.

	Hohenemser et al. [23]	Merkhofer [36]	Vlek & Keren [26]
1.	Human needs	Risk source	Need arousal, goal specification
2.	Human wants	Exposure processes	Design of relevant activities
3.	Choice of technology	Ultimate effects	Evaluation of alternatives
4.	Initiating events	Consequence valuation	Choice of activity
5.	Energy/materials' release		Implementation of chosen option
6.	Exposure to energy/ materials		Monitoring and control of activity
7.	Human/environmental effects		Emergency situation
8.			Accident occurrence
9.			Feedback towards above components

In an attempt to answer these questions, the Health Council of the Netherlands [8] has adopted a multi-stage model picturing risk generation and risk management as a function of the social context, human needs and preferences, activity design and planning, and the choice of a specific goal-directed activity. Once selected, an activity may be implemented according to plan and yield the intended benefits as well as some anticipated negative side-effects. Or the activity may develop into a "failing realization", whereby unanticipated quantities of energy (as in an explosion) and/or hazardous materials (as in gaseous or liquid emissions) are released. The spreading and the eventual harmful effects of any energy and/or materials' release depend upon situational characteristics such as the vicinity of people, weather conditions, or accident-mitigating activities by rescue workers. The splitting up of a single initial part of the process into two later parts – one intended and probable, the other undesired and improbable, also emphasises the fact that risk evaluation and risk-taking involve a weighing of benefits (from "planned realization") against costs and risks (under "failing realization").

In connection with the multi-stage process model of risk generation and risk management, the Dutch Health Council [8] provides a listing of 44 different "risk attributes" which refer to relevant aspects of the various process stages. Examples are: availability of choice alternatives (a "context" attribute), technical possibilities for a safe planning of an activity, problem complexity (an attribute of strategic decision-making), perceived controllability (important for both planned and failing realization of an activity), and a variety of consequence-attributes such as different kinds of intended benefits and diverse possible negative effects (e.g., fatality, morbidity and function losses).

Conclusions on blood transfusion

Clearly, the riskiness of a particular blood transfusion (donation or reception) extends well beyond the supreme hour itself. Both before and after that hour things have been done or are being undertaken, which have a greater or lesser bearing upon the overall probability of ultimate negative effects. Donors as well as patients may have a limited view on the total process embedding their particular involvement. But when they get to think about it, they may gradually widen their perspective on the total business of blood collection, processing, storage, distribution and patient administration. Through his or her activated imagination, any person involved may end up applying the initial question: "How risky is this (for me)?" to the entire process of which blood donation and blood reception are just separate components. Hence, it seems prudent to consider the main aspects of the various process stages for their impact on the overall riskiness (or safety) of the whole business. This would also facilitate one's understanding of any client's "perceived" risk of his or her involvement in blood transfusions.

Multi-attribute risk characterization

Following any risk assessment procedure, it is desirable to arrive at a compact and sufficiently comprehensive description of the risks inherent in a given activity or situation. Such a summary characterization may be needed for public deliberation, for political judgement and decision-making, for the communication of decisions made, and for the justification of safety policies. Given the large number of potentially relevant risk attributes, it seems obvious to attempt to carry out a *multi-attribute risk characterization*. Briefly, this would involve two basic steps: 1) identification and selection of relevant risk attributes; and 2) the scoring of a given activity or situation with respect to each attribute so as to obtain a multi-attribute risk profile. If one were to go further on the way towards full risk quantification, two additional steps would be: 3) assignment of importance-weights to each relevant attribute; and 4) weighted aggregation of all attribute scores in order to obtain one single numerical risk figure for the activity or situation under consideration (for basic models and methods of multi-attribute evaluation see 37-39).

Following the above four steps may seem simpler than it is. Properly making step 1 requires to generate relevant risk attributes. This may be done following the multistage model briefly discussed above [8]. Or one may determine risk attributes by systematically comparing various different activities or situations for their distinguishing characteristics. Or one may perform a hierarchical multi-attribute analysis of desired overall "safety", which may be laid out as a concept involving subgoals, each to be differentiated into various specific safety objectives. But then you would have to select the *relevant* ones, i.e., those that are both important and nonredundant or nonoverlapping. And one would not want to end up with too many ones, in view of the scoring task of step 2. Also, each risk attribute must be concrete and specific enough to be able to assess its value for a given activity or situation. For step 2, the scoring itself, one may have different kinds of information available. This may allow to score some risk attributes "objectively" and others by "expert judgement" or "public perception". Whatever the scoring is done, the end result should be an informative risk profile telling its observer what kind of risk one is dealing with and how high or low an activity or situation scores on its relevant attributes.

Full quantification of a multi-attribute risk into a one-dimensional number may serve the purpose of allowing to *numerically* compare different risky alternatives, and/or to weigh a multi-attribute risk against a similarly quantified multi-attribute benefit. However, the importance-weighting of individual risk (or benefit) attributes presupposes that these are commensurable. That is, equal scores on each weighted attribute scale should reflect comparable contributions to overall riskiness. Otherwise, weighted aggregation of attribute scores would not be allowed, and a one-figure risk quantification would be meaningless. But commensurability may be too much asked, if one is dealing with a subset of risk attributes as variable in meaning as discussed in the above. We may therefore conclude that a multi-attribute risk characterization in itself may be necessary and useful, but that a full-fledged weighted aggregation of attribute scores may be impossible or unwarranted, and that it may (therefore) turn out to be counterproductive in any risk management context.

Conclusions on blood transfusion

Linking up with the "conclusions" in the three sections above, we may state that a compact, multi-attribute "risk profile" of any blood transfusion (donation or reception) may be a useful tool for considering its riskiness, for understanding the process components – and aspects thereof – which are underlying riskiness, for making the decision to go ahead with transfusion or choose an alternative course of action, and for selecting the possible safety measures that seem most appropriate. If carefully conducted, a full-fledged multi-attribute risk quantification could be performed, which yields a numerical estimate of the seriousness of the risk. However, given the difficulty of doing this in a justifiable manner, for most cases it would seem wiser to stop at the multi-attribute profile itself, and to leave the judgemental aggregation of the various – objective as well as expert-subjective – assessments to those responsible for final decisions.

Decision-making on risk acceptance

From empirical research on the dimensions of perceived risk (see Table 2 plus text above) an early conclusion ventured by Vlek and Stallen [17] was that risk acceptance seemed to revolve around three key questions concerning a particular activity or situation: 1) Are the benefits large enough?; 2) Is the maximum credible accident (or: the catastrophe-potential) low enough?; and 3) Is the activity or situation sufficiently controllable? Let us more generally consider how one might proceed when multi-attribute risk characterization has taken place.

Decision-theoretically, when a multi-attribute risk profile has been established, a decision-maker may follow roughly two general models. The first one, labelled "maximizing", implies a comparison of two or more alternative options and a rank ordering of these on the basis of their multi-attribute risk profile. This yields a conclusion about which alternative is the "riskiest" and which the "safest", or – more modestly perhaps – which alternative seems to have the "best" risk profile.

The comparison and rank ordering required may be done on qualitative, i.e., judgemental grounds, as when one critically considers each multi-attribute profile (without any explicit numerical statements). Or the comparison and rank ordering may be done on the basis of some weighted-aggregate risk score which numerically summarises a multi-attribute profile. A maximizing approach is most suitable for *strategic* decision problems involving risk.

The second model of decision-making, labelled "satisficing", involves a consideration of one multi-attribute risk profile at the time, and testing its actual scores against pre-set acceptance criteria on the various risk attributes. This amounts to testing a given course of action against available risk standards, and it requires that such (reasonable and valid) standards have been adopted *a priori*. There are three submodels of "satisficing", viz. the conjunctive, disjunctive and compensatory-weighting model. Applying these would yield an acceptance decision when all, or a subset, or some weighted combination of risk attribute standards have been met, respectively. A satisficing approach is most suitable for *tactical* decision problems. Because of its special suitability and popularity for practical policy making, we will come back to it immediately below.

A third general way of making decisions, frequently used in everyday life, involves the application of simple choice-production rules, of the type "if this and that, do such and so". Due to their pre-programmed and often automatic character, risk-acceptance choices made in this way may hardly be called decisions. But they nevertheless are very effective, as well as effort- and time-saving, and sufficiently rewarding in many practical contexts. Choice-production rules are effective for solving *operational* decision problems. Table 4 summarises the three general ways of making decisions and it also indicates the type of decision problem and the quality of the decision going along with them.

Table 4. Three general ways of making decisions on risk acceptance.

Type of problem	**Decision approach**	**Nature of decision**
Strategical	Analytic: maximizing	"Best alternative"
Tactical	Standardized: satisficing	"Acceptable course"
Operational	Automated: rewarding	"Positive outcome"

In many practical cases, the risk problem is "tactical", i.e., there is a single course of action, or a given situation, which is being questioned as regards its "acceptability". Thus the decision-maker may consider a satisficing approach for which risk attribute standards are needed and valid attribute scores have to be assessed. Standards setting and standards testing constitute a practicable and convincing approach towards decision-making on risk acceptance. Its application, however, is limited to well-defined categories of activities or situations, which are more or less comparable amongst each other. Comparability may obviously be determined on the basis of multi-attribute risk profiles. And, obviously (but not so for some), standards monitoring and enforcement should necessarily follow in the wake of any standards-testing decision on risk acceptance [see especially 40].

Although it may seem as if decision-making on risk acceptance implies comprehensive decisions of a "go/no go" character, actually such decision-making may differentially apply to separate stages in the total process of risk generation. For example, decisions – of either a maximizing or a satisficing, i.e., standards-testing character – may pertain to goals and preferences, design and planning, feasible courses of action, differing ways of implementing a chosen alternative, and various safety measures. Any set of stage-specific decisions may well start from a careful consideration of a multi-attribute risk profile, and they may greatly contribute to reducing the riskiness of the overall process by which a given activity or situation emerges and is being managed.

The decision approaches summarized in Table 4 seem to be mutually-exclusive and self-contained. More often than not, however, risk acceptance is the result (or even the by-product) of a dynamic process of assessment, decision-making and control, in which several management principles may be successively applied. Inspired by the safety policy of the International Commission on Radiological Protection (ICRP-26) [41], a sequential decision-making scheme may be followed, in which *risk limitation*, the *ALARA principle* (risks should be As Low As Reasonably Achievable), trading-off of risks against benefits ("*justification*"), and comparison of options (*maximization*) are put forward as logically successive evaluation grounds for "acceptable risk"; see Vlek [42] for the complete diagram.

According to this approach, evaluation of a given activity or situation against risk standards may form an early and provisional part of the decision-making process. As an exclusive evaluation ground this can only be sufficient under limiting conditions, namely when the activity stays below the risk limit and the risk is characterized as "ALARA", while no alternative can be found that would be safer yet. If the activity or situation is above the risk limit, a more comprehensive assessment of benefits and risks is undertaken, unless in the meantime the risk can be successfully reduced or a safer alternative is found. After this satisficing approach aimed at a single option, a comparative maximizing evaluation may be performed when there is more than one "acceptable" option. This would yield a choice for the "best" available option.

The strength of this sequential decision-making scheme lies in the fact that inherent problems surrounding risk assessment and evaluation may be absorbed by the later steps, which deal with risk reduction, the search for safer options and risk-benefit trade-offs. This means that decision makers could allow themselves a provisional or even "wrong" outcome of testing against risk limits. A decision to reject a proposed activity or situation could only be made if: a) there are no inherent significant benefits; or b) the benefits do not sufficiently offset the (irreduceable) risks. Rejection cannot therefore simply take place because the risk or riskiness is considered too high.

Conclusions on blood transfusion

Acceptable risk of blood transfusion depends only partly on the seriousness of the risk involved. It strongly depends also upon the benefits involved and upon the safety precautions one may take following any decision. Given that these major components of acceptable risk can be handled (characterized, formalized, controlled) in various ways, "acceptable risk" also is a function of the overall approach taken to arrive at an answer to the questions: "Is this safe enough?". It is tempting to state that – like risk itself – "acceptable risk" is a process characteristic rather than a single-dimensional concept. Hence, it would be in the nature of the process of risk assessment, decision-making and risk control, that one should seek to convince either oneself or other persons (donors, patients) that any "risk" involved could be an "acceptable" risk. This would make risk communication an essential activity.

Risk communication

The question "Why risk communication?", has been answered variously by different authors. Covello, Von Winterfeldt and Slovic [43, p.72] conclude that risk communication is needed: a) to inform and educate risk-involved persons and groups; b) to specify and support behaviour change and protective action; c) to adequately provide disaster warnings and emergency information; and d) to aid joint problem solving and conflict resolution. Wiedemann, Rohrmann and Jungermann [44, p.5] follow this set of major risk communication objectives but add a fifth one: the analysis of risk conceptualizations ("Risiko-Verständnisse") and risk evaluations by various interest groups. Cvetkovich, Vlek and Earle [45, p.255] propose that "hazard communication" is: "to improve the public's ability to make appropriate decisions in view of technological hazards (and benefits)". Stern [46, p.100] warns that: "It is dangerous to misunderstand risk communication because effective decision-making about risks depends on it". The decision function of risk communication is also emphasized in the review on health risk perception and communication by Fischhoff et al. [5, p.184]: "To make such decisions wisely, individuals need to understand the risks and the benefits associated with alternative courses of action".

Common to all risk communication objectives listed above is its decision-making and behaviour- (or system-) regulating function. This does not need to be restricted to "the public" (whoever they are) but may generally apply to risk-taking actors or organizations, risk-exposed individuals or groups, and risk-regulating government officials. In general, risk communication should be supportive of some overall assessment-decision-and-control process, which may cover as much as planning and design, acceptance decision-making, safety management, emergency control and accident (effects) mitigation. Two additional functions may be anxiety reduction and learning to manage risks, an affective and a cognitive by-product of risk communication, respectively.

Hence, effective risk communication should serve one or more of six distinct functions. It should stimulate or lead to: a) appropriate planning and design of risky activities or products; b) good decision-making on risk acceptance; c) adequate safety management concerning a chosen course of action; d) proper accident handling and effects mitigation, if necessary; e) anxiety reduction in exposed persons; and f) improved insights into risk management among all parties involved.

Conclusions on blood transfusion

From a process-perspective on overall risk management, transfusion risk communication is a broad-ranging set of activities involving various different parties. Risk communication (mostly among experts) may concern the optimal design of procedures for safe-donor recruitment and maintenance of an adequate donor population. It may also deal with proper decision-making (e.g., between doctor and patient) about the administration of blood products to potential recipients. And it may be focused on the very moment of blood donation or reception, when the possibility of negative health effects may be most salient. Any message about transfusion risks cannot be properly understood if it is not tuned towards the intended receiver. Some prior diagnosis of the background knowledge, values and skills of the people addressed may therefore be necessary. Also, it is useful to specify beforehand what purposes one's risk communication is to serve, so that the latter may be optimally designed to achieve adopted goals. For one thing, written donor information accompanied by requests to read it and behave accordingly, may not be as effective as personal interviews that fit the receiver's individual background for an empirical study on AIDS risk communication [see 47]. Transfusion risk communication may best be aimed at developing (further) confidence or trust [48], since anyone involved in risk-taking needs confidence: in the achievement of intended benefits, in the avoidance of irrepareable disaster, and in the skills and the safety motivation of the experts who are responsible for most of the risk management process, of which the subject is a crucial but just a single component.

Some general conclusions and suggestions

This paper has been written by a psychologist who does not know much about the ins and outs of blood transfusion. That may be bad for a full understanding, but it may be good for a detached view of the major issues. The author's assignment, and his aim, have been to present a systematic overview of concepts, models and methods of risk management in complex situations. Risk management is here conceived as a process comprising risk assessment, decision-making and risk control. The main direct implications of the present framework for the business of blood transfusion have been briefly indicated at the end of each separate section. To conclude, it seems useful to emphasize a few general points and formulate some suggestions.

"Risk" is not a uni-dimensional concept which can be easily quantified. This is mainly due, firstly, to the multi-attribute nature of any risky activity or situation which may engage the subject in a decision problem. Secondly, it is due to the multi-stage character of risk generation and risk management in dynamic, multi-actor situations, such as exist around blood transfusions. Thus, optimal risk management – which may involve a maximization of relative benefits – should come close to "total quality management" which covers documentation, validation, regulatory laws, licensing, teaching and training of staff, standards, record keeping, and quality control of products and their distribution [49].

Clients of the blood transfusion system: blood donors and recipients, but also intermediate administrators, should trust total quality and risk management. Due to almost every actor's limited view, obligations and influence vis-à-vis the entire organization of blood collection, processing, storage, distribution and administration, trust in others' knowledge, skills and (safety) motivation is indispensable for the acceptance of any risk, however minute, in any stage or component of the process as a whole. Thus, risk communication should be focused on "trust-building", and the latter should be undertaken in an honest, valid manner. Blood donors as well as blood recipients come in to provide, or to obtain certain (potential) benefits from blood transfusion. They should be able to trust the technical-social-organizational system for delivering what they are hoping for, and for preventing what they are fearing. So, again, trust – like risk – seems to cover the whole process involving blood transfusion rather than a single "gambling" moment in time.

Finally, we should perhaps be aware of the fact that blood donors are facing a fundamentally different risk-benefit situation than do blood recipients. Donors are expected to provide a future (potential) benefit to an anonymous person, at some immediate cost (of showing up and delivering blood) and risk of infection or other negative health effect. Their special sensitivity to risks may well be related to the remoteness and obscurity of the associated benefits of transfusion to others. Providing donors with a tangible direct benefit might obviously suppress some of their anxieties. In contrast, blood recipients are patients in need, who expect an immediate personal benefit (at some cost and risk) from administered blood made available by anonymous risk-bearing donors.

This asymmetry makes the donor position particularly sensitive to questions about altruism and social responsibility, which the recipient in turn may not wish to care much about. It should not be surprising that potential donors are less likely to be willing to deliver their blood for others' benefit, as society individualises and tends to find common goods and collective responsibilities less important. This conclusion would imply that the whole blood transfusion system is continually to be presented and discussed as a "common good" requiring numerous individuals' loyal cooperation, because everyone is actually or potentially benefitting from its adequate functioning.

References

1. Slovic P, Fischhoff B, Lichtenstein S. Cognitive processes and soietal risk taking. In: Carroll JS, Payne JW (eds). Cognition and social behavior. Potomomac MD: Erlbaum L. Also in Jungermann H, de Zeeuw G (eds). Decision making and change in human affairs. Reidel, Dordrecht/Boston 1976.
2. Slovic P, Fischhoff B, Lichtenstein S. Behavioral decision theory perspectives on risk and safety. Acta Psychologica 1984;56:183-203.
3. Vlek Ch, Stallen PJ. Rational and personal aspects of risk. Acta Psychol 1980;45:273-300.
4. Yates JF (ed). Risk-taking behavior. Wiley, Chichester UK/New York 1992.
5. Fischhoff B, Bostrom A, Quadrel MJ. Risk perception and communication. Ann Rev Public Health 1993;14:183-203.
6. Krimsky S, Golding D (eds). Social theories of risk. New York, Plenum 1992.
7. Bayerische Rück (eds). Risk is a construct; perceptions of risk perception. Knesebeck, Munich 1993.
8. Gezondheidsraad. Risk is more than just a number. Health Council of The Netherlands, The Hague, 1996, 120 pages. (Complete Dutch version: Risico, meer dan een getal, also available).
9. Lowrance WW. Of acceptable risk; science and the determination of safety. W. Kaufmann, Los Altos (CA) 1976.
10. Rowe WD. An anatomy of risk. Wiley, New York 1977.
11. Kaplan S, Garrick BJ. On the quantitative definition of risk. Risk Anal 1981;1:11-27.
12. Coombs CH. A review of the mathematical psychology of risk and risk taking. University of Michigan, Michigan Mathematical Psychology Program Report MMPP 1972:72-76.
13. Libby R, Fishburn PC. Behavioral models of risk taking in business decisions: A survey and evaluation. J Account Res 1977;Autumn:272-92.
14. Vlek CAJ. Beslissen over risico-acceptatie/Decision making about risk acceptance. Rapport in Hoofdlijnen/Executive Summary. 1990, 52 pp. Gezondheidsraad/Health Council, The Hague. Report nr A 90/10H, abt. 80 pages. (Main report nr. A 90/10, 236 pp in Dutch).
15. Fischhoff B, Slovic P, Lichtenstein S, Read S, Combs B. How safe is safe enough? A psychometric study of attitudes toward technological risks and benefits. Policy Sciences 1978;9:127-52.
16. Slovic P, Fischhoff B, Lichtenstein S. Facts and fears: Understanding perceived risk. In: Kahneman D, Slovic P, Tversky A. Judgement under uncertainty: Heuristics and biases. Cambridge Univ. Press, London/New York, 1982:463-89.
17. Vlek Ch, Stallen PJ. Judging risks and benefits in the small and in the large. Organizational Behavior and Human Performance 1981;28:235-71.
18. Renn O. Technology, risk and public perception. J Appl System Anal/Zeitschrift für Angewandte Systemanalyse 1983;4:50-65.
19. Kuyper H, Vlek Ch. Contrasting risk judgments among interest groups. Acta Psychol 1984;56:205-18.
20. Kraus NN, Slovic P. Taxonomic analysis of perceived risk: Modeling individual and group perceptions within homogeneous hazard domains. Risk Anal 1988;8:435-55.
21. Gardner GT, Gould LC. Public perceptions of the risks and benefits of technology. Risk Anal 1989;9:225-42.
22. Otway HJ, von Winterfeldt. Beyond acceptable risk: On the social acceptability of

technologies. Policy Sciences 1982;14:241-46.
23. Hohenemser C, Kates RW, Slovic P. The nature of technological hazard. Science 1983;220:378-84.
24. Hansson SO. Dimensions of risk. Risk Anal 1989;9:107-12.
25. Jungermann H. Inhalte und Konzepte der Risiko-Kommunikation. In: Jungermann H, Rohrmann B, Wiedemann PM (eds). Risiko-Konzepte, Risiko-Konflikte, Risiko-Kommunikation. Forschungszentrum Jülich GmbH, Jülich 1990:309-27.
26. Vlek Ch, Keren GB. Behavioral decision theory and environmental risk management: Assessment and resolution of four 'survival' dilemmas. Acta Psychol 1992;80: 249-78.
27. Buss DM, Craik KJ. Contemporary world views: Personal and policy implications. J Appl Soc Psychol 1983;13:259-80.
28. Peri-operative red blood cell transfusion. NIH Consensus development conference. Bethesda (MD), National Institutes of Health. JAMA 1988;260:2700-05.
29. Dodd RY. Adverse consequences of blood transfusion: Quantitative risk estimates. In: Nance ST (ed). Blood supply: Risks, perceptions and prospects for the future. American Association of Blood Banks, Bethesda, MD 1994:1-24.
30. Kalbfleisch JD, Lawless JF. Estimating the incubation time distribution and expected number of cases of transfusion-associated acquired immune deficiency syndrome. Transfusion 1989;29:672-76.
31. Bove JR. Statement on AIDS and blood transfusion. Hearings before the Subcommittee on Intergovernmental Relations and Human Resources of the House Committee on Government Operations. Government Printing Office, Washington, DC 1993.
32. Vlek CAJ, Wagenaar WA. Judgment and decision under uncertainty. In: Michon JA, Eijkman EG, de Klerk LFW (eds). Handbook of psychonomics. Vol II. North Holland, Amsterdam 1979.
33. Hendrickx L, Vlek Ch, Oppewal H. Relative importance of scenario information and frequency information in the judgment of risk. Acta Psychol 1989;72:41-63.
34. Howell WC, Burnett SA. Uncertainty measurement: A cognitive taxonomy. Organizational Behavior and Human Performance 1978;22:45-68.
35. Kahneman D, Tversky A. Variants of uncertainty. Cognition 1982;11:143-57.
36. Merkhofer MW. Decision science and social risk management. Reidel, Boston/ Dordrecht 1987.
37. Edwards W, Newman JR. Multi-attribute evaluation. Sage, Baverly Hills (CA) 1982.
38. Von Winterfeldt D, Edwards W. Decision analysis and behavioral research. Cambridge University Press, New York/Cambridge (UK) 1986.
39. Yoon KP, Hwang C-L. Multiple attribute decision making; an introduction. Sage Publications Series, London/New Delhi 1995;7:104.
40. Fischhoff B. Setting standards: A systematic approach to managing public health and safety risks. Management Science 1984;30:823-43.
41. ICRP. Recommendations of the International Commission on Radiological Protection. Pergamon, Oxford. Annals of the ICRP 1 1977;26.
42. Vlek CAJ. A multi-level, multi-stage and multi-attribute perspective on risk assessment, decision-making and risk control. Risk, Decision and Policy 1996;1(in press).
43. Covello VT, von Winterfeldt D, Slovic P. Risk communication: A review of the literature. Risk Abstracts 1986;3:171-82.
44. Wiedemann P, Rohrmann, Jungermann H. Das Forschungsgebiet 'Risiko-Kommunikation'. In: Jungermann H, Rohrmann B, Wiedemann P (eds). Risiko-Konzepte,

Risiko-Konflikte, Risiko-Kommunikation. Monographien des Forschungszentrums Jülich, Programmagruppe Mensch, Umwelt, Techniek, 1990;Band 3.
45. Cvetkovich G, Vlek Ch, Earle TC. Designing technological hazard information programs: Towards a model of risk-adaptive decision making. In: Vlek Ch, Cvetkovich (eds). Social decision methodology for technological projects. Kluwer Academic Press, Dordrecht/Boston 1989.
46. Stern PC. Learning through conflict: A realistic strategy for risk communication. Policy Sciences 1991;24:99-119.
47. Los APM, Achterhof L, Tijmstra TJ, Suurmeyer TPBM, Smit Sibinga CTh. Informing blood donors about AIDS and risk factors: Reactions to information provided in a regional blood bank in The Netherlands. AIDS 1989;3:439-41.
48. Menitove JE. Perception of risk. In: Nance ST (ed). Blood supply: Risks, perceptions and prospects for the future. American Association of Blood Banks, Bethesda, MD 1994:45-59.
49. Smit Sibinga CTh, Das PC, Heiniger HJ (eds). Good manufacturing practice in transfusion medicine. Kluwer Academic Press. Dordrecht/Boston 1994.

SURGICAL CRITERIA FOR BLOOD TRANSFUSION: HOW FAR SHOULD WE GO?

H.J. ten Duis

In surgery and traumatology, blood loss is and always will be unavoidable. Despite the use of surgical and anaesthesiolocal blood saving techniques, such as isovolaemic haemodilution, preoperative donation and intraoperative blood salvage, the availability of sufficient quantities of high quality donor blood remains a primary condition for the performance of modern surgery. Obviously, the demand for donor blood strongly depends on the type of patients being treated, the type of operation performed, the skill of the surgeon, but above all on the transfusion trigger level, which is defined as the haematocrit or haemoglobin value, at which it is decided to transfuse a patient with red cells. It is the doctor's decision whether or not to transfuse a patient and the policy followed elucidates indirectly his or her knowledge about modern transfusion medicine and should reflect the awareness of balancing the pros and cons of a tissue transplantation, which a blood transfusion is.

In contemporary clinical practise, the rationale for replacing blood loss is not always clear and any written indications for transfusion are often ill-defined. Blood is frequently requested and transfused in arbitrary quantities to achieve undefined clinical or physiological outcomes, such as improving the colour of the patient. This is a description of red cell transfusion practise at the majority of surgical clinics in Western Europe in 1995. If we realize that the situation is far from optimal and admit that decision-making is still often rather speculative, then the consequence is that we should wonder what the progress is we have made about the indications for red cell transfusion since Landsteiner discovered the ABO blood group system in 1900? It is of major interest to study the indications used in the first half of this century to decide whether to compensate for blood loss in a given patient.

In 1921 [1] the indications for blood transfusion in surgical patients were described as follows (Figure 1a):

- all severe post-haemorrhage anaemias whether or not accompanied by shock
- certain cases of shock and
- all kinds of untamed bleeding.

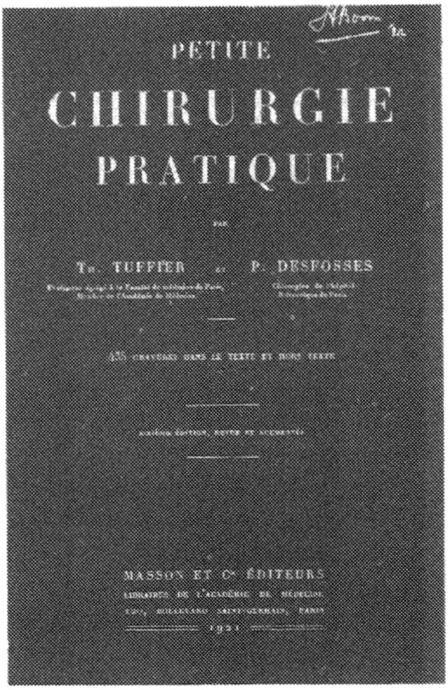

PETITE

CHIRURGIE

PRATIQUE

TH. TUFFIER et P. DESFOSSES

MASSON ET Cie ÉDITEURS

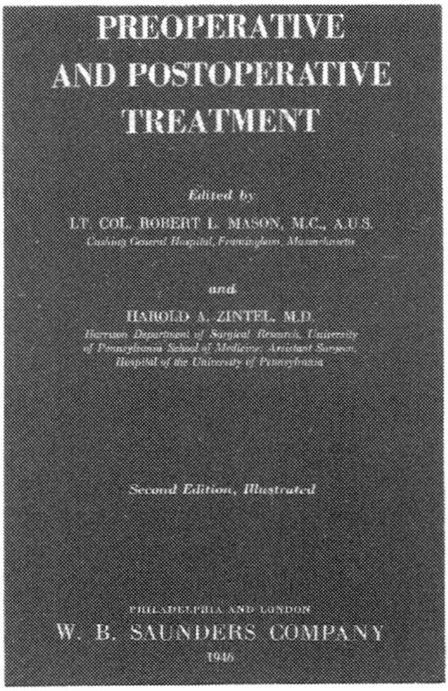

PREOPERATIVE

AND POSTOPERATIVE

TREATMENT

Edited by

LT. COL. ROBERT L. MASON, M.C., A.U.S.

Cushing General Hospital, Framingham, Massachusetts

and

HAROLD A. ZINTEL, M.D.

Second Edition, Illustrated

PHILADELPHIA AND LONDON

W. B. SAUNDERS COMPANY

1946

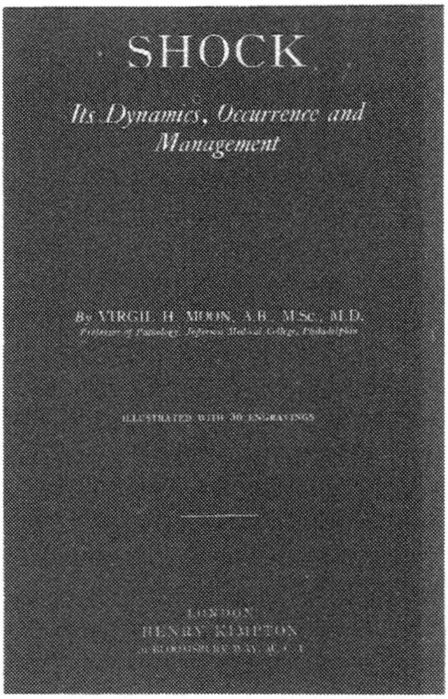

SHOCK

Its Dynamics, Occurrence and Management

By VIRGIL H. MOON, A.B., M.Sc., M.D.

ILLUSTRATED WITH 30 ENGRAVINGS

LONDON

HENRY KIMPTON

Figure 1. Title pages of the respective publications about indications for blood transfusion.

Most remarkably, the authors don't mention a word about the severity of the blood loss or the extent of the anaemia.

Even in 1946, 25 years later, the indications for blood transfusions in surgical patients were still ill-defined.

In: "Preoperative and postoperative treatment" by Mason and Zintel [2], the indications for blood transfusion included (Figure 1b):

- shock;
- hypoprothrombinaemia;
- hypoproteinaemia;
- intestinal obstruction; and
- blood dyscrasia.

Again no hard and sharp criteria were given and the authors were very vague about the transfusion indications.

The following sentence in "Shock, its dynamics, occurrence and management" (Figure 1c) by Virgil Moon also published in 1946 explains [3]: ".... infusions of plasma or serum are highly effective in restoring the blood volume and plasma proteins after severe haemorrhages and transfusions of whole blood are needed only when the haemoglobin content and erythrocytes are below 40 or 50% of the normal". Converted into haemoglobin levels, this means a haemoglobin level of 6 to 8 gm/dl or a haematocrit value of between 20 and 25%. It demonstrates the very restrictive policy that clinicians were following in those days.

What is the present clinical situation?

Numerous, recently held, consensus meetings on red cell transfusions have failed to indicate a trigger haemoglobin level at which a blood transfusion should be given to surgical patients. Nevertheless, the only generally accepted and objective indices available which influence the decision to transfuse are the haemoglobin level and haematocrit value. Indicators of the need for transfusion, such as mixed venous oxygen saturation and tissue oxygen concentration, might be determined in intensive care patients, but it is not always feasible to perform these tests on every surgical patient who undergoes an operation.

This brings us to the central theme: surgical criteria for blood transfusion, how far should we go? Unfortunately, a uniform answer cannot be given. In an attempt to answer this question, it is easier to explain what we are not aiming at. We can easily identify the undesirerable extremes, haemoglobin levels which we will never accept in our patients, lower as well as upper levels. We all recognize the emotional feelings when we see the pink coloured liquid drawn from the veins of a Jehovah's Witness, who is being resuscitated with cristalloids and artificial colloids or recognise the anger of being confronted with a surgical patient who has been transfused to a haemoglobin level, equally high or even higher than the preoperative value.

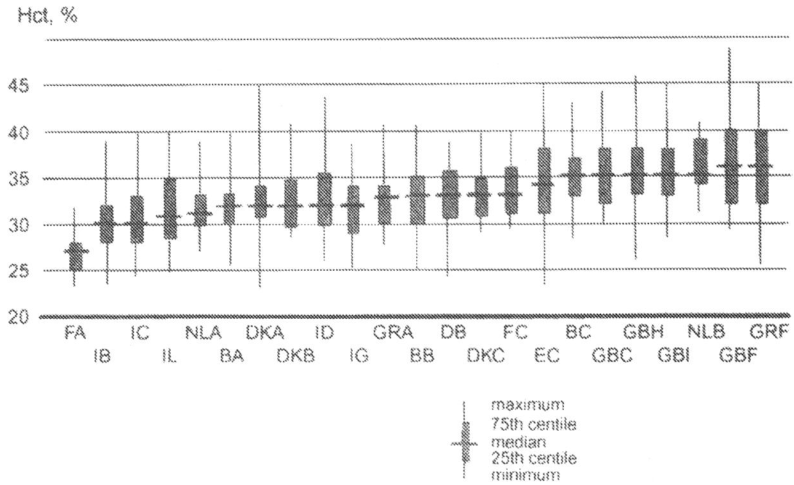

Figure 2. Last recorded Hct values in patients who underwent total hip replacement (THR). From SANGUIS publication EUR 15398 EN, ISBN 92-826-4118-X.

Many studies on young trauma patients and Jehovah's Witnesses have shown that major blood loss is well-tolerated. In various articles, although often casuistic presentations, the survival of patients with extremely low haemoglobin levels is mentioned [4-7]. In exceptional cases haemoglobin levels of 1 gm/dl are reported. It is clear that these patients will have to pay the price of undertransfusion. If they survive, the lack of all essential blood components will result in severe pathophysiological disturbances, including clotting disorders, decubitus of the skin and vocal cords, ischaemia of the liver, ischaemia of the heart, eventually resulting in prolonged ventilation times, prolonged intensive care periods and numerous other complications. It is clear that no doctor in his or her right mind is out to aim this situation.

On the other hand, there are still clinicians who transfuse surgical patients towards haemoglobin levels comparable to or even higher than preoperative values. Neither the oxygen transport capacity, nor the erythrocyte rheology justify the maintenance of such high haemoglobin levels. Under these circumstances, being exposed to one or more units of donor blood, means that the patient "benefits" fully from the disadvantages of blood transfusion.

So, as can be expected, the trigger haemoglobin level for surgical patients will lie somewhere between these extremes.

The physical and physiological responses to a decrease in circulating haemoglobin include an increase in the cardiac output and the haemoglobin oxygen extraction rate, as well as improvement of the rheological properties of the blood. Today the majority of transfusionists and clinicians agree that if the blood viscosity decreases and cardiac output increases along the path of haemodilution, and an optimal oxygen transport capacity is reached at haemoglobin levels of about 10 gm/dl, there is seldom an indication to transfuse red cells in patients with a haematocrit of over 30%. Recent major studies in Europe as well as the United States have shown that nowadays a haematocrit level of around 30% to 33%, as an upper transfusion level, is generally accepted, even in the elderly. The SANGUIS Study, presented in 1992, gives numerous examples [8]. Figure 2 shows the haemoglobin levels at discharge of patients who underwent a total hip replacement at 23 European hospitals. These are all elderly patients with a mean age of 66 years. As can be observed, most hospitals discharged their patients at haematocrit values of 30-35%. At 8 of these 23 hospitals, patients could be identified with a haemoglobin level of less than 25% at discharge. The fall in haematocrit in patients not transfused with red cells is presented in Figure 3. In some hospitals a fall in haematocrit of 10% is accepted.

We often have the feeling that even a trigger haemoglobin level of 10 gm/dl or a haematocrit level of 30% is much too high. The body's compensatory mechanisms to blood loss are tremendous, especially in young patients, and are usually sufficient to clinically accept haemoglobin levels of between 6 and 8 gm/dl for longer periods without being confronted with any signs or symptoms related to

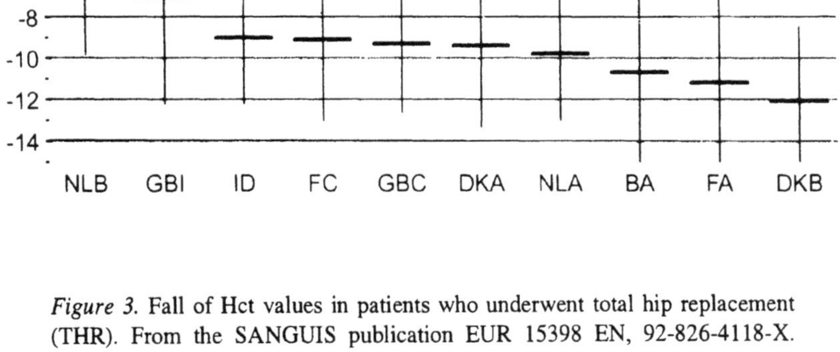

Figure 3. Fall of Hct values in patients who underwent total hip replacement (THR). From the SANGUIS publication EUR 15398 EN, 92-826-4118-X.

undertransfusion. In previous presentations, the results of trauma patients who underwent open reduction and internal stabilisation of fractures of the spinal column were shown. These physically healthy patients were aged between about 20 and 40 years. The surgical procedure was accompanied by an average blood loss of about one and a half to two litres, and was performed under controlled conditions of blood loss, infusion of cristalloids and artificial colloids. During the operation and in the postoperative period a haemoglobin levels of 8 gm/dl was accepted (Figure 4). The absence of any cardiovascular and/or pulmonary complications indicated that even under the circumstances of significant blood loss and without the use of intraoperative blood salvage or preoperative haemodilution, it is safe to perform major operations on young and middle aged patients without using donor blood transfusions. This illustrated that we have developed a very restrictive policy of indications for red cell transfusions. We can even go a step further in our attempts to minimize the use of blood products in surgical patients. If we are performing good surveyable operations and we are dealing with young healthy patients, we can easily accept haemoglobin values of 6 gm/dl without becoming nervous. Admittedly they may look very pale, but that per se is no reason to transfuse.

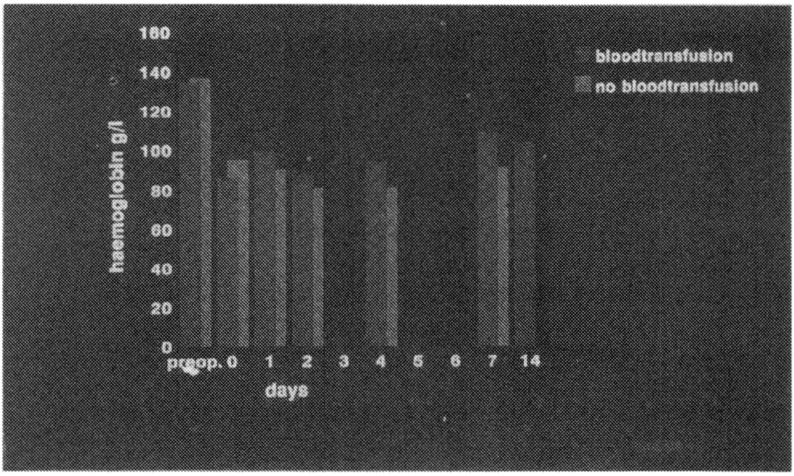

Figure 4. Haemoglobin values in patients with instable fractures of the spinal column. Pre- and postoperative values.

How do we monitor the perioperative blood loss and circulatory state of the patient in practise?

It is obvious that we determine the amount of blood loss by measuring the amount of aspirated blood and by weighing all the gauzes. However, this is a rather inaccurate measurement. When the patient is under general anaesthesia and the operation is in progress, relatively simple physiological parameters are used to detect symptoms of undertransfusion: blood pressure, heart rate and paleness. What we don't do, is draw blood samples every ten minutes to measure the haemoglobin level, but we will clinically follow the patients reaction to blood loss. This means for example that if a patient shows a compensatory increase in heart rate of more than 15-20 beats per minute induced by bloodloss and we are sure that the patient is normovolaemic and not in pain, we will determine his haemoglobin or haematocrit level. This implies along that in one patient we will measure a haemoglobin level of as low as 4 gm/dl and in another a haemoglobin level of 8 gm/dl before we decide to transfuse. In general, the young surgical patient seldom forms a problem in terms of transfusion policy.

In contrast, we all except to be confronted with problems if we withhold red cell transfusion from elderly patients. Everyone will agree that a decreased oxygen transport capacity forms a potential risk in elderly patients, because their cardiovascular and pulmonary reserves may be limited. Here lies the threatened risk of undertransfusion. However, signs related to undertransfusion seldom become evident under conditions of general anaesthesia or in the recovery room where oxygen delivery to the patient is guaranteed and the circulation is fully supported. Only in exceptional cases are we confronted with a preoperative or direct postoperative problem related to a lack of oxygen transport capacity. Undertransfusion becomes evident by signs of ischaemia on the ECG or the development or aggravation of arrhythmia which, if necessary can be corrected by the immediate infusion of red cells. That is the reason why we always have available at least one unit of red cells for these patients. Most problems related to undertransfusion manifest themselves on the hospital ward. A lack of oxygen transport capacity becomes evident when mobilisation therapy is started. These patients may complain of dizziness or show signs of extreme weariness. If these symptoms prevent the rehabilitation of the patient, one should consider adjustment of the haemoglobin content.

Other symptoms related to undertransfusion include swelling and oedema in the operated area. A shortage of colloid osmotic pressure may result in wound healing disturbances and even infection. These complications may indicate the transfusion of a plasma product.

If we consider transfusing a blood product to an elderly patient, we must realize that by withholding a blood product, the risk of undertransfusion must equal the risk related to the transfusion of that product, like for example, viral infections. In this respect, we should realize that transfusion-related hazards are of less importance in the elderly than in children and young adults, because many elderly patients will not have the opportunity to become ill if a transfusion-related disease has a long latency period.

To illustrate the transfusion policy followed in the elderly, some retrospectively obtained transfusion data on 100 patients who were operated on between 1991 and 1995 are presented. All the patients were injured and had broken their hip. They were treated by removal of the femoral head and hemiarthroplasty. The male/female ratio was 24/76 and their mean age was 81.3 years.

The 100 patients were divided into 4 groups according to the lowest accepted haemoglobin level in the period from the start of the operation to one week after the operation. Four levels of postoperative haemoglobin value were distinguished:

- group 1 > 12 gm/dl
- group 2 10 - 12 gm/dl
- group 3 8 - 10 gm/dl
- group 4 < 8 gm/dl

To compare these groups, it was necessary to know whether the patients were otherwise comparable. Elderly people are known to have limited cardiopulmonary reserves and the incidence of accompanying cardiopulmonary disease is high. Obviously, these are reasons for clinicians to transfuse the elderly at an earlier stage than they would in young surgical patients. We also needed to know the physical condition of the patients in the separate groups. Therefore their age as well as their ASA scores[1] were compared. The score grades the gravity of an illness. Score 1 means healthy, 2 means accompanying disease under control, like regulated hypertension, 3 means accompanying disease, not regulated and 4 means dangerously or terminally ill.

The four groups were compared in terms of age, ASA score, mortality rate, complication rate, duration of hospitalization and number of red cell transfusions. Table 1 shows data about age and patient numbers.

Table 1.

	n	**mean age (years)**
Group 1: Hb >12	14	79.4
Group 2: Hb 10-12	44	82.7
Group 3: Hb 8-10	38	81.2
Group 4: Hb <8	4	79.0

About half of the patients were discharged home with a haemoglobin level of less than 10 gm/dl.

1. The ASA score stands for the American Society of Anaesthesiologists.

How did the patients reach their postoperative haemoglobin level?

In group 1 (haemoglobin > 12 gm/dl) (Table 2) the preoperative haemoglobin value was 14.3 gm/dl and it decreased to 12.6 gm/dl in the postoperative period. 86% of these patients did not receive a blood transfusion. Per patient operated, not per patient transfused, the quantity of red cells given was 128 ml.

Table 2.

	pre/post Hb (gm/dl)	ml tr red cells per oper pat	% not tr pat
Group 1: Hb >12	14.3-12.6	128	86%
Group 2: Hb 10-12	13.2-10.9	157	81%
Group 3: Hb 8-10	12.3- 8.8	100	78%
Group 4: Hb <8	12.5- 7.6	300	50%

The haemoglobin level of the patients who had a postoperative level of between 10 and 12 had a preoperative maximum of 13.2 and dropped to a minimum of 10.9 in the postoperative period. 18% of them received a red cell transfusion, while 82% did not. Calculated for the entire group of transfused and not transfused patients, the average quantity of red cells administered was 157 ml.

In the group that ended with a haemoglobin level of between 8 and 10, group 3, the operation could be performed without a transfusion in 78% of the patients, with an average transfusion quantity of 100 ml per operated patient. In group 4, 50% of the patients were discharged home without being transfused with red cells. Calculated per patient operated, they received 300 ml of red cells.

Were these patient groups comparable in terms of accompanying disease?

In Table 3 the comparison of the ASA scores, complication rate and duration of hospitalisation is given. There was no in-hospital mortality.

Table 3.

	ASA	IC	Hospitalization
Group 1	2.14	0	19 days
Group 2	2.5	2	16 days
Group 3	2.83	10	23 days
Group 4	2.0	0	19 days

These data show that the patients in group 3 had the poorest preoperative condition; 10 out of the 38 were treated for a short interval in the intensive care unit and had an accepted low haemoglobin level of between 8 and 10 gm/dl. It is not clear whether there is a relation between the low haemoglobin level and admission to intensive care. The intensive care period was probably related to the severity of the cardiovascular condition of these patients. The mean length of hospitalization seemed to be related to the number of patients treated in the intensive care unit, rather than to the low haemoglobin level, as evidenced by group 4 who had no intensive care admissions and a relatively short hospital stay.

Conclusion

What we can learn from the past, from the recently held consensus meetings and the presented data, is that we should not aim for a lowest possible trigger haemoglobin level. It does not exist. Clinicians should follow the physiological reaction to blood loss in a given patient. If this reaction is considered or expected to be harmful for the patient, then red cells should be given. Red cells should be transfused in the smallest quantity, necessary to balance the pathophysiological reactions observed.

References

1. Tuffier Th, Defosses P. Petite Chirurgie Pratique. Masson et cie, editeurs. Paris, 1921:350.
2. Mason RL, Zintel HA. Preoperative and postoperative treatment. W.B. Saunders, Philadelphia, London 1946:157-59.
3. Moon VH. Shock. Henri Kimpton, London 1946:275.
4. Howell PJ, Bamber PA. Severe acute anaemia in Jehovah's witness. Anaesthesia 1987;42:44-48.
5. Brimacombe J, Skipper P, Talbutt P. Acute anaemia to a haemoglobin of 14 g/l with survival. Anaesthesia and Intensive Care 1991;19:581-83.
6. Law EJ, Still JM, Gattis CS. The use of erythropoietin in two burned patients who are Jehovah's witnesses. Burns 1991;17:75-77.
7. Ott DA. Cardiovascular surgery in Jehovah's witnesses. JAMA 1977;238:1256-58.
8. Sirchia G, Giovanetti AM, McClelland B, Fracchia GN. Safe and good use of blood in surgery, SANGUIS. Bruxelles, Luxembourg, 1994. Eur 15398 EN. ISBN 92-826-4118-X.

TRANSFUSION POLICIES AND CLINICAL PRACTICE IN A TERTIARY ACADEMIC MEDICAL CENTER: ROLE OF PROTOCOLS AND DOCUMENTATION

M. Petrides, E.L. Snyder

Introduction

In the last five years several consensus guidelines for blood product usage have appeared in the literature [1-13]. The guidelines can be used to form the framework from which individual institutions can design criteria for the appropriate use of blood and blood components, while taking into account the preferences of physicians at the institution. Some aspects of these guidelines are generally accepted by most physicians. Reflecting the ever-evolving nature of transfusion practice, however, some of the guidelines which are more controversial are less widely accepted. Establishing a set of audit criteria for blood component usage should be considered as just the first step in improving the quality of care. To be truly effective, audits must be accompanied by feedback to the clinicians. Audits and guidelines should also reflect continued awareness of the changes taking place in clinical transfusion practice. We will discuss some of these published guidelines, playing particular attention to the portions which are either controversial or currently in evolution. Additionally, we will focus on the approach taken by our tertiary academic medical center and some of our experiences with audits and our attempts to control blood product utilization.

Consensus guidelines for blood product usage

Red Blood Cells

There is general consensus that red blood cell (RBC) components are indicated only when there is a need to improve oxygen carrying capacity. RBCs should not be used for other purposes such as providing a source of colloid osmotic pressure, substituting for administration of haematinics such as iron or vitamin B_{12} for improving wound healing or enhancing a patient's subjective sense of well-being. Despite general agreement on these principles, however, the definition of a trigger point for transfusion of RBCs remains elusive.

For years, based upon experience with combat causalities in otherwise healthy soldiers, a haemoglobin level of 10 gm/dl was generally regarded as an acceptable trigger for red cell transfusion [4]. However, the 1988 NIH Consensus Conference on use of Red Cells, failed to find good evidence to support the "10/30" rule (10 gm/dl of haemoglobin or a haematocrit of 30%). The NIH panel noted experimental data which showed that in healthy humans, cardiac output did not increase dramatically until the haemoglobin fell below 7 gm/dl [1]. Both the NIH Consensus Conference guideline and guidelines published by the American College of Physicians (ACP), stressed that red cell transfusion should be based on clinical assessment of the individual patient and his/her response to the level of anaemia present [1-3]. Thus, duration of anaemia is an important variable to consider. Chronically anaemic patients, such as those with sickle cell anaemia, are more likely to tolerate lower levels of haemoglobin without significant symptoms than are patients who have not compensated to an underlying chronic anaemia. On the other hand, in the presence of coexistent illness such as coronary artery disease, congestive heart failure, COPD, cerebral and/or peripheral vascular disease, transfusion of red cells might be necessary at much higher levels of haemoglobin than would be needed in otherwise healthy young persons. Finally, the ACP stressed that in the acutely anaemic patient, one should attempt, whenever possible, to relieve symptoms by correcting intravascular volume depletion with crystalloid infusion before using red cells.

Most physicians would likely agree on several points: that transfusion to a haemoglobin level above 10 gm/dl is rarely indicated; that symptomatic anaemia unresponsive to other measures, such as volume repletion, necessitates red cell transfusion, especially in the setting of underlying cardio/pulmonary/vascular disease; and that even healthy patients may require transfusion if their haemoglobin falls much below 7 gm/dl. It is the range between 7 gm/dl and 10 gm/dl of haemoglobin which remains a gray zone, particularly in the perioperative period, which is when the majority (approximately two thirds) of red cell transfusion takes place [1]. However, while the acceptable range of haemoglobin for transfusion criteria in the asymptomatic patient will vary from institution to institution, one should attempt to reduce the size of this gray zone within an institution as much as possible. This strategy should decrease areas of confusion and controversy. For example, more progressive Hospital A may define 6.5 gm/dl as an acceptable haemoglobin below which red cell transfusions are not subject to audit and a level of 8.0 gm/dl as a level above which transfusion without other clinical indication is subject to review. Conservative Hospital B, however, may use levels of 7.0 gm/dl and 9.2 gm/dl, respectively, for the same purposes. To improve transfusion practices at Hospital B, one can resort to lobbying the hospital medical staff with data and educational programmes, or by having the medical board impose a stricter guideline by fiat. Clearly, the former approach is more collegial and far more preferable. Once a trigger is set, even if it believed to be too liberal, efforts at improving the quality of the transfusion guideline can begin. The first step, however, is in defining a set of criteria for transfusion.

Fresh Frozen Plasma

Most consensus documents agree that FFP is indicated to correct deficiency of coagulation proteins for which no specific factor concentrates are available [5-7, 10]. Whenever possible, however, alternative therapies should be tried first [8]. Such manoeuvres include use of vitamin K for reversal of coumarin effect or infusion of desmopressin (DDAVP) for treatment of von Willebrand's disease. If FFP is to be given, an adequate amount should be administered and transfusion should be timed to achieve the desired effect. For example, if correction of a markedly prolonged PT or PTT is desired prior to a surgical procedure, FFP should be given just prior to surgery, not the night before. Because the half-life of several coagulation proteins, notably factor VII, is in the range of eight hours, giving FFP too early, such as the night before surgery, will allow the levels of these factors to markedly decay before surgery. At Yale - New Haven Hospital, depending on the dose needed, we recommend that FFP be started 2-3 hours before surgery and that the infusion be continued intraoperatively to maximize the efficacy of the FFP infused. Therapy should be monitored with screening or specific coagulation assays.

Published triggers for use of FFP revolve around a PT and/or PTT value of greater than 1.5 times the midpoint of the reference range on patients who are either actively bleeding or scheduled for surgery or invasive procedures [5,6]. Justification for this trigger arises from early studies, albeit with small sample sizes, dating back to the 1950s and 1960s, which showed that certain types of surgical procedures could be safely performed on patients taking coumarin with a PT in the therapeutic range [14]. Other studies, however, call into question the utility of in vitro clotting times such as PT and PTT for predicting haemorrhage following liver biopsy [15]. Burns et al. provide a possible explanation for the lack of correlation between bleeding and mild to moderate elevation in PT/PTT. In their 1992 study, they noted that mixtures of factor-deficient plasma paradoxically showed a PT and PTT more prolonged than one would have expected based on the actual factor levels measured [16].

The figure of 1.5 times normal is consistent with a study which demonstrated no increased bleeding following paracentesis and thoracentesis in patients with a PT or PTT up to 1.5 to 2 times the midpoint normal range [17]. Another study also found the PT and PTT to be good predictors of bleeding in massively transfused trauma patients but only when the PT and PTT were greater than or equal to 1.5 times the control value [18].

Beyond the correction of markedly prolonged PT and/or PTT in bleeding patients or in patients scheduled for surgery or invasive procedures, other generally accepted indications for FFP include emergent reversal of warfarin therapy; massive transfusion in patients with a dilutional coagulopathy; replacement of antithrombin III, protein C or protein S; and treatment of thrombotic thrombocytopenic purpura, usually in conjunction with plasma exchange [5-7, 12]. It can reasonably be said that a well accepted indication for use of FFP should be chosen and documented in the chart. Indiscriminant use of FFP is likely to lead to legal liability. Transfusion of FFP to a patient purely for volume expansion or a source of protein may, in some areas, be considered to border on the edge of unacceptable medical practice.

Cryoprecipitate

There is a little controversy regarding the use of cryoprecipitate. "Cryo" is generally indicated for correction of hypofibrinogenaemia, usually defined as fibrinogen < 80-100 mg/dl, and for replacement of von Willebrand's factor in patients unresponsive to desmopressin (DDAVP) [5, 6, 12]. Another increasingly common request for cryoprecipitate relates to its use for production of "fibrin glue". The use of cryoprecipitate has sparked civilian as well as military interest. Indeed, a recent symposium was held on this topic sponsored by the United States military. Ironically, many clinicians fail to realize that 5 bags of cryoprecipitate for use as "glue" also provides 5 donor exposures to a recipient who may have donated autologous red cells for his/her surgery which was highlighted by use of intraoperative blood salvage. Hence, auditing the use of cryoprecipitate is very appropriate in today's clinical/legal environment. This is especially true in light of the number of donor exposures associated with ordered "doses" of cryoprecipitate of 20 units or more.

Platelets

A widely quoted trigger for prophylactic platelet transfusion is a platelet count of 20.000/μL trigger, which is often traced back to a paper from 1962 by Gaydos et al. in which gross haemorrhage (haematuria, melena or haematemesis) was noted to occur rarely in patients with platelet counts above an arbitrarily selected level of 20,000/μL [19]. Although this paper is frequently cited in support of the 20,000/μL trigger, the authors themselves specifically and repeatedly state that, while it would be desirable to find a threshold platelet count above which haemorrhage is unlikely to occur, in their study "no 'threshold' platelet level was observed." [19]. Furthermore, the data in the Gaydos study was generated at a time when aspirin was widely used and when the effects of ASA on platelet function were not recognized. These data, therefore, may be of limited applicability today [20, 21].

Today there is increased awareness of the risks of transfusion-transmitted diseases as well as concern that prophylactic platelet use may result in platelet refractoriness which could potentially result in poor platelet increments [22]. This has resulted in reevaluation of the 20,000/μL trigger. In 1991, Gmur et al. studied 102 consecutive patients with acute leukaemia and concluded that, in the absence of fever or bleeding, a trigger platelet count of 5,000/μL can safely be employed. In the presence of fever or bleeding, they found that a platelet count of 10,000/μL was sufficient. For patients with concomitant disorders of the coagulation cascade, including those on heparin, and patients with anatomical lesions, a trigger of 20,000/μL was considered justified [21].

Some published guidelines reflect the higher threshold derived from the Gaydos paper, listing platelet counts of 10 to 20,000/μL as appropriate prophylactic triggers [5], whereas other consensus guidelines list 5,000/μL as a threshold for strictly prophylactic use and levels of between 5,000 and 30,000/μL for prophylaxis in patients with significant bleeding risks, including those with headache, GI blood loss, petecchiae or continuous bleeding from a wound or other site [6, 20]. For patients undergoing surgery or invasive procedures as well as those with DIC with diffuse microvascular bleeding, a trigger of 50,000/μL may be appropriate [5]. Neurosurgery or ophthalmologic surgery may require platelet counts of 100,000/μL [6] because the consequences of bleeding into closed spaces such as the eye or brain can be so devastating. Likewise, bleeding in the setting of cardiopulmonary bypass with normal coagulation values justifies a platelet trigger of 100,000/μL to some experts [6]. This relates to the consensus opinion that bleeding in a patients with a qualitative platelet defect, whether congenital, acquired or iatrogenic, merits platelet transfusion, regardless of the platelet count [5, 6].

Granulocytes

The use of granulocyte transfusions in severely neutropenic patients is regarded as controversial by some physicians. Others believe, however, that granulocytes can be beneficial when used in an appropriate setting. These include patients with bacterial sepsis unresponsive to appropriate combination antibiotic therapy and patients with persistent, severe neutropenia associated with continuing bone marrow failure [23-25]. Strauss et al. [23, 24] reviewed the literature on granulocyte transfusion, focusing particularly on seven controlled studies. Three of these seven studies showed overall benefit from granulocyte transfusion in infected, neutropenic patients, while another two demonstrated benefit in certain subgroups only. One of these, the first controlled study on granulocyte transfusion, indicated that transfused PMNs are likely to benefit patients with persistently severe neutropenia but not those with resolving marrow function [23, 24]. Most acute leukaemics who develop bacterial sepsis following induction chemotherapy show bone marrow recovery in the early days of sepsis and respond to antibiotic therapy alone with little additional benefit derived from granulocyte transfusion. On the other hand, septic bone marrow transplant patients, whose marrow may take three weeks to recover, may benefit from granulocyte transfusion coupled with aggressive antibiotic therapy [24]. Granulocyte transfusion may also be beneficial in neonates with fulminant bacterial sepsis [9, 23], in life-threatening fungal or yeast infections in patients with chronic granulomatous disease [23], and in severely neutropenic patients with disseminated fungal or yeast infections. It should be noted, however, that the efficacy of granulocyte transfusion in yeast and fungal infections is insufficient to reach a definitive conclusion at this time [24].

Consensus indications for granulocyte transfusions include: bacterial infections unresponsive to appropriate antibiotic therapy in patients with absolute neutrophil counts < 500/μL, and bacterial or progressive fungal infection in patients with neutrophil dysfunction [5, 9, 23, 24].

The quality and quantity of transfused PMNs is an important factor and may account for the lack of efficacy seen in early studies of granulocyte transfusion. Current clinical recommendations are for a minimum of 2 to 3×10^{10} PMNs per dose. HLA-matched or leukocyte crossmatch-compatible units are preferred, at least on theoretical ground, but a definite benefit has yet to be established [23, 24]. Once begun, granulocyte transfusion should be continued on a daily basis until either the infection resolves or the absolute neutrophil count (ANC) remains above 500/μL for 48 hours [9].

An area of emerging interest is the use of recombinant growth factors (G-CSF and GM-CSF) in accelerating recovery following chemotherapy and also in improving granulocyte yield from healthy donors, which appears very promising at this time with reported yields as high as to 14.4×10^{10} granulocytes per collection [24, 26]. The long term effects of recombinant growth factors on healthy donors remains to be studied, as does the properties of the granulocytes collected by this technique. It is possible that larger doses of HLA matched granulocytes will provide a greater clinical benefit than does the current PMN transfusion product which only requires 1 x 10^{10}/bag [27]. Due to the cost and difficulty in obtaining apheresis donors of granulocytes for transfusion, it is prudent to audit requests for this product. At Yale - New Haven Hospital requests for granulocytes must be audited and approved by the blood bank before a donor is recruited.

Special Products

CMV-safe Cellular Blood Products

CMV is a DNA virus of the Herpesvirus family. It is ubiquitous in nature, with prevalence estimates varying regionally from a low of 20% to a high of 80% or higher [28-30]. These estimates are based primarily on sero-positivity rates for CMV antibody which may actually underestimate the true exposure rate. CMV, an intracellular pathogen, can be transmitted in the latent, non-infectious state in cellular blood products, presumably via carriage in leukocytes [29, 30]. The term "CMV-safe" has been used to describe both CMV-seronegative cellular blood components and cellular blood products that have been filtered through a third-generation leukoreduction filter. Currently, there is not yet universal agreement concerning the equivalence of these two methods.

While CMV-seronegative cellular blood products remain the standard of care in many institutions, there have been numerous reports suggesting that leuko-depleted cellular components are comparable to seronegative units. In 1994, Hillyer et al. reviewed a number of studies comparing leukocyte filtration for CMV and concluded that 3 $\log_{10}$ leukocyte depletion is at least as effective as CMV-seronegative components for prevention of transfusion-transmitted CMV infection. Bowden et al. [31] showed that in bone marrow transplant recipients, the incidence of CMV infection was equivalent in a group receiving filter-leukoreduced blood components and in a group receiving CMV seronegative blood. Disturbingly, however, all the fatalities due to CMV disease occurred only in the filter arm. No explanation is readily apparent for why the filtered arm should have a rate of development of active disease that is so much higher than that seen in the CMV seronegative arm.

The sensitivity and specificity of CMV serotesting has been called into question by PCR data which revealed the presence of CMV viral genomic material in CMV seronegative individuals. In a study of 313 normal donors Zhang et al. found that 44% of CMV seronegative individuals had demonstrable CMV RNA, which may represent latent CMV infection in the leukocytes of these CMV-seronegative donors [32]. Theoretically removal of the leukocytes which harbour latent CMV infection should diminish the risk of transmission of the virus. In fact, Smith et al. [33] were able to demonstrate that leukoreduction filtration was successful in eliminating CMV DNA from blood samples from 5 donors previously shown to have CMV DNA demonstrable by PCR. While it is not yet definitively known whether CMV antibody-negative (seronegative) blood is capable of causing transfusion-transmitted CMV infection, these data would suggest that leukodepletion may, in fact, be preferable in reducing the risk of CMV infection.

While exposure to the virus determines whether one becomes infected by CMV, the recipient's immune status is a major determinant of whether or not the individual develops symptomatic CMV disease [30]. Thus, although most CMV infections in normal, immunocompetent hosts are asymptomatic, infection in neonatal, oncology or other immunocompromised patients can present significant problems [31]. Congenital CMV infection can be associated with deafness and neurological problems in the neonate. Preterm neonates infected after birth can present with respiratory depression, hepatosplenomegaly and lymphocytosis which is usually self-limited but which has been felt to have contributed to some deaths; full-term neonates appear to be at less risk [29]. Transplant patients, particularly bone marrow transplant recipients, are at risk not only from reactivation of latent infection (recipients seropositive prior to transplant) but also to newly acquired infection from a seropositive marrow or solid organ or from transfusion of seropositive cellular blood products [29, 30]. The majority of HIV infected patients are CMV seropositive. CMV infection in the setting of HIV can be associated with significant morbidity and mortality, including chorioretinitis, encephalitis and enteritis [29, 30].

There is general consensus about the need for CMV-safe product in seronegative pregnant women, low birth-weight seronegative neonates (<1100g) born of CMV-seronegative mothers, and in other seronegative immunocompromised populations. The latter includes seronegative recipients of allogeneic bone marrow and solid organ transplants and the rare seronegative patient with HIV infection [5]. Consensus has not been reached on the utility of CMV-safe cellular products in seropositive persons and in seronegative individuals receiving allografts from seropositive donors. In the latter case, where recipients are either already seropositive or are receiving seropositive organs, questions have been raised about the degree of likelihood and clinical effects of infection with a second strain of CMV [29, 30].

There remains significant controversy about some of the indications for CMV-safe blood components and, more importantly, the relative efficacy of leukodepletion versus seronegativity in the prevention of infection and infectious complications due to CMV. Other considerations on which consensus has not yet been reached include whether bedside filtration is as effective as laboratory prestorage leukodepletion. At Yale - New Haven Hospital all request for CMV negative blood products are audited and require Blood Bank approval. All CMV-safe blood is provided as CMV seronegative. If type compatible CMV sero-negative blood is unavailable and there is urgent need, leukoreduced blood components will be substituted. Thus, although consensus has not yet been reached, even the current level of agreement on the efficacy of leukoreduced blood products is sufficient to provide guidance for clinical transfusion practice.

Irradiated Blood Products

In immunocompromised patients, irradiation of cellular blood products prevents replication and engraftment of transfused donor lymphocytes and thus development of transfusion-associated graft-versus-host disease (GvHD) [34]. A dose of 2,500 rad (cGy) is generally utilized and there appears to be consensus that 2,500 cGy irradiation has no deleterious effect on red cells [34-36].

The use of 2500 rad (cGy) irradiation for blood products known to contain viable lymphocytes is generally considered indicated for transfusion of: bone marrow transplant recipients; neonates – especially following intrauterine transfusion; recipients of directed donations from family members; patients with Hodgkin's disease and those with congenital immune deficiency syndromes. Other less widely accepted indications for irradiation of blood products include: patients with leukaemia and non-Hodgkin's lymphoma and patients with solid tumors undergoing either chemotherapy and/or radiation therapy [5]. While GvHD is well known in solid organ transplantation, this had previously been felt to be caused by donor lymphocytes residing in the transplanted organ. An emerging concern, however, is transfusion-associated GvHD in solid organ transplant recipients. Recently, a fatal case of transfusion-associated acute GvHD was described in a cardiac transplant recipient in whom the post-transplant HLA type of the recipient's lymphocytes could only have come from one of several units of blood transfused either intraoperatively and postoperatively and not from the donor heart [37]. A factor which may play a role in the criteria a hospital will use to determine whether or not to irradiate blood is the availability of a blood irradiator in the blood bank. While convenience must not play a role in this decision, in those patient conditions for which there is a lack of consensus, convenience and financial constraints may tend in some institutions, to begin to play a role. All request for irradiated blood are audited at Yale - New Haven Hospital as a means of monitoring to ensure appropriate use.

Leukocyte-depleted Blood Products

In addition to the role of transfused white cells in transmission of CMV infection and in graft-versus-host disease, leukocytes present in cellular blood products have been implicated in febrile non-haemolytic transfusion reactions and in refractoriness to platelet transfusion due to HLA-alloimmunization [38].

Prevention of febrile Reactions

Most febrile reactions tend not to recur [39]. Also, febrile reactions can be due to a number of different causes. For patients with single febrile reactions, in the absence of concerns about platelet refractoriness, some clinicians thus feel that leukodepletion of subsequent units is not required. Although, leukocytedepletion by filtration eliminates the majority of febrile non-haemolytic transfusion reactions, these reactions are not totally eradicated. This is probably due in part to the generation of cytokines in stored blood products [40, 41].

Platelet Refractoriness

In patients who are already alloimmunized, there is no evidence that leukodepletion results in improved platelet increments. Therefore, some would advocate the prophylactic use of third-generation leukodepletion filters (>3 $\log_{10}$ reduction in white cells), for transfusions of cellular products to all patients in whom platelet refractoriness may become a problem, especially those undergoing treatment for haematologic/oncologic malignancies. Others regard the magnitude of the benefit to be derived from prophylactic leukodepletion in this setting to be controversial and expensive, citing small sample sizes and heterogeneity of patient population as problems with currently published reports. A United States multicenter randomized (TRAP) trial is currently underway to assess the impact of leukodepletion on platelet (HLA) refractoriness in acute leukaemia patients. Results are pending as of this writing.

Guidelines for Leukocyte Depletion

Despite an extensive number of meetings and a large number of published materials, there is surprisingly little real consensus that leukodepletion is required for almost any indication [42]. This lack of agreement includes use of leukoreduction filters for prevention of febrile non-haemolytic transfusion reactions and for preventing or delaying alloimmunization and resulting platelet refractoriness [43]. Curiously, there is consensus that leukocyte reduction is not effective in prevention of graft-versus-host disease and that it should not be used for this purpose [5]. Probably the main area of controversy with regard to leukocyte depletion, namely its efficacy on preventing CMV disease transmission, has been discussed above.

Implementation of guidelines

As one can see from the preceding discussion, arriving at a consensus for appropriate blood product usage, even at a single static point in time, is not a trivial task. In order for a set of guidelines to be effective, however, the majority of physicians at the institution must first agree on the appropriateness of the criteria involved. Many physicians believe fervently in what, from their perspective, may simply be described as "not fixing what ain't broke." This clinical inertia and lack of willingness to change can be a major impediment to improving physician blood product ordering practices. Indeed, it took a global catastrophe of the proportion of the AIDS epidemic to even draw physician attention to the issue of blood product utilization.

An effective way to change transfusion ordering practices is by firmly implementing guidelines. To attain general agreement, these guidelines must be developed by representatives of the various services which use blood products in their daily clinical practice. At our institution, as at many others, this is accomplished via the Transfusion Committee which is comprised of representatives from blood bank, medicine, surgery, paediatrics, haematology/oncology, anaesthesiology, nursing, legal/risk management, quality assurance, neurology, cardiothoracic surgery, and plastic surgery. The committee meets formally on a quarterly basis and, after reviewing the indications for each product and discussing current controversies, the committee establishes a set of guidelines which are then subject to periodic review and revision.

In any set of guidelines, provision must be made to allow deviation from published criteria based on exigencies of a particular patient's clinical condition. The Blood Bank Director has a major role to play in any such discussion. He or she is usually the ultimate arbiter of transfusion practice and frequently the individual held responsible for establishing good transfusion practices in the institution and held accountable if something goes wrong with the system.

Auditing for compliance

Once a set of guidelines is established the real work of auditing to insure adherence to the criteria can proceed. There are a variety of approaches to this problem but they fall into three broad categories: prospective, concurrent and retrospective audit [5, 12].

Prospective Audit

In prospective review, clinicians are asked to specify the indication(s) at the time blood products are ordered. Product requests which do not meet the criteria set forth in the institution's guidelines are audited prior to product release and product is issued only if the request is deemed appropriate by the blood bank physician. This approach has many advantages not the least of which is the opportunity to interact with and educate clinical staff about risks of which they may not be aware. For example, while most clinicians are aware of the risk of transfusion-transmitted disease associated with transfusion of FFP, many are not acutely aware of the risk of transfusion-related acute lung injury (TRALI). In cases such as these, not only can this help reduce inappropriate use of FFP, but this can also insure that clinicians are alerted to consider the diagnosis of TRALI as well as fluid overload when a patient receiving FFP suffers respiratory decompensation.

Some educators feel that prospective audit is the most effective way of modifying blood ordering behaviour. The downside of prospective review lies in the delay in product issuance that is inherent in the process. In addition, some clinicians may view being questioned about product use prior to issue as undue interference with, and criticism of, their management of a patient who is ultimately their primary responsibility. The concern about delay can be addressed by providing a fail-safe mechanism to allow product release in critical situations, such as when the patient is in the operating room, emergency room, or the ICU. The interference concern often requires a diplomatic approach to the clinician and emphasis on the educational aspect of the interaction. This is best accompanied by assurance that if the clinician still feels product is needed that it will be issued and the usage reviewed later by the Transfusion Committee. Prospective audit can also be a very time-consuming process. Thus, it is amenable to use in an academic setting where pathology/laboratory medicine house staff can be involved in the early stages and can learn a considerable amount about transfusion practices from their involvement in the approval process.

Concurrent and Retrospective Audit

Concurrent and retrospective review also begin with the requirement that a clinical indication be specified at the time product is ordered. At Yale - New Haven Hospital for example, specific blood component requests are reviewed monthly by senior blood bank technical personnel. Those cases in which the clinical indication and/or laboratory data do not meet the specified criteria are referred for further audit by a blood bank physician, who gathers additional information from both the patient's chart and the clinicians who cared for the patient. Timing of the review process is the main difference between concurrent and retrospective review, with a concurrent audit taking place within one or two days of the issuance of product and a retrospective audit taking place, perhaps, weeks or months after transfusion.

The advantage of concurrent audit over retrospective is that review occurs and feedback can be given to clinicians at a time when the clinical circumstances associated with the request for product are still fresh in the clinician's mind. Also. further blood ordering may still be taking place. So while the concurrent review is technically retrospective, it can still have an immediate impact on further blood ordering for the same patient. This approach is also time consuming, although perhaps less so than prospective review.

Retrospective audit has the advantage of taking place at a time most convenient for the blood bank staff and transfusion medicine physician. It is generally less time consuming, although difficulties in obtaining charts on patients discharged some time in the past may diminish this benefit. It is certainly the least intrusive upon patient care and the least likely to be viewed as interference on the part of the clinician. It is also the least likely to result in modification of behaviour, although consistent feedback can not help but make physicians more aware of the ways in which their blood ordering practices depart from the norm among their peers. It is the peer review aspect which should be stressed, as this is often a strong motivating force for recalcitrant physicians. Again, if the educational aspect of the interaction is stressed, the potential to significantly modify practice remains.

Regardless of the timing of the audit process, the physician performing the audit must remain alert to the special features of each individual patient's clinical situation which may necessitate a transfusion trigger different from those specified in the guidelines. For example, patients with sickle cell anaemia are often chronically compensated to a low haematocrit and may even suffer from hyperviscosity problems when transfused to a "normal" haematocrit. Likewise, a healthy 18 year old trauma victim may tolerate loss of 15 to 20% of his total red cell volume, dropping his haemoglobin to 7 of 8 gm/dl, whereas an elderly cardiac patient may develop angina if his haemoglobin falls below 9 of 10 gm/dl. Similarly, the presence of fever or a concomitant abnormality in the coagulation cascade or platelet dysfunction, may necessitate maintaining higher platelet counts than would be required in the absence of these clinical factors. It should be remembered that guidelines are intended to be just that – guidelines, not fixed indications for transfusion which must be applied to all patients in all clinical situations.

The Yale - New Haven Hospital Experience

The manner in which we set guidelines at our institution and then monitor adherence to the established criteria is, in many ways, an amalgam of the preceding methods. Certain requests, such as those for CMV-seronegative components, irradiated blood products, requests for leukoreduction filters, uncrossmatched blood and single donor platelets, are reviewed prospectively. Those requests which do not meet the specified criteria are referred to the laboratory medicine resident covering the blood bank for clearance. At Yale - New Haven Hospital this can be assisted by the computer screens used for ordering blood products. These screens ask a series of questions which are answered while placing an order for blood products or for special services such as irradiation. The indication for blood products orders and relevant laboratory values (haemoglobin/haematocrit for RBCs, PT/PTT for FFP, etc.) are monitored by hospital quality assurance staff. These are non-blood bank employee members of the audit staff from the Office of Clinical Quality Assurance. They are trained to review patient records, comparing indications specified in the chart against the established guidelines. This office uses two linked computer systems to monitor transfusion practices. All platelets and FFP, and 30% of all red cell transfusions which do not meet the Yale-specified criteria are subjected to chart review. Those out of compliance with Yale criteria are referred to the Audit Review Committee, a subcommittee of the Transfusion Committee, as part of the retrospective audit review process. If quantities of requested blood products are excessive, such as 32 units of platelets, or if the order is unusual, such as an order for washed plasma, the blood bank physician is notified and, in consultation with the ordering physician, determines whether the product should be issued by the blood bank. In exceptional cases where the indication is marginal but the clinical staff firmly believes that good patient care demands the product, the component in question may be released with the proviso that the request will be honoured but referred to the Transfusion Committee for review.

Once the resident has obtained information regarding the clinical indication for the requested product, he/she makes a determination as to whether the use is appropriate and either approves or disapproves the request. If time is an issue and if clinical events warrant, the resident will review the case with the blood bank attending immediately. If time is not an issue, the request whether approved by the resident or not is reviewed by the blood bank attending and senior technical staff at daily transfusion medicine rounds and a decision is made at that time as to whether further requests for similar products for that patient will be deemed justified.

Prospective audit also takes place in cases where the product requested appears reasonable but is actually contraindicated given the patient's diagnosis. For example, platelets are never issued to patients who carry a diagnosis of thrombotic thrombocytopenic purpura without the approval of a blood bank physician. Approval in these cases usually occurs only after consultation with the clinicians caring for the patient discloses that TTP is no longer considered a working diagnosis.

Concurrent component audit is frequently performed at Yale - New Haven Hospital follow-up the next day at clinical blood bank rounds. Retrospective audits are performed much more often. One type of retrospective audit, in particular is helpful. On a day chosen at random once during each month, utilization of one blood product is reviewed retrospectively, in depth. All requests for the component chosen for audit which were signed out and transfused on that day are audited for compliance. The product to be audited rotates in three month cycles, with red cells being audited one month, platelets the next and FFP/cryoprecipitate the third. This one day audit cycle repeats quarterly. In a year red cells are thus reviewed four times, as are FFP/cryo and platelets. All requests which were received on "audit day" for the product being audited are reviewed by a senior blood bank technologist. Those which do not clearly meet the specified hospital criteria are referred to a blood bank physician, either the resident or fellow, who obtains the chart on the patient and ascertains whether product usage falls within the guidelines. Those instances in which usage falls outside the criteria are reviewed with a member of the blood bank attending staff. If the usage does indeed appear inappropriate the case is sent to the Transfusion Committee, Audit Review Subcommittee.

This group reviews the case and if found to be inconsistent with current guidelines, a letter is sent to the physician of record requesting further information, including a request for delineation of any extenuating factors present in the patient. The Transfusion Committee reviews the clinicians comments and then arrives at a final determination as to whether the usage is regarded as appropriate or inappropriate. If inappropriate, a letter is sent to the attending informing him/her of the decision of the Committee with suitable copies to the Chair of the appropriate Department, Chief of the Medical Staff and Office of Risk Management/Legal Affairs. Repeat infractions with no mitigating circumstances could result in the Hospital Medical Board removing the physician's admitting privileges. While such a "doomsday" scenario has never been played out to completion at Yale - New Haven Hospital, the process, while lengthy and convoluted, does exist. There is little doubt that should a physician be a chronic severe offender, harsh action could indeed be taken. The driving factor first and above all, is concern for the good patient care. The Hospital's accreditation which affects third party reimbursement does play a minor role in this as well. The ripple effect of this concern has a beneficial impact on clinical transfusion practice.

The main thrust of the audit process should be an attempt to educate the physician as to why the transfusion request was unacceptable. To do this via letter is easiest but also least likely to be effective. A telephone call is better, but a friendly face to face meeting on the wards or even in the parking lot is, in our experience, more likely to modify behaviour. The personal touch while most time consuming is much more effective. If it does change ordering practices, in the long run, probably saves time. Diplomacy is required. A "slash and burn" approach to human relations is not likely to work here – it will only serve to alienate the physician. Change is difficult and some physicians have more trouble than others in adapting to the alterations in blood ordering practice which audits impose. Audits are here to stay, however, and the physician should be encouraged, firmly but gently, to get "on the bus".

Continual Evolution

Modification of existing behaviour to reduce needless product usage is a noble goal. If we are truly seeking to minimize unnecessary use of blood components, however, then we must engage in continual assessment of our practices, the assumptions on which they are based and the ways in which they can be improved. At Yale - New Haven Hospital, one way in which we improve our understanding of the problems associated with blood transfusion is by encouraging the reporting of possible transfusion reactions. We aggressively follow up on the reported transfusion practice, which may be suggested by these reaction reports. In our institution, as in most other hospitals, transfusion reactions are reported to the blood bank. Immediately, (within an hour of receipt), the blood bank resident is apprised of the serological data and gathers clinical information by speaking with the staff taking care of the patient and/or reviewing the patient's chart. The resident reports his/her findings at blood bank rounds if it is a "routine" reaction. If it is a serious clinical reaction involving high fever, shock, intravascular haemolysis, anaphylaxis, sepsis, or other life-threatening condition a blood bank attending is immediately notified day or night.

In this way, transfusion reactions are used to provide feedback and education for both clinicians and for the blood bank. For example, attention to the potential for diagnosing transfusion-related sepsis is stressed when reviewing febrile reactions in which dyspnoea, rigors, hypotension and sustained shock are reported in response to transfusion of a blood component, especially platelets and red cells. This has several effects: 1) by interacting with clinicians in the process of investigating such reactions we can heighten their awareness of the risk of septic transfusion reaction and facilitate the initiation of appropriate therapy; 2) we can also get a better sense of the incidence of this complication which some feel is grossly under-reported at present.

In one recent instance, two episodes of severe febrile reactions occurred, one of which was indeed attributable to transfusion of an infected unit of platelets. Following this we began to see a plethora of requests for culture of blood products involved in any type of febrile reaction - even those of minimal intensity which clearly resolved within minutes following cessation of the transfusion.

We used this situation as an opportunity to educate the house staff and refine our transfusion practices. First we concluded that all requests for culture of blood products must be approved by a blood bank resident/attending; we established guidelines for this decision including minimum temperature elevations and guidelines for changes in pulse and blood pressure. Second, we decided to culture the blood bag only if the patient was cultured, as well. This was to minimize the chance that inadvertent contamination of the blood bag would be confused with patient sepsis. If both the patient and the blood bag had the same organism of the same serotype, a diagnosis of a septic transfusion reaction would be cleared. Third, we arranged for a series of presentations at teaching conferences and clinical rounds to educate the staff on transfusion-induced sepsis. Fourth, we were able to closely review the transfusion practices surrounding transfusion accompanied by febrile responses and found that in several cases the most likely etiology of the febrile reaction was that the unit was infused much too rapidly for the clinical setting. Since febrile reactions, even with leukoreduction filtration are rate and dose related, many suspected septic reactions were found instead to be rate-related reactions from too rapid infusion of sterile blood components. In-services to house and nursing staff helped to improve this aspect of clinical transfusion practice by discouraging infusion of platelets "as fast as tolerated."

We also helped the Nursing Department revise their Guidelines for Blood Product Administration. Lastly, we developed a Standard Operating Procedure (SOP) for evaluation of reports of septic transfusion reactions which the blood bank technologists and residents follow. This plan has improved clinical transfusion practice among the housestaff, improved nursing blood administration protocols, provided a systematic approach to handling a difficult situation which permits good medical care to co-exist with fiscal responsibility. Thus, by auditing all requests for work-up of septic transfusion reactions, we were able to improve transfusion practice at our institution. Some centers are now recommending a Gram stain and/or a culture of all transfusion reactions with a report of any fever and/or chills.

Another example of how audits can be used to improve clinical care and educate the medical staff arose from a case in which a reaction of dyspnoea, rash, nausea/vomiting and fever was reported in response to a plasma unit. Review of the patient's chart revealed that, immediately prior to transfusion of the FFP, a unit of additive solution red blood cells had been given. On questioning the house officer about the details of the reaction, it became apparent that this house officer had erroneously assumed that the red cell unit could not possibly have accounted for the reported reaction since the red cells were not actually being infused at the time the reaction occurred. This provided the opportunity to review the symptoms and signs of haemolytic transfusion reactions and TRALI with the house officer in question and to reinforce the fact that transfusion-related symptomatology can still occur hours after the transfusion is completed. The fact that the discussion took place within hours of the reported reaction (concurrent review) provides a clinical correlation which will hopefully make the lessons involved more memorable.

Conclusion

Transfusion triggers can provide a starting point for dialogue within an institution and, with appropriate allowances for patient clinical factors, can provide a means to greatly improve the quality of transfusion practice.

Despite the lack of consensus on all issues, usage criteria can still be established in those areas where consensus has been achieved. As experience with institutional auditing grows, the process can be refined and the non-consensus areas can be brought into consensus. We have discussed methods by which one can improve the quality of transfusion practice through both component usage audits and evaluation of transfusion reactions. Improvement in transfusion practices involves an entire Quality Plan, coupled with attention to current good clinical practice (cGCP) [44]. The 90's is the decade of regulation. While the criticism that regulations are more concerned with form rather than substance may be true in some instances, we can nonetheless use today's regulatory climate to our patients' advantage by developing effective auditing practices and implementing them.

References

1. Consensus conference. Perioperative red cell transfusion. JAMA 1988;260:2700-03.
2. Welch HG, Meehan KR, Goodnough LT. Prudent strategies for elective red blood cell transfusion. Ann Intern Med 1992;116:393-402.
3. Audet AM, Goudnough LT. Practice strategies for elective red blood cell transfusion. Ann Intern Med 1992;116:404-6.
4. Halsey PB, Lave JR, Kapoor WN. The necessary and the unnecessary transfusion: A critical review of reported appropriateness rates and criteria for red cell transfusions. Transfusion 1994;34:110-15.
5. Stehling L, Luban NLC, Anderson KC, et al. Guidelines for blood utilization review. Transfusion 1994;34:438-48.
6. Lundberg GD (ed). Practice parameter for the use of fresh-frozen plasma, cryoprecipitate, and platelets. JAMA 1994;271:777-81.
7. Consensus conference. Fresh-frozen plasma: Indications and risks. JAMA 1985;253: 551-53.
8. Metz J, McGrath KM, Copperchini ML, et al. Appropriateness of transfusions of red cells, platelets and fresh frozen plasma: An audit in a tertiary care teaching hospital. Med J Aust 1995;162:572-77.
9. Blanchette VA, Hume HA, Levy GJ, Luban NLC, Strauss RG. Guidelines for auditing pediatric blood transfusion practices. AJDC 1991;145:787-96.
10. National blood resource education program expert panel on the indications for the use of red blood cells, platelets and fresh frozen plasma. Transfusion alert: Indications for the use of red blood cells, platelets and fresh frozen plasma. Aug 1993. National

Institutes of Health (NIH Publication No. 93-2974a).
11. Mintz PD. Quality assessment and improvement of transfusion practices. Hemat/ Oncol Clin Nrth Amer 1995;9:219-32.
12. American Association of Blood Banks Transfusion Practices Quality Assurance Committee, 1992-1993 Committee. Guidelines for blood utilization review. Bethesda, MD, American Association of Blood Banks, 1994.
13. Consensus conference. Platelet transfusion therapy. JAMA 1987;257:1777-80.
14. Rustad H, Myhre E. Surgery during anticoagulant treatment. Acta Med Scand 1963;173:115-19.
15. Ewe K. Bleeding after liver biopsy does not correlate with indices of peripheral coagulation. Digestive Diseases and Sciences 1981;26:388-93.
16. Burns ER, Goldberg SN, Wenz B. Paradoxical effect of multiple mild coagulation factor deficiencies on the prothrombin time and activated partial thromboplastin time. Am J Clin pathol 1993;100:94-98.
17. McVay PA, Toy PTCY. Lack of increased bleeding after paracentesis and thoracentesis in patients with mild coagulation abnormalities. Transfusion 1991;31:164-71.
18. Counts RB, Haisch C, Simon TL, Maxwell NG, Heimbach DM, Carrico CJ. Hemostasis in massively transfused trauma patients. Ann Surg 1979;190:91-99.
19. Gaydos LA, Freireich EJ, Mantel N. The quantitative relation between platelet count and hemorrhage in patients with acute leukaemia. N Engl J Med 1962;266:905-9.
20. Beutler E. Platelet transfusions: The 20,000/μL trigger. Blood 1993;81:1411-13.
21. Gmur J, Burger J, Schanz U, Fehr J, Schaffner A. Safety of stringent prophylactic platelet transfusion policy for patients with acute leukemia. Lancet 1991;338:1223-26.
22. Pisciotto PT, Benson K, Hume H, et al. Prophylactic versus therapeutic platelet transfusion practices in hematology and/or oncology patients. Transfusion 1995;35:498-502.
23. Strauss RG. Granulocyte transfusion therapy. Hemat/Oncol Clin Nrth Amer 1994; 8:1159-66.
24. Strauss RG. Therapeutic granulocyte transfusions in 1993. Blood 1993;81:1675-78.
25. Huestis DW, Glasser L. The neutrophil in transfusion medicine. Transfusion 1993;34: 630-46.
26. Bensinger WI, Price TH, Dale DC, et al. The effects of daily recombinant human granulocyte colony-stimulating factor administration on normal granulocyte donors undergoing leukapheresis. Blood 1993;81:1883-88.
27. Klein H (ed). Standards for blood banks and transfusion services. 16th ed. American Association of Blood Banks, Bethesda, MD, 1994:13.
28. Hillyer CD, Emmens RK, Zago-Novaretti M, Berkman EM. Methods for the reduction of transfusion-transmitted cytomegalovirus infection: Filtration versus the use of seronegative donor units. Transfusion 1994;34:929-34.
29. Preiksaitis JK. Indications for the use of cytomegalovirus-seronegative blood products. Trans Med Rev 1991;5:1-17.
30. Bowden RA. Transfusion-transmitted cytomegalovirus infection. Hemat/Oncol Clin Nrth Amer 1995;9:155-66.
31. Bowden RA, Slichter SJ, Sayers M, et al. A comparison of filtered leukocyte-reduced and cytomegalovirus (CMV) seronegative blood products for the prevention of transfusion-associated CMV infection after marrow transplant. Blood 1995;86:3598-603.
32. Zhang LJ, Hanff P, Rutherford C, Churchill WH, Crumpacker CS. Detection of human cytomegalovirus DNA, RNA, and antibody in normal donor blood. J Infect Dis 1995;171:1002-6.

33. Smith KL, Cobain T, Dunstan RA. Removal of cytomegalovirus DNA from donor blood by filtration. Br J Haematol 1993;83:640-42.
34. Leitman SF, Holland PV. Irradiation of blood products: Indications and guidelines. Transfusion 1985;25:293-300.
35. Huestis DA, Bove JR, Case J. Practical Blood Transfusion. Boston: Little, Brown and Company, 1988.
36. Center for Biologics Evaluation and Research; FDA. Recommendations regarding license amendments and procedures for gamma irradiation of blood products. Rockville, MD, July 22, 1993.
37. Sola MA, Espana A, Redondo P, et al. Transfusion-associated acute graft-versus-host disease in a heart transplant recipient. Brit J Derm 1995;132:626-30.
38. Lane TA. Leukocyte reduction of cellular blood components. Arch Pathol Lab Med 1994;118:392-404.
39. Menitove JE, McElligott MC, Aster RH. Febrile transfusion reactions: What blood component should be given next? Vox Sang 1982;42:318-21.
40. Stack G, Snyder EL. Cytokine generation in stored platelet concentrates. Transfusion 1994;34:20-25.
41. Heddle NM, Klama L, Singer J, et al. The role of the plasma from platelet concentrates in transfusion reactions. N Engl J Med 1994;331:625-28.
42. Heddle NM, Blajchman MA. The leukodepletion of cellular blood products in the prevention of HLA-alloimmunization and refractoriness to allogeneic platelet transfusion. Blood 1995;85:603-6.
43. De Wolf JThM, Westerterp A, Smit Sibinga CTh, Halie MR. Prestorage leukocyte depletion is not necessarily required for the prevention of refractoriness to platelet transfusion. Blood 1995;86:3263.
44. Nevalainen DE, Lloyd HL. ISO-9000 quality standards: A model for blood banking? Transfusion 1995;35:521-24.

CHOICE OF SINGLE DONOR AND RANDOM DONOR PLATELET TRANSFUSION - ITS COSTS

A. Westerterp-Maas, J.Th.M. de Wolf[1], P.C. Das, C.Th.Smit Sibinga, M.R. Halie[1]

The use of platelets transfusion has not only doubled between 1980 and 1985 in the USA [1-5], but seems to be still continuing to grow in most industrialized countries (Figure 1). Most commonly platelets have been used prophylactically, in chronically thrombocytopenic patients in the haemato-oncology departments. Platelets play a crucial role in transfusion practice, not only because of the short shelf life but also because there is no available growth factor to replace it yet in the clinical practice [6-8].

Most platelet supports are given by random blood donations, and pooling the donor platelets into multi-donor concentrates (RDP). Alternatively apheresis platelets derived from a single donor (SDP) may be used. Following the emergence of AIDS, the demands for SDP have grown especially in the USA where 25% of increased use of platelets was carried by SDP (Figure 2). But future estimates suggest that these proportions might increase to 60 to 100%, while critical issues such as the clinical justification, HLA-alloimmunization, risk of infection and availability, remain still to be defined.

In this paper we discuss the triggering of choice of platelets products (SDP versus RDP) in the clinic, and its financial and logistical consequences. For this study we surveyed the platelets use in the University Hospitals and district hospitals in the entire Netherlands (Figure 3) over a 10 years period [9,10] (1984-1993). In addition we surveyed the norther region in greater detail. This region (1.1 million population supported by 5,000 acute beds in 12 hospitals) is supplied by our blood bank. In our University Hospital the major disciplines of medicine, surgery, obstetrics and paediatrics are present; specialized units such as haematology and oncology are situated in the department of internal medicine. The blood bank receives 60,000 annual blood donations from which 15,000 RDP are made. By cytapheresis machines we also produce about 300 SDP annually. Both types of platelets could be stored for 5 days.

For comparison we investigated the platelets transfusion in seven University Hospitals providing specialized and supra regional services, and also in the district hospitals.

1. Dept. of Haematology, University Hospital Groningen, NL.

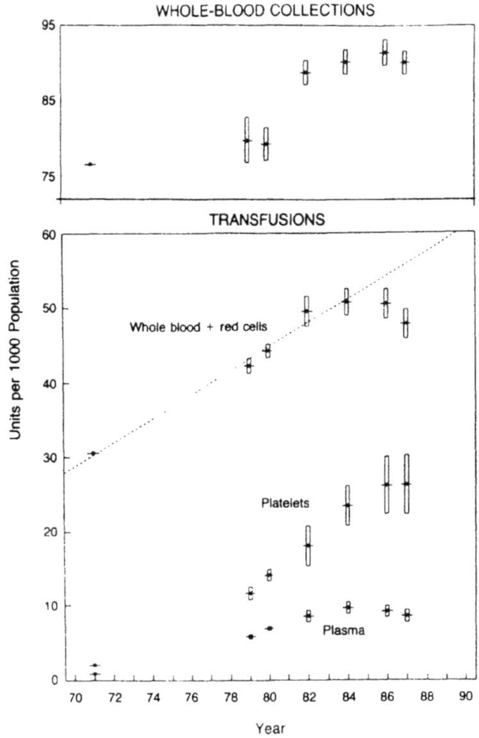

Figure 1. Rates of blood collection and transfusion in the United States. 1971-1987. (Courtesy of the N Engl J Med 1990;322:1646-51)

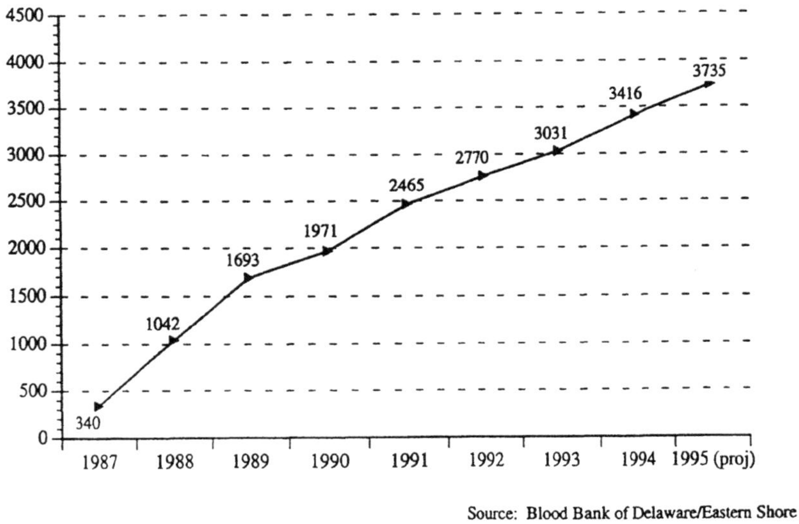

Figure 2. Relative growth of single donor platelets (SPD). (Courtesy of the AABB Newsbrief 1 July 1995)

For better analysis we also compared the platelets use per hospital bed at different points of time. In addition further analysis was made in different clinical departments with regards to their growth and intensity of platelets use in our University Hospital. In the Netherlands one unit of RDP costs about Dfl. 15.- and six of them are generally pooled to provide an adult dose, while one SDP costs about Dfl. 600,-. Comparative American prices quoted are US$100.- for RDP and US$500.- for SDP.

Results

The number of platelets transfusions in the Netherlands over the 10 years has nearly doubled (Figure 4). Understandably their use in the University Hospitals is considerably higher than that of the district hospitals. However, there are considerable and marked differences of platelets use per bed among the University Hospitals (Figure 5). Our own hospital while following the national trend, had much lower platelets transfusions per bed. The main increase occurred in the department of internal medicine where haematology and oncology patients are treated; a small increase is also seen in the surgical department that has cardiac bypass and liver transplantation units (Figure 6). Most of the increase was met by RDP, and SDP remains to about 300 per year for this entire period. This may be due to voluntary restriction imposed on SDP (with or without HLA matching) for multiply transfused patients, not responding to RDP therapy, rather than

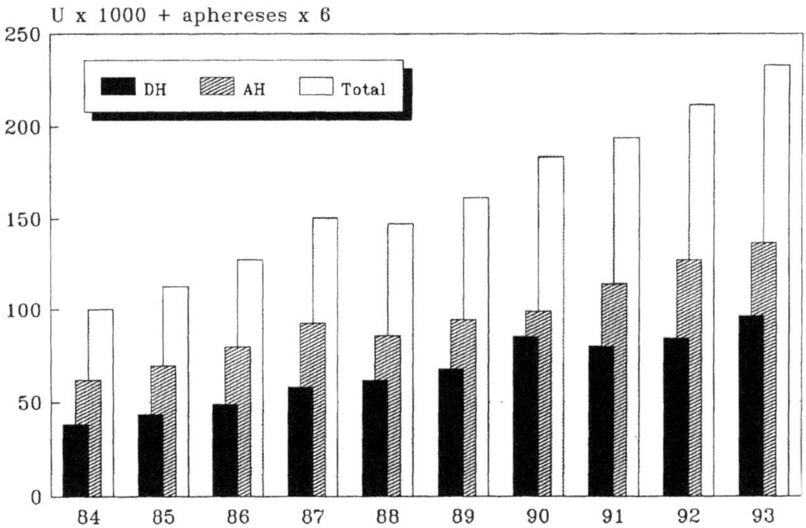

Figure 3. Platelets transfusions in the academic hospitals (AH) and district hospitals (DH) in the Netherlands (1984-1993.

supplying SDP on demands, which is always considered and discussed in clinical consulation.

The costs of platelets transfusions, both SDP and RDP are shown in the Figure 6. In 1993 for example, in three academic hospitals 3% to 14% of the platelets are transfused as SDP. This represented 16 to 52% of the total platelet costs. Regarding the platelet transfusion costs in our University Hospital, SDP represented 37% in clinical haematology, compared to 93% in oncology. There was a sustained rise in the total SDP use in the Netherlands over the last 10 years, in 1993 it still only represented 4% of the total platelets transfusions. However, there are exceptions as shown in the figure when a blood bank supplying only district hospitals had incurred 99.5% of the total platelets transfusion costs due to SDP.

Some parts of the USA had shown 25% of the platelets transfusion due to SDP. Such a change sofar has not occurred in the Netherlands. Responding to such a change at the blood bank level is logistically possible. However, aside the issues of its indication and patients' clinical outcome or development of alloimmunization, which would not be discussed here, the crucial question must be – what would be the costs of such a policy?

With a modest 25% increase of SDP use, the total platelets transfusion costs would not only be doubled to Dfl. 8.4 million where SDP represent 70% of the total platelets budget (Table 1). This somewhat surprised us. The current estimated

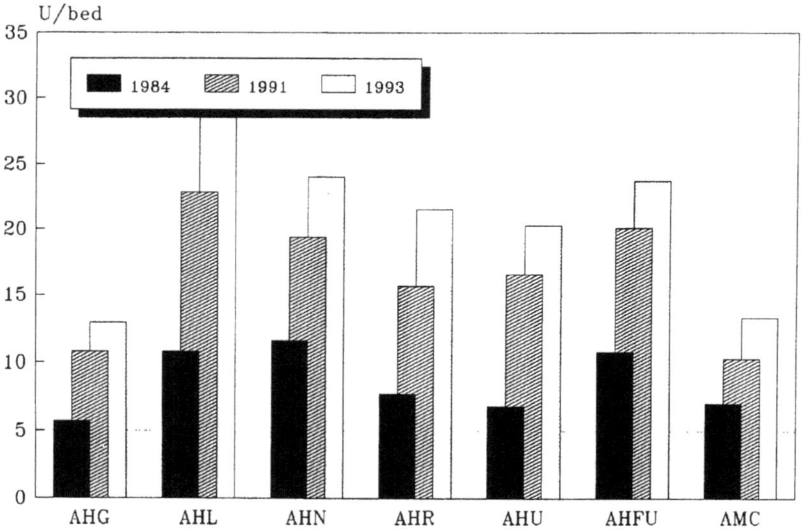

Figure 4. Per bed platelet transfusions in 7 academic hospitals [AHG (Groningen), AHN (Nijmegen), AHL (Leiden), AHU (Utrecht), AMC (Amsterdam), AHR (Rotterdam) and AHFU (Amsterdam)] in 1984, 1991 and 1993.

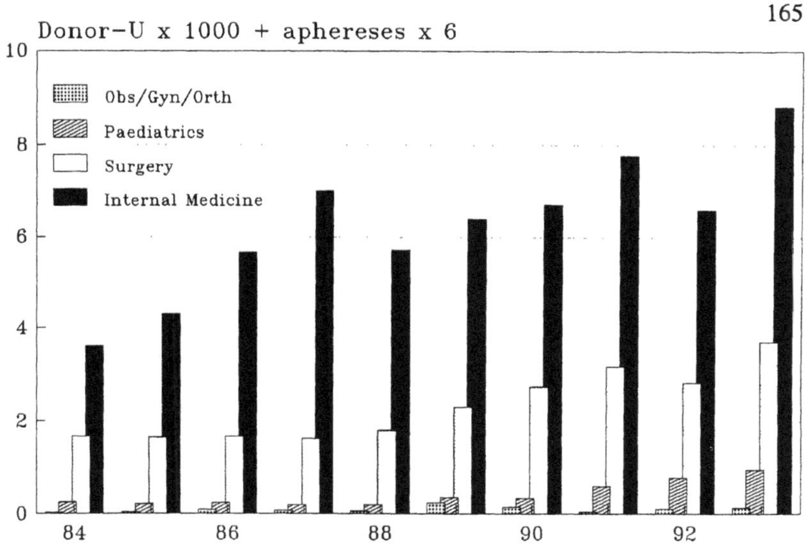

Figure 5. Platelets transfusions in the different clinical departments of the Academic Hospital Groningen (AHG) during 1984-1993.

annual costs for platelets support in a multiply transfused patient in our haematology unit is about Dfl. 616.- using mainly RDP. However, this figure will enormously increase to Dfl. 4,622.- per patient if the transfusion is provided entirely by SDP. Thus it should be noted that agressive growth of SD platelets

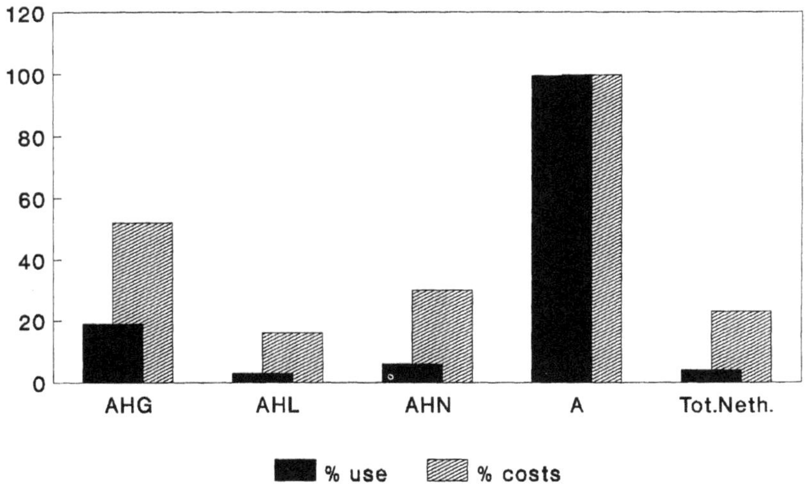

Figure 6. Analysis of the proportion of single donor platelets (SDP) use and its relative cost to the total platelet budget in 3 different academic hospitals [AHG (Groningen), AHL (Leiden), AHN (Nijmegen)] and one blood bank A supplying district hospitals (Red Cross Blood Bank Arnhem)] in 1993.

use, possibly due to benevolent but inappropriate use, could result in a minority of platelets transfusion taking excessive share of the platelets budget.

This study also demonstrates that there is considerable difference in the use of platelets transfusions per bed in different University Hospitals. Such variation is recognized nationally and internationally [11,12], indicating a variation in clinical perception of its appropriateness, and variation of trigger mechanism for platelets transfusion [13]. Critical study of such trigger mechanisms at the bedside could allow optimal use of platelets demonstrating its costs effectiveness for the benefit of the patient care.

Table 1. Costing (in US$) of platelets transfusions in the Netherlands with an estimated 25% support through SDP.

	4% of platelets as SDP	**25% of platelets as SDP**
Random platelets (6 U) (US$45.-)	US$ 1,672,035.-	US$ 1,311,127.-
Single donor platelets (US$300.-)	US$ 507,600.-	US$ 2,913,600.-
Total	US$ 2,179,635.-	US$ 4,224,727.-

References

1. Surgenor DM, Wallace EL, Hale SG, Gilpatrick MW. Changing patterns of blood transfusion on four sets of United States hospitals, 1980 to 1985. Transfusion 1988; 28:513-18.
2. Sherma LA. The implications of trends in transfusion (editorial). Transfusion 1988;28:511-12.
3. McCullough J, Steeper TA, Connely DP, Jackson B, Huntington S, Scott EP. Platelets utilization in a University Hospital. JAMA 1988;259:2414-18.
4. Surgenor DM, Wallace EL, Hao SMS, Chapman RH. Collection and transfusion of blood in the United States 1982-1988. N Engl J Med 1990;322:1646-51.
5. Consensus Conference (1987). Platelet transfusion therapy. JAMA 1987;257:1777-80.
6. Winearls CG, Oliver DO, Pippard MJ, Reid C, Dowmug KR, Cotes PM. Effect of human erythropoietin derived from recombinant DNA on the anemia of patients maintained by chronic haemodialysis. Lancet 1986;ii:1175-78.
7. Peters WP. Use of cytokines during prolonged neutropenia associated with autologous bone marrow transplantation. Rev Infect Dis 1991;13:993-96.
8. Kaushansky K. Thrombopoietin: The primary regulation of platelet production. Blood 1995;862:419-31.
9. Central Medical Blood Transfusion Committee. Overzicht van het bloedtransfusie gebeuren 1984 [report]. Amsterdam, NL.
10. Council on Blood Transfusion of the Netherlands Red Cross. Overzicht van de bloedtransfusie in Nederland 1993 [report]. Amsterdam, NL.
11. Thomson A, Contreras M, Knowles S. Blood component treatment, a retrospective audit in five major London hospitals. J Clin Pathol 1991;44:734-37.

12. Goodnough LT, Johnston MFM, Shah T, Chernosky A. Two-institution study of transfusion practise in 78 consecutive adult elective open-heart procedures. Am J Pathol 1989;91:468-72.
13. Beutler E. Platelet transfusion: The 20,000/μL trigger. Blood 1993;81:1411-13.

ETHICAL ASPECTS OF THE TRANSFUSION OF BLOOD: RESTRICTIVE OR JUSTIFYING?

C.R. Macpherson

Donors come first

It should be understood that the dilemmas to be discussed are not the exclusive concern or responsibility of physicians. Others share them, but in many issues, particularly patient care, final responsibility cannot be delegated or avoided by the physician. The primary focus may appear to shift to and fro because obligations are frequently complex and overlapping, not single and either/or. For example, when a donor unit is processed and every effort is being made to avoid harm to the donor and to meet his wishes, this does not of course reduce in any way the imperative to minimize risk to the recipient. Possibly the most difficult and persistent dilemma involving donor ethics was quoted by Busch and Alter recently [1]. If p24 antigen testing is available only in blood banks, donors who have consistently reported that they donate blood to obtain Human Immunodeficiency Virus (HIV) testing will probably continue this behaviour, and nobody seems to have much idea of how to prevent it. It is postulated that only about 17% of HIV-infected units donated during the window period will be detected by the p24 antigen test, since the window is reduced from 42 days to around 35 days, but is not eliminated. The increased yield projected by adding the p24 test is small, about 6 infected units per year in the United States, so it is possible, though not likely, that an influx of high-risk donors seeking more sensitive testing could actually increase the hazard to the blood supply since those units will theoretically be infectious, but undetectable for 35 days. If this is documented to have occurred in the follow-up of p24 antigen testing, it will certainly complicate decisions about adding new tests to narrow the window even more. This illustrates that primary ethical imperatives for donors, apart from being altruistic and charitable, are to tell the truth and to refrain from high-risk behaviour, or at least not to donate afterwards. On the other hand the recipient's moral obligation to support the organization that has provided his blood and blood-products seems to suffer when blood banking is perceived as a major business rather than as a public service or charitable activity.

Blood bank physicians

One dilemma for blood bank physicians arises when there is need to call on a donor more often than usual, whether for red cells or single-donor platelets, and raises both medical and ethical questions. The procedure requested should be very likely to be tolerated by the donor, even though serious sequelae are unlikely. Ethically, the unusual request should have been fully explained to the donor. This should not be just an explanation of the urgency of the patient's needs, which may be interpreted as an appeal for generosity and suspension of normal caution on the part of the donor, who must have a clear understanding of the chances of ill-effects from the donation before giving permission. In other words, in this situation as in many others, consent should be truly "informed", if the United States (US) concept of "Informed Consent" is in place and is followed. However this is not universal practice, and even in the US there are suggestions that we may be pressuring some people to become more autonomous than they really wish to be [2].

In the less common situation of considering transfusion of incompletely tested blood, or of blood that is not wholly compatible the issue of Informed Consent becomes paradoxically less urgent and less achievable. The patient is usually in a very grave condition, possibly in a coma or under anaesthesia. It is difficult enough for the average patient in good condition to fully understand the options involved, so the tendency is for discussion and decision-making to be confined to blood bank and patient physicians. Relatives and patient representatives should be involved, and informed as fully as possible, even if it is not felt to be a legal necessity.

Still another problem is related to testing autologous units for infectious markers. In the US, Federal regulations are clear, if not altogether logical. An interesting discussion of the ethical issues involved appeared recently, outlining possible hazards to staff and other patients, but also to the autologous donor [3].

Theoretically, shortages are a simple problem, with an equally simple solution, "draw, borrow or buy", though details of how to achieve this can be vastly complicated and frustrating. Ethical issues are involved in how scarce resources are allocated to certain hospitals and patients, and sometimes are the focus of intense debate. Possibly surprisingly, regular or frequent over-supply can also raise ethical concerns. If surpluses result in a profit, should the proceeds not go to the community, at least in part? The rationale for retaining them in the blood centre is to found research or something else which will benefit the community, but if "Informed Consent" was not obtained from the relevant groups before that decision was made, it can be difficult to explain (and to justify) after the fact. This is often perceived as another manifestation of Paternalism in that the Director of the blood bank knows what is best for the community, or so it appears.

In the more common situation where surpluses are not regular but intermittent, and are used to help other parts of the blood transfusion community so that they will return the favour when the need arises, this is so logical that questions do not commonly arise, and if they do, are easily answered.

Let us next consider a more complicated scenario for the blood bank physician, who is aware that some of the hospitals served are consistently using more blood per patient and per procedure than is the norm elsewhere. The supply is fortunately equal to the demand, with periodic surpluses, which are exported. The Blood Bank governing body is happy, as are the local physicians. What obligation, if any, is there on the blood bank physician to address this situation, at the least with the medical community? An ethicist who favours the Utilitarian approach might very well say that nothing need be done - let well alone.

A Deontologist in the other hand, reasons from the position that if there are relevant principles they should be honoured. There are three at least in this situation. First, if more donors are being drawn than are actually required, one must not ignore the (admittedly infrequent) severe adverse reactions that can result - issue being non-maleficence. Second, some patients are being given more transfusions than they need. Since these are unavoidably hazardous to the recipient in some unpredictable degree, non-maleficence applies again. Third, obtaining more blood than is necessary from the community of donors, without their understanding that this is a deliberate policy, violates the principles of truthtelling and fairness. Should something be done? The ethical principles involved seem to suggest that action should be taken.

The Utilitarian perspective would suggest to some, "laissez faire" or "do not rock the boat." It is always difficult to justify interfering with, or trying to change a system that is successful, especially when success is so hard to achieve. On the other hand, although it was a long time ago, I remember doing autopsies, close together, on two patients who died of hepatitis B. Both had received a single unit of red cells. In one patient there was no good reason, in the other a very questionable justification for the transfusion. Does the marked improvement in detection of infectious markers since those days justify a more relaxed attitude about unnecessary transfusions? The statistics are certainly better, and the sense of urgency will understandably be less for most people, but statistics for other adverse events such as contamination or transfusing the wrong person have not improved as markedly. The Deontological approach has to be favoured if one accepts that there is still a need to try and correct overusage.

It is not generally advocated that such dilemmas must always be decided on a purely ethical basis. Ethicists as individuals, ethics committees and other groups reviewing clinical decisions prospectively or after the fact, act as advisors, not judges. They also act as facilitators, helping decision-makers to consider all points of view and hear all those who have legitimate interests. It is unfortunate when ethics are not included in discussions nor weighed in the final decision. It is a perception, shared by many, that better decisions are likely to result when ethics are viewed as an important component leading to better and fuller understanding of situations, rather than as an obstruction. This of course tends to be a self-fulfilling prophesy. If one expects inclusion of ethics to cause confusion and delay it is very likely to do so.

Patient physicians

In decisions whether or not to transfuse, as in most other clinical settings, the primary obligation of the patient physician is unquestionably to the patient, involving both beneficence and non-maleficence. This has been a standard for many years, and in many, though by no means all, societies. Overall there are basically three choices or patterns governing decision making of this type. The first is where the physician makes decisions without much input from others, an approach which has been much criticized under the label of "Paternalism". In reaction to this, "Autonomy" has caused much decision-making to shift to the patient, or to appropriate surrogates. Recently it has been suggested that neither of these may suit significant numbers of people and that the extended family as the decision-maker is a valid third option, even though it may sometimes withhold information which the family feels could be harmful to the patient [4].

The patient should always be transfused in accordance with physiologic needs, not because of custom nor for cosmetic reasons, but it is also important that they should not be given more transfusions, allogeneic or autologous, than are needed, based primarily on non-maleficence to the patient, but conservation of community resources can also be involved. Especially in the US such decisions are increasingly associated with careful cost-benefit analysis, especially where the "gate-keeper" role is part of the physician's contract. If such an analysis invokes the term "Transfusion Trigger" to define when a specific patient should be transfused, this is reasonable. The term however, has been more commonly been applied to groups. I do not know how widespread the application of the "10GmHb/30%Hct" trigger or threshold was in Europe, but in the US alone the number of units unnecessarily transfused because of this uncritically applied criterion must be measured in the hundreds of thousands.

While we are all familiar with refusal to accept transfusion, most commonly by Jehovah's Witnesses [5, 6] there has been less experience with patients (or their families) demanding treatment which we may not agree is appropriate. A particularly difficult aspect of the beneficence/non-maleficence equation has recently become better defined and more widely discussed under the heading of "Futile Care". Essentially this means that there is no therapy which is curative or can provide significant benefit to the patient at the current stage of the disease - commonly leukaemia or other malignancies. Futile care can also be viewed as prolonging death rather than providing additional days or weeks of what the average observer would agree was useful, valuable or worth-while life. An ethics committee can play a very useful role here, not only by clarifying the issues and facilitating discussion, but also in helping to understand the patient and family's attitude to death and dying, their religious perspective and therefore their attitude to such decisions as withholding food, water and medications [7, 8].

In many cases obtaining a consensus on when care has become futile, and should be withheld or withdrawn, can be very difficult. While the usual parties are the health-care team and the patient, physician and family, the institution and its administration may perceive that they have a significant interest in the outcome of the discussion, often because of legal liability or jeopardy. The crux of this dilemma is that while there is widespread agreement on the patient's right to refuse any treatment at any time, there is little support for the thesis that patients have a right to demand, and receive, any therapy they choose. When patients or families believe that there is such a right, it can lead to a very difficult situation.

Ethics committees and similar bodies

Ethical considerations can undoubtedly be restrictive in settings where a rapid answer is needed, since they represent an additional step, one which can be quite time-consuming, for example fully informing patients and families about a complex decision or choice, especially if it involves a meeting of the interested parties - physicians, nurses, patient and relatives. However in an emergency, omitting steps which would be judged essential in non-emergent situations is a well-accepted principle, so delaying or complicating clinical decisions should not be a major, nor a frequent issue.

Inclusion of ethical considerations in routine discussions can lead to sounder decisions and policies, whether the topic is patient care, daily operations or organizational relationships to business partners and the community. It is critical that there be groups or committees charged with these tasks, whose members have been given (or have taken) sufficient time to become thoroughly familiar with basic principles of ethics and with each other, so that discussions can be both searching and comfortable, and therefore productive.

Bioethics committees often have broad concerns about ethical problems apart form health care itself, but even when the agendas and discussions focus on patient care the committee should be multidisciplinary, not exclusively physicians. Non-physicians, especially nurses, bring backgrounds and perspectives to patient care discussions which are vital, so do clergy, social workers and others who have direct patient interactions. All of them can and do greatly improve the scope and effectiveness of such committees, provided that the setting is what has been described as a "Save Haven". This is a place where views and opinions can be freely expressed and are valued for their worth and insight, not the seniority, rank or discipline of the speaker. The effectiveness of such committees is commonly derived from mutual respect, common goals and a shared awareness of the urgency and importance of so many of the issues that are brought to them.

Establishing an Ethics Committee and giving it enough time to educate its own members and develop the necessary skills is one approach which has been shown to be workable, worthwhile and attainable [9]. This is not to suggest that the process is either cheap or easy. To put it in place will take a year, optimistically, but probably more than that. There are many strategies and instruments that are commonly used, often some variant of an "Ethical Work-up". Components and emphasis vary slightly, but usually include determining all the relevant facts, followed by identifying legal and ethical perspectives, conflicts, possible courses of action, and finally being prepared to defend the chosen option [10].

Members of new ethics committees often bring with them little or no ethics experience. If a year or more for them to become functional is felt to be an excessive investment, consider how many years of transfusion experience the members of a typical Transfusion Committee bring to the task. How long does it take the average Transfusion Committee to "get up to speed" and become a force to be reckoned with in the hospital? A year would probably be considered a remarkable achievement.

A more recent development is the emergence of what are termed "Organizational Ethics". This involves such concerns as truth in advertising, ethical relationships with suppliers of goods and services, avoiding conflicts of interest for Board members and administrators and living up to commitments to the community.

Again, an educational program for the Board or its designated committee, and time to develop the necessary skill, are critical [11].

Probably the worst approach to incorporating ethics as a real and beneficial component of clinical problem-solving is "Crisis Management". This means that a committee is hastily formed because of sudden acute need, or that an inactive committee is galvanised into action to provide rapid solutions to problems which might well baffle a competent, well-prepared group of people who are already educated and comfortable with each others ways and opinions.

Ethical discussions and approaches to facilitate and improve patient-care decisions and policies will achieve what is desired only when those involved are well-trained, dedicated to the task involved and represent as many different segments of the health professions as is reasonable and feasible. If these conditions are not met there is a real possibility that their ethical discussions will be frustrating, divisive and misleading.

Conclusion

Ethics can add to the quality of decisions in the field of Transfusion Medicine provided that the focus is upon those most directly affected - patients, donors and the community - and that every effort is made to ensure that the outcome is what they chose, and expected, based on previous understanding of what was offered and what alternatives were available.

References

1. Busch MP, Alter HJ. Will human immonodeficiency virus p24 antigen screening increase the safety of the blood supply and, if so, at what cost? Transfusion 1995; 35:536-39.
2. Veatch RM. Abandoning informed consent. Hastings Center Report 1995;#2,25:5-12.
3. Domen RE. Infectious disease marker testing of autologous blood donor. Arch Path Lab Med 1995;119:807-10.
4. Blackhall LJ, Murphy ST, Frank G, et al. Ethnicity and attitudes toward patient autonomy. JAMA 1995;274:820-25.
5. Vercillo AP, Duprey SV. Blood transfusion in Jehovah's witnesses. Lab Medicine 1991;22:170-72.

6. May L. Challenging medical authority: The refusal of treatment by Christian Scientists. Hastings Center Report 1995,#1;25:15-21.
7. Schoenberger CI. Medical futility: An evolving ethical and clinical concept. Federation Bulletin 1995;82:72-9.
8. Capron AM. Medical futility: Strike two. Hastings Center Report 1994;#3:42-3.
9. Thomasma DC. Education of ethics committees. Bioethics Forum 1994;10#4:12-8.
10. Macpherson CR. The ethical workup: Definition and process. In: Smith DM, Carlson KB (eds). Current ethical/scientific dilemmas in blood banking. Bethesda MD, American Association of Blood Banks 1987:1-13.

WHAT TRIGGERS THE INITIATIVE OF DEVELOPMENTS IN TRANSFUSION MEDICINE: ADVANCES IN EX VIVO HAEMATOPOIETIC CELL THERAPY AND NEXT GENERATION TRANSFUSION PRODUCTS.

D.E. van Epps

Transfusion medicine and blood banking have evolved over the years from the collection and use of whole blood to the fractionation of blood into plasma and cell components including red blood cells, platelets and granulocytes (Figure 1). Plasma has been further refined and fractionated into specific components of significant therapeutic value including albumin, immunoglobulin and coagulation components such as Factor VIII. The evolution of molecular biology and recombinant protein technology has had a significant impact on the field and resulted in ways to generate therapeutic proteins which are functionally equivalent to proteins derived directly from the plasma. The best example of this is Factor VIII for the treatment of haemophilia. The therapeutic form of the protein has moved from being a plasma fraction to affinity purified Factor VIII using monoclonal antibody technology to the recombinant form of this protein which was introduced commercially in 1993. Many other basic plasma proteins have now been cloned and it is anticipated that many of these will be produced cost-effectively and applied clinically. It can also be anticipated that there will be a need for specific antibody therapy for infectious disease, autoimmune disease, transplantation, and cancer therapy. Such antibodies may augment or even replace the use of immunoglobulin fractions from plasma in situations where broad spectrum activity is not required.

The therapeutic use of blood cell components has increased dramatically over the years to the point where over 29 million red blood cell products and 4 million platelet products are utilized annually worldwide. This has been driven by an increased need for cell replacement as a result of increases in chemotherapy for cancer, organ and marrow transplantation, renal disease, surgical intervention and immune deficiency disease. We are currently at a point in time where dramatic changes in the field of transfusion medicine and blood banking are inevitable. Advances in molecular and cellular technology will potentially change both the nature and demand for plasma-based transfusion products as well as the types of cell products that will be used for therapy.

Although recombinant plasma components and hybridoma antibodies may have some impact on transfusion medicine, major changes in transfusion medicine will come from the evolution and use of novel ex vivo cell therapies requiring cell processing and the development and extended use of haematopoietic growth factors for both in vivo and ex vivo use. Erythropoietin (EPO) is an excellent example of a growth factor that has now been commercialized and used clinically to drive in vivo red cell production, reducing the need for red blood cell transfusions. The primary use of EPO is in renal disease, although it is also being applied to a variety of other anaemic conditions including AIDS. Thrombopoietin (TPO) is another example of a growth factor that has the potential to reduce the need for platelet transfusions. Although this growth is not approved for clinical use, data from animal studies indicate that it has significant therapeutic potential with limited adverse effects [1-4]. Although both EPO and TPO have the potential to reduce the need for transfusion products, several cytokines such as G-CSF and GM-CSF have increased the need for transfusion products as a result of enabling a more efficient harvest of stem cells from the peripheral blood by apheresis [5-7]. This has contributed dramatically to the use of high dose chemotherapy and blood stem cell transplantation which in turn has enhanced the need for blood cell transfusion products and apheresis products. The primary driver for the use of peripheral blood stem cells has been the reduction of both the time to platelet recovery following transplantation and the consequent, cost reduction associated with this. It has been demonstrated that the use of peripheral blood stem cells as

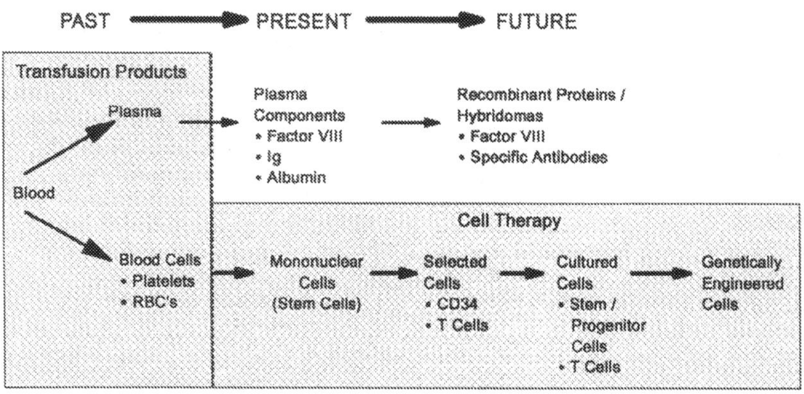

Figure 1. Evolution of blood products. Shaded area represents those processes that are carried out in blood banks or cell processing centres.

opposed to bone marrow results in enhanced haematopoietic recovery as evidenced by the reduction in patient days to 50,000 platelets (15 days with peripheral blood versus 30 to 50 days with bone marrow). This has led to a 2/3 reduction in the use of platelets in the transplant procedure, and a consequent reduction in hospital days. This has resulted in an overall cost reduction of transplantation in the U.S. from a range of approximately US$150,000 to US$200,000, to US$60,000 to US$80,000 per transplant [8, 9]. It is this therapeutic benefit and cost reduction as well as the trend towards autologous stem cell transplantation that has pushed the field of bone marrow transplantation towards the use of peripheral blood. It is estimated now that there are approximately 20,000 stem cell transplants per year with 50% of those being autologous. About a half of these autologous transplants are peripheral blood transplants. The number of transplants is increasing at approximately 20% per year and will probably reach well over 100,000 per year world wide. It is also likely that allogeneic transplants will be performed utilizing growth factor mobilized apheresis products from normal donors. Several studies in the U.S. and Europe have demonstrated that this is possible [10-12] and barring any unforseen adverse effects, allogeneic peripheral blood transplants will likely be used widely in the future.

Indicators and drivers for development of cell therapies and cell transfusion products

There are a variety of indicators that point to the future development of ex vivo cell therapies and their use as "transfusion products". One of significance is the response form Dr. David Kessler of the U.S. F.D.A., who has provided this definition for somatic cell therapy "somatic cell therapy is the administration to humans of living somatic cells that have been manipulated or processed to change their biological characteristics" [13]. Gene therapy is considered to be a subset of somatic cell therapy. This statement and the article by Kessler suggest that in the U.S. this cell product will be regulated and that guidelines for somatic cell products will be established, much like other blood cell transfusion products. It will remain to be seen whether other countries will follow suit. Other indicators of advancement in the field of cell therapy include the dramatic increase in the number of scientific papers, meetings, meeting sessions and conferences dedicated to the subject of cell therapy, and ex vivo gene therapy. In addition, over 120 gene therapy trials incorporating ex vivo cell manipulation have been approved by the Recombinant Advisory Committee (RAC) in the United States, and regulatory bodies or committees in other countries.

The primary drivers for ex vivo cell therapies include both clinical need and economic parameters. The initiation of clinical research in these areas is driven primarily by clinical need including:

– A need to enhance a currently practiced therapy and make it more effective. An example of this would be the use of bone marrow or peripheral blood stem cell transplantation to allow the use of higher doses of chemotherapy in the treatment of malignancy;

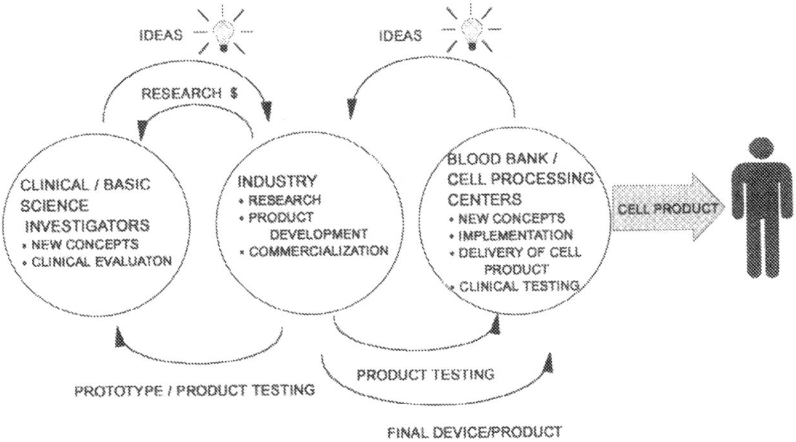

Figure 2. Interactions of basic and clinical scientists, industry, blood banks and cell processing centres.

– A need to reduce the morbidity and mortality of an existing therapy. Simple platelet transfusions in chemotherapy patients would be an example of this. A more technically advanced example would be the use of culture expanded haematopoietic stem cells of neutrophil progenitor cells as a supplement to high dose chemotherapy and stem cell transplantation to further enhance post transplant recovery [14-18]. Another example incorporating gene therapy would be the insertion of a multi-drug resistance gene into the transplanted stem cells making them resistant to chemotherapy [19];

– A final clinical need would be to develop a totally new therapy where no effective treatment exists. An example of this would be gene therapy using stem cells or other cell types as target cells for genetic engineering to replace a defective gene.

Although clinical need is the primary driver to trigger research into new therapies, cost reduction is rapidly becoming a factor in developing new treatments and technology. Even though innovative science and technology is a critical first step in developing and implementing new technology, the reduction to practice and commercialization of the final cell product or technology is directly dependent upon several additional components. All of these serve as triggers to the broad therapeutic use of cell products and include clinical efficiency, safety, cost, reimbursement potential, regulatory approval and simplicity to practice. Failure in any of these may severely limit or prevent the common practice of any cell therapy. Success in these areas will trigger the broad applications of these therapies.

The future of transfusion medicine is rapidly becoming more sophisticated and complex with the advances in cell and molecular biology and the implementation of ex vivo cell therapies. Implementation of effective cell therapies will require close collaboration of clinical and basic scientists who will define the new cell therapy approaches, industry which will develop the products that allow the therapy to be practiced in a wide spread and efficient manner, and blood centres and cell processing facilities which will work closely with clinical practitioners and industry to define and implement the cell processing procedures and deliver the final standardized cell product (Figure 2).

Industry relies on both the clinical and basic scientist for novel ideas, innovative science and therapeutic approaches. It also relies on blood banks and cell processing centres for new or practical ideas for new products as well as how to best implement these novel concepts. In this respect, the clinical scientists, blood banks and cell processing centres are the customers for industry, providing input on what products are needed or how to improve the current products to meet their needs and the needs of the patient. The primary drivers for clinical and basic scientists are discovery, innovation, improved patient treatment, publication and research support. For blood centres and cell processing centres, the drive is to deliver safe, efficacious, cost-effective and consistent cell products that meet a high standard. Industry on the other hand has a goal to produce and commercialize new products that support the blood and cell processing industry, improve the quality of patient care, and justify the investment made in research and development. As shown in Figure 2, industry also depends on the clinical scientist and blood centres for evaluation of new products and obtaining data to obtain approval for new products. In addition, industry can also be seen as a source of research support for new ideas that address unmet clinical needs, and lend themselves to commercialization. The blood centres and cell processing centres not only provide a testing site for new products, but are also a primary customer for these new products once they are developed. The blood centre on the other hand has the clinicians and hospitals as its major customer and is the provider of the final cell product. In some centres this may differ with blood banks and cell processing centres playing a much more active role in patient treatment and interfacing with the practicing physician to jointly define the appropriate treatment. All three of these organizations or groups are dependent upon each other and when successful in these interactions have the opportunity to raise the standard of medical practice and efficacy of patient treatment to their mutual benefit and to the benefit of the patient.

Ex vivo cell therapies

All ex vivo cell therapies will likely involve one or more of the following processes: 1) harvest of the primary cells from the patient, 2) selection of the

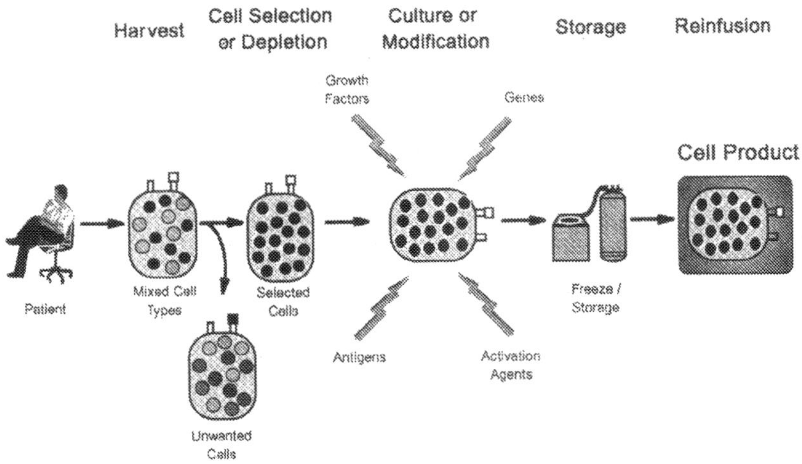

Figure 3. Common steps involved in therapeutic ex vivo cell processing.

appropriate cell type, 3) culture of the cell population, 4) modification of the cell population, and 5) storage of the cell population prior to infusion (Figure 3). These procedures are applicable to almost any ex vivo cell therapy whether it involves haematopoietic stem cells, T cells, or gene therapy. These procedures can be viewed as a manufacturing process with the final cell preparation being the infusible products. In many ways ex vivo cell therapy parallels what is currently done in the blood banking business with red blood cells and platelets, but with more sophisticated technology. The difference is primarily in the ways in which the cells are manipulated. For example, isolated cell populations can be cultured to 1) produce more of the cell population, 2) activated to produce a more efficient therapeutic cell population, or 3) be modified genetically to correct defects or create a cell resistant to infection or drug toxicity. It can be assumed that ultimately the final cell products may be regulated much like the current red cell and platelet cell products, but with different release criteria. Estimates of the overall use of cell therapies including gene therapy indicate that in 10 years there will be nearly 250,000 cell processing procedures per year performed worldwide with the bulk of these involving some aspect of stem cell transplantation.

Safety is a primary issue with cell therapies which will need to be addressed before these cell products become universally accepted and approved. This includes both safety for the patient and safety for the technician performing the process. One aspect that lends itself well to maintaining a safe and sterile cell population and potentially eliminates the need for costly sophisticated clean rooms is the incorporation of closed system technology into the cell manufacturing process. Closed system technology simply refers to the technology that can be incorporated into cell processing that allows the manipulation and transfer of cells from start to finish without breaching the sterile culture or fluid path. Sterile connect technology that allows for this is now available or under development and can potentially be implemented into many cell processing procedures in the future. These procedures could then potentially be done under laminar flow hoods with less stringent clean room requirements.

Cell processing and stem cell transplantation

Although ex vivo cell therapies are not being practiced routinely and are still at the exploratory phase there are many approaches to harvesting and modifying blood and marrow cells for therapeutic use. LAK (lymphokine activated killer cells) and TIL (tumor infiltrating lymphocytes) cell therapies were the forerunners of what will likely be an expanding approach to the treatment of malignancy, infectious disease, autoimmunity and congenital deficiencies. These novel treatments are likely to gain greater acceptance as more is learned about the generation and activity of antigen specific T cells in tumor and infectious disease and technical hurdles in gene therapy are overcome. At this point in time, the best example of cell therapy is bone marrow transplantation. Although this began as a process for simply harvesting and reinfusing marrow into allogeneic recipients with deficient marrow it has evolved into an accepted practice to support the use of high dose chemotherapy. As previously indicated it is anticipated, pending the clinical success of high dose chemotherapy as a treatment for solid tumors, the number of stem cell transplants for this purpose will expand to well over 100,000 per year. The majority of these transplants will likely be done using peripheral blood apheresis products and ultimately may involve both autologous and allogeneic peripheral blood.

In spite of the rapid expansion in the use of stem cell transplantation there still remain a number of issues with processing stem cells that will directly impact the way that transplantation will be performed and the way that cell processing centres will handle and process these cells. Some of these are listed in Table 1 which shows both the issues and potential solutions. One of the primary issues that applies to both autologous stem cell transplantation and allogeneic stem cell transplantation is stem cell purity. In the autologous transplant setting, several studies have demonstrated in patients with solid tumors, that tumor cells can be found in both bone marrow and peripheral blood apheresis products [20-25]. Whether these are clonogenic and capable of forming tumors when reinfused is still not clear. However, data from several laboratories utilizing gene marking and PCR technology have suggested that reinfusion of tumor cells in neuroblastoma patients and lymphoma patients leads to reoccurrence of tumor cell expressing the gene marker [21-26]. In allogeneic transplants the issue of T cell contamination is a problem and can mediate graft vs. host disease. This is complicated further by the fact that some T cells may be required to assure engraftment and that T cells may also be required for a graft versus leukemia effect [27-30]. One potential solution to the problem of contaminating cell populations is to select the population of cells that are responsible for engraftment, namely the CD34$^+$ cell population. This would then eliminate the majority of tumor cells or T cells in the graft. Several technologies have been or are in the process of development to do just this.

Table 1. Clinical/technical issues in stem cell transplantation.

Issue	Potential solution
– Tumor free cells in autologous setting – T cell reduction (GvH) in allogeneic setting	CD 34 cell selection or contaminant depletion
– Stem cell dose – Cell recovery post transplant	Harvest efficiency Culture expansion – stem cells – precursor cells
Open system cell processing	Closed system processing

Magnetic cell separation technology has been developed by Baxter (Isolex® system) and Miltenyi for the selection of CD34 cells based on specific CD34 antibody recognition. A column-based system has been developed by CellPro (Ceprate™) and a flow cytometry system is under development (Systemix). Finally, a flask and panning system for CD34 selection has also been pursued by Applied Immune Science (CELLector™). The Isolex® system and the Ceprate™ system have been utilized extensively in clinical trials world wide and have demonstrated that haematopoietic recovery occurs after transplantation of CD34$^+$ cells with minimal adverse effects. One of the better examples of this is a study by Traycoff et al using the Isolex® system where patients underwent a double stem cell transplant [31]. In these studies, the same patient received either marrow mononuclear cells of selected CD34$^+$ cells on the first transplant and the opposite product for the second transplant. Studies showed that neutrophil and platelet recovery under either scenario were comparable.

One of the primary reasons to do CD34 selection is to reduce contaminating cell populations in the final infusion product. Figure 4 shows a summary of results from several sites demonstrating the selection of CD34 cells with final purities averaging 66.3% for marrow and 90.7% for peripheral blood. This selection provides a significant reduction in T cells which is most apparent with peripheral blood T cells where over a 3 log reduction in T cells delivered to the patients was observed. Similar levels of tumor cell depletion have been observed following CD34$^+$ cell selection. The alternative approach to selection of CD34$^+$ cells is the "removal" of tumor cells or T cells. Such approaches incorporate anti-tumor cell

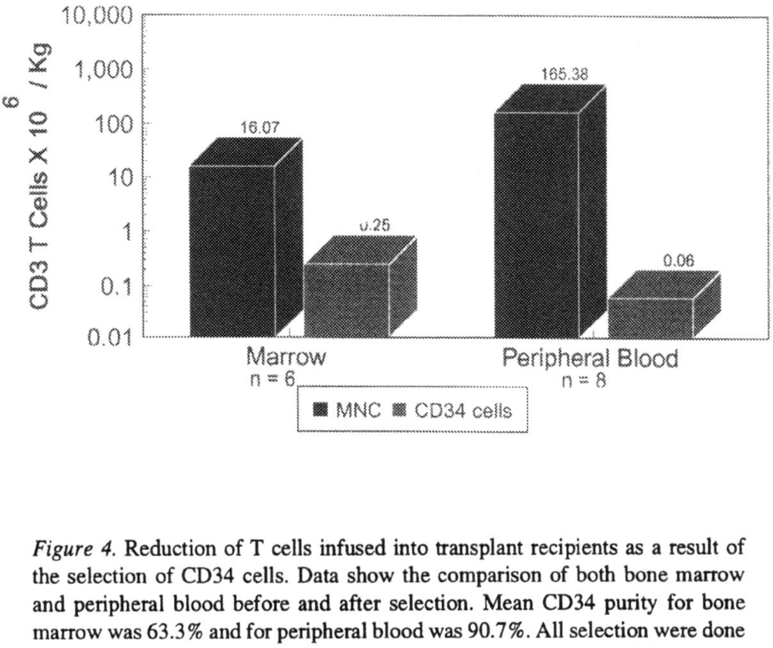

Figure 4. Reduction of T cells infused into transplant recipients as a result of the selection of CD34 cells. Data show the comparison of both bone marrow and peripheral blood before and after selection. Mean CD34 purity for bone marrow was 63.3% and for peripheral blood was 90.7%. All selection were done using the Isolex® 300 magnetic bead based cell selection system with lymphoma or breast cancer patient bone marrow or periopheral blood apheresis products.

or T cell antibodies to either remove cells physically or lyse them with complement. Magnetic bead approaches have been used and are being evaluated in a current European Bone Marrow Transplant group protocol in non-Hodgkin lymphoma [32-34] and for breast cancer cell depletion [22]. Similarly, magnetic and panning techniques have been used to deplete T cells in allogeneic transplants. Depending on the success of these studies, this type of technology or combination of positive selection of CD34 cells and depletion of contaminating cells may ultimately be employed in cell processing centres to deliver tumor free or T cell free $CD34^+$ cell preparations for therapy. In addition, the enrichment of $CD34^+$ cells may also provide a means to isolate target cells to ensure a more efficient gene transfer to appropriate cell in gene therapy procedures.

A second area of stem cell transplantation which may have an impact on transfusion medicine is the area of stem and progenitor cell expansion. Two clinical needs in stem cell transplantation that can potentially be addressed by stem cell cultures include: 1) obtaining enough cells for transplantation in patients where mobilization is poor or marrow is damaged and 2) providing larger numbers of cells of the appropriate lineage and stage of maturation to enhance recovery. The latter is an issue in virtually all transplants since the time for neutrophil and platelet recovery can only be reduced to approximately 8-10 days at best for neutrophils and 12-15 days for platelets [5-7, 35]. This has been the case regardless of how many $CD34^+$ cells or CFU-GM have been returned to the patient or how much G-CSF or GM-CSF is used post infusion [6]. It is believed this threshold is due to the fact that the cells being delivered to the patient are sufficiently immature and that it takes a significant amount of time to divide, mature and appear in the circulation. It is also theorized that if sufficient neutrophil precursors (post-CFU-GM, promyelocytes, myelocytes, etc) can be provided to the patient, that these cells may fill this gap. Studies of cultured cell supplements for stem cell transplantation have been pursued by many investigators [14, 15, 17, 18, 36, 37] and it is clear now that human CD34 cells can be generated under serum free conditions [15, 17, 18]. Studies by Brugger et al [15] have utilized only these culture expanded CD34 cells for transplantation and have shown that neutrophil and platelet recovery times are similar to uncultured mononuclear cells. In our own studies we have developed a serum free culture system to produce a population of predominantly myeloid precursors from $CD34^+$ cells selected from mobilized peripheral blood [17, 18]. These cells have been used as a supplement to peripheral blood mononuclear cells in patients with breast cancer receiving high dose chemotherapy and an autologous peripheral blood stem cell transplant. Phase I studies to date show that the infusion of these cells is without toxicity and that there may be a tendency for more rapid neutrophil recovery in those patients receiving the higher doses of cultured cells (Figure 5). These cultured cells were prepared under totally serum free conditions with PIXY321 (IL3/GM-CSF fusion protein, Immunex, Seattle, Washington) in gas permeable blood bags which are conducive to a standardized process as it may be performed in a cell processing facility. The final cell product after 12 days of culture of $CD34^+$ cells from a single apheresis product produced up to 10^{10} cells containing very high percentages of myelocytes and promyelocytes. This cell product was washed and resuspended in a blood bag much like any other transfusion product. We can anticipate that gene therapy approaches using $CD34^+$ cells will require similar cell processing and culture, although procedures may be a little more complex given the need for gene transduction. However, the final cell product again will be a blood cell transfusion product and ultimately will likely have to meet at least the requirements now applied to other transfusion products.

The final issue for cell processing is that of safety. The manipulation required in processing and culturing cells for cell therapy is a level of complexity higher than that currently required for platelet and red cell processing. As ex vivo gene therapy evolves, the level of complexity increases even further. As the degree of cell manipulation increases, the potential for contamination of the cell product also increases. This is turn triggers a need for a highly controlled environment to accommodate the level of complexity. This has been addressed primarily by the use of clean rooms for cell processing procedures. Some of the need for expensive clean room facilities may be reduced by advances in closed system technology and instrumentation which will allow the technician to manipulate and transfer cells and fluid and sterile conditions without exposure to the outside. As we look to the future we can anticipate that there will be a greater emphasis on cell processing and hence a greater need to develop the technology to do so under safe, efficient, and cost effective conditions.

Future of transfusion medicine and blood centres

Although we anticipate that the need for red cells, plasma and platelets will not disappear, it is clear that there may be a new role for centres that have the capabilities and skills to handle and deliver the next generation of cell products. As shown in Figure 6, cell processing laboratories will evolve as the therapies evolve. At this point in time the primary demand for cell therapies will be mononuclear cells for transplantation. These may come from bone marrow or peripheral blood, but will require standardized procedures of harvesting,

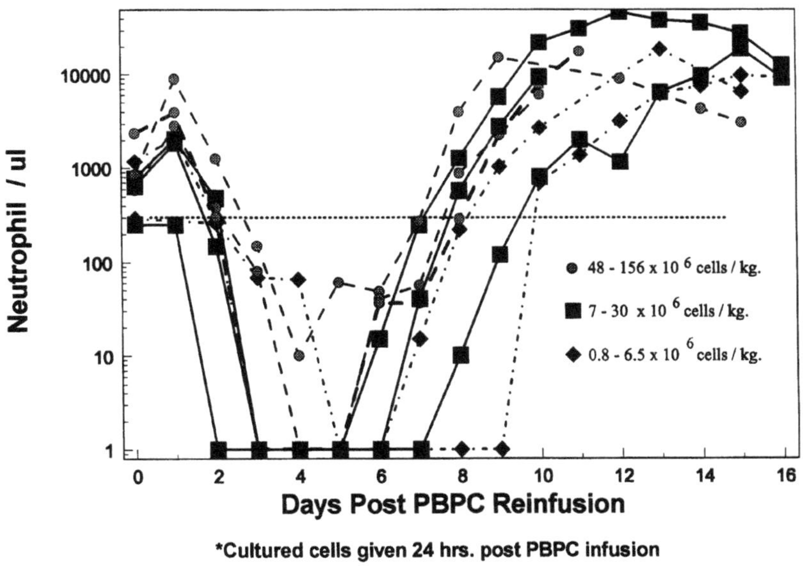

Figure 5. Neutrophil recovery following peripheral blood stem cell transplantation supplemented by infusion of 12 day cultured CD34 cells to produce committed neutrophil progeny. Data show recovery with different concentrations of culture derived neutrophil progenitors. CD34 cells were cultured for 12 days under serum free conditions with PIXY321 to stimulate growth and differentiation of CD34 cells down the neutrophil pathway. Historical controls show recovery of neutrophils at an average of 10 days to 500 neutrophils. Peripheral blood mononuclear cells were given 48 hours after high dose chemotherapy withcultured neutrophil precursors delivered 24 hours later. Details are presented elsewhere [17, 18].

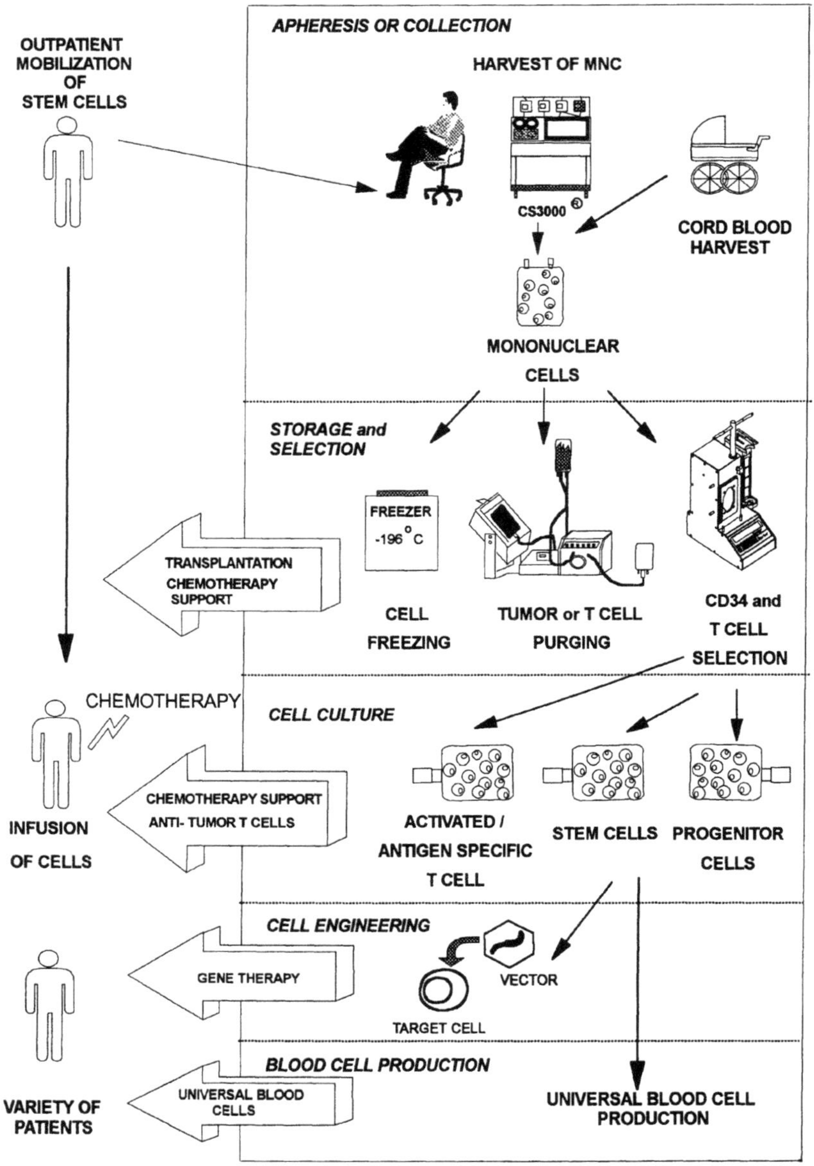

Figure 6. Future of cell processing centres. The various types of cell processing that are being done or will likely be done in the future.

processing and storage. There has also been a trend toward using neonatal cord blood cells for transplantation [38-41]. Although this is still an experimental procedure with less than 100 transplants done at this time, significant resources are being put into developing cord blood banks for allogeneic transplantation [38,

39]. If these cells prove to be more effective than other sources of stem cells and show reduces graft vs host disease and if the limited sample size can be overcome by cell culture, this approach to transplantation may become a valid alternative.

As we look to the future, the next level of sophistication for cell processing and ex vivo cell therapy will rely on cell selection (Figure 6). Instruments are being developed that will allow for safe and efficient selection of various cell populations. Although the emphasis has been on $CD34^+$ cells, it is anticipated that other cell types with therapeutic value will evolve. The most likely candidate will be T cells which can be used for graft vs. tumor, infectious disease applications, or replenishment of T cells in T cell deficiency diseases such as AIDS. Although much of this work is experimental it can be assumed that at least a few of these novel therapies will make their way into common practice. The next level of sophistication in cell processing that is rapidly approaching reality is the ex vivo expansion of cells for therapeutic use. Both stem cells and T cells fall into this category and many of the requirements for final cell product release will be the same although the nature of the cell product and the growth conditions and manufacturing process to produce such cells may differ substantially. Following the use of cultured cells, genetically engineered cell processing will likely be implemented into cell processing centres. Criteria for release of these cell products and the requirements and guidelines for using viral vectors are still evolving. Ultimately, when this technology becomes common practice, release criteria and standardized procedures for production of the final cell product will need to be in place. The ultimate advance in transfusion medicine, namely the in vitro production of universal blood cells is still far off and it will likely be many years before these cells can be generated in vitro cost-effectively and in sufficient quantity to make them competitive with blood products produced in vivo and simply harvested and processed. At some point, however, with significant technical breakthroughs, this may ultimately become possible, again changing the nature of blood banking and cell processing.

References

1. Farese AM, Hunt P, Boone T, MacVittie TJ. Recombinant human megakaryocyte growth and development factor stimulates thrombocytopoiesis in normal primates. Blood 1995;86:54-9.
2. Lok SI, Kaushansky K, Holly RD, et al. Cloning and expression of murine thrombopoietin cDNA and stimulation of platelet production in vivo. Nature 1995;369:565-68.
3. De Sauvage FJ, Hass PE, Spencer SD, et al. Stimulation of megakaryocytopoiesis and thrombopoiesis by the c-Mpl ligand. Nature 1994;369:533-38.
4. Kaushansky K, Lok S, Holly RD, et al. Promotion of megakaryocyte progenitor expansion and differentiation by the c-Mpl ligand thrombopoietin. Nature 1994;369:568-70.
5. Ho AD, Gluck S, Germond C, et al. Optimal timing for collections of blood progenitor cells following induction chemotherapy and granulocyte-macrophage colony-stimulating factor for autologous transplantation in advanced breast cancer. Leukemia 1993;7:1738-46.

6. Bender JG, To LB, Williams S, Schwartzberg LS. Defining a therapeutic dose of peripheral blood stem cells. J Hematother 1992;1:329-41.
7. Dreger P, Marquardt P, Haferlach T, et al. Effective mobilisation of peripheral blood progenitor cells with 'Dexa-BEAM' and G-CSF: Timing of harvesting and composition of the leukapheresis product. Br J Cancer 1993;68:950-57.
8. Uyl-de Groot CA, Ossenkoppele GJ, van Riet AAPM, Rutten FFH. The costs of peripheral blood progenitor cell reinfusion mobilised by granolocyte colony-stimulating factor following high dose melphalan as compared with conventional therapy in multiple myeloma. Eur J Cancer 1994;30A:457-59.
9. Faucher C, le Corroller AG, Blaise D, et al. Comparison of G-CSF-primed peripheral blood progenitor cells and bone marrow auto transplantation: Clinical assessment and cost-effectiveness. Bone Marrow Transplant 1994;14:895-901.
10. Körbling M, Przepiorka D, Huh YO, et al. Allogeneic blood stem cell transplantation for refractory leukemia and lymphoma: Potential advantage of blood over marrow allografts. Blood 1995;85:1659-65.
11. Bensinger WI, Weaver CH, Appelbaum FR, et al. Transplantation of allogeneic peripheral blood stem cells mobilized by recombinant human granulocyte colony-stimulating factor. Blood 1995;85:1655-58.
12. Schmitz N, Dreger P, Suttorp M, et al. Primary transplantation of allogeneic peripheral blood progenitor cells mobilized by filgrastim (granulocyte colony-stimulating factor). Blood 1995;85:1666-72.
13. Kessler DA, Siegel JP, Noguchi PD, Zoon KC, Feiden KL, Woodcock J. Regulation of somatic-cell therapy and gene therapy by the food and drug administration. N Engl J Med 1993;329:1169-73.
14. Williams SF, Bender JG, Zimmerman T, et al. Selection and expansion of $CD34^+$ cells: Their clinical utility for the treatment of cytopenias. Bone Marrow Transplant 1995;15(Suppl 2):S41[Abstract].
15. Brugger W, Heimfeld S, Berenson RJ, Mertelsmann R, Kanz L. Reconstitution of hematopoiesis after high-dose chemotherapy by autologous progenitor cells generated ex vivo. N Engl J Med 191995;333:283-87.
16. Koller MR, Bender JG, Miller WM, Papoutsakis ET. Expansion of primitive human hematopoietic progenitors in a perfusion bioreactor system with IL-3, IL-6, and stem cell factor. Bio/Technology 1993;11:358-63.
17. Zimmerman T, Williams SF, Bender JG, et al. Clinical use of selected and expanded peripheral blood $CD34^+$ cells: A preliminary report of feasibility and safety. J Hematother 1995;4:527-29.
18. Bender JG, Zimmerman T, Lee WJ, et al. Large scale selection of $CD34^+$ cells and expansion of neutrophil precursors in PIXY321 for clinical application. Blood 1994;84: 542a[Abstract].
19. O'Shaughnessy JA, Cowan KH, Nienhuis AW, et al. Retroviral mediated transfer of the human multidrug resistance gene (MDR-1) into hematopoietic stem cells during autologous transplantation after intensive chemotherapy for metastatic breast cancer. Hum Gene Ther 1994;5:891-911.
20. Simpson SJ, Vachula M, Kennedy MJ, et al. Detection of tumor cells in the bone marrow, peripheral blood, and apheresis products of breast cancer patients using flow cytometry. Exp Hematol 1995;23:1062-68.
21. Brenner MK, Rill DR, Moen RC, et al. Gene-marking to trace origin of relapse after autologous bone-marrow transplantation. Lancet 1993;341:85-6.
22. Shpall EJ, Bast RC, Joines WT, et al. Immunomagnetic purging of breast cancer from

bone marrow for autologous transplantation. Bone Marrow Transplant 1991;7:145-51.
23. Brugger W, Bross KJ, Glatt M, Weber F, Mertelsmann R, Kanz L. Mobilization of tumor cells and hematopoietic progenitor cells into peripheral blood of patients with solid tumors. Blood 1994;83:636-40.
24. Moss TJ, Sanders DG, Lasky LC, Bostrom B. Contamination of peripheral blood stem cell harvests by circulating neuroblastoma cells. Blood 1990;76:1879-83.
25. Craig JIO, Langlands K, Parker AC, Antony RS. Molecular detection of tumor contamination in peripheral blood stem cell harvests. Exp Hematol 1994;22:898-902.
26. Gribben JG, Freedman AS, Neuberg D, et al. Immunologic purging of marrow assessed by PCR before autologous bone marrow transplantation for B-cell lymphoma. N Engl J Med 1991;325:1525-33.
27. Butturini A, Gale RP. Clinical trials of T-cell depletion: Current controversies, future directions. Bone Marrow Transplant 1989:495-509.
28. Kolb H, Mittermuller J, Clemm C, et al. Donor leukocyte transfusions for treatment of recurrent chronic myelogenous leukemia in marrow transplant patients. Blood 1990;76:2462-65.
29. Frassoni F, Fagioli F, Sessarego M, et al. The effect of donor leucocyte infusion in patients with leukemia following allogeneic bone marrow transplantation. Exp Hematol 1992;20:712a[Abstract].
30. Porter D, Roth M, McGarigle C, Ferrara J, Antin J. Induction of graft-versus-host disease as immunotherapy for relapsed chronic myeloid leukemia. N Engl J Med 1994;330:100-6.
31. Traycoff CM, Broun ER, Burgess J, et al. Evaluation of the hematopoietic potential of CD34 enriched autologous bone marrow grafts prepared with the Baxter Isolex 300. Exp Hematol 1994;22:824[Abstract].
32. Straka C, Drexler E, Mitterer M, et al. Autotransplantation of B-cell purged peripheral blood progenitor cells in B-cell lymphoma. Lancet 1995;345:797-98.
33. Dreger P, von Neuhoff N, Suttorp M, Loffler H, Schmitz N. Rapid engraftment of peripheral blood progenitor cell grafts purged with B cell-specific monoclonal antibodies and immunomagnetic beads. Bone Marrow Transplant 1995;16:627-29.
34. Kvalheim G, Jakobsen E, Holte H, et al. Autologous bone marrow transplantation of non-Hodgkin's lymphoma patients with marrow purged using immunomagnetic beads. Adv Bone Marrow Purging/Processing: Fourth Intl Symp 1994:133-38.
35. Wodinsky HB, Dillman RO, MacDonald SA. Assessing peripheral blood stem cell transplant technology. J Oncol Manage 1994:22-7.
36. Smith SL, Bender JG, Maples PB, et al. Expansion of neutrophil precursors and progenitors in suspension cultures of $CD34^+$ cells enriched from human bone marrow. Exp Hematol 1993;21:870-77.
37. Haylock DN, To LB, Dowse TL, Juttner CA, Simmons PJ. Ex vivo expansion and maturation of peripheral blood $CD34^+$ cells into the myeloid lineage. Blood 1992; 80:1405-12.
38. McCullough J, Clay ME, Fautsch S, et al. Proposed policies and procedures for the establishment of a cord blood bank. Blood Cells 1994;20:609-26.
39. Rubinstein P, Rosenfield RE, Adamson JW, Stevens CE. Stored placental blood for unrelated bone marrow reconstitution. Blood 1993;81:1679-90.
40. Gluckman E, Broxmeyer HE, Auerbach AD, et al. Hematopoietic reconstitution in a patient with Fanconi's anemia by means of umbilical cord blood from an HLA-identical sibling. N Engl J Med 1989;321:1174-78.

41. Wagner JE, Broxmeyer HE, Byrd RL, et al. Transplantation of umbilical cord blood after myeloablative therapy: Analysis of engraftment. Blood 1992;79:1874-81.

DISCUSSION

J.Th.M. de Wolf and W.G. Murphy – moderators

K. Sazama (Philadelphia, PA, USA): Dr. Snyder, in reviewing your practices for audits a couple of points strike me and I wonder if you could address them specifically. The first is that in the US for accrediting organizations we have a new requirement to look for the possibility of underutilization of blood. I just wondered if you could say a word or two about what you are doing with respect to establishing a monitoring of that kind of activity.

E.L. Snyder (New Haven, CT, USA): Well, we are not actively looking at underutilization. We would need to reconsider the way we would determine underutilization. An adverse outcome would have to be called to our attention and be part of the investigation to look at underutilization. You have to turn the system around a little bit to do that, but we have not started doing that yet.

K. Sazama: A second observation to which you may or may not choose to respond that we have a lot of system support in place for responding to the request. It seems to me that in the current situation of blood transfusion it may be useful to prospectively define what the need probably should be, and then we can use our systems of monitoring to ensure that requests are actually following the scheme. Let us use as example, identifying the groups of patients who might be eligible for leukoreduction. One can establish the prospective nature of what the audits are going to be based on the real need for the component that you have, and then establish your review or audit practice to be concurrent and/or in accordance with that policy. I am wondering if those kind of practices are what you put in place: you start first by saying to the clinicians, "These are the components we ought be using because we know that every red cell is not like every other red cell, and every patient's need is not like every other patient's need". Start first by establishing which the policy should be with respect to some of these components and then do your audit to see if it is concurrent with that.

E.L. Snyder: What dr. Sazama is describing is really moving towards this total quality plan that we talked about, I guess that it sort of incorporates ISO 9001 concepts of planning quality at the beginning. The answer to your question is no, we do not do that. We are reactive. We would find the problem and then investigate it. In order for us to do what you are saying, we would need to have a person whose job it would be to prospectively plan to do quality audits of patients before there is a problem, to identify an issue – this used to be called "looking for trouble" – but that is not called that any more, it is now called ISO 9001. You go out and you prospectively audit knowing what you are looking for seeing if the practices fit in that guideline and if it does not change your practices to fit into what you think should be a good outcome. Dr. Sazama is one of the leaders in this field and what she basically is asking me is how far along are we. We are not that far along for a major medical centre. We should be doing more, we are going to have to be doing more. I welcome this kind of a conference because it brings to all of our attention how much further we have to go. Not only am I talking about triggers, but we are talking about targeting appropriate blood component use which is a new concept for us. The points that dr. Sazama has raised are excellent. While you were talking for the second question I figured out how we would do the first one, which is doing prospective checks for undertransfusion. The way we would do that is we could look for patients who have haematocrits under 22% or platelet counts under 10,000/μl or whatever and if they were not transfused, find out why not.

P.V. Holland (Sacramento, CA, USA): I have another question for dr. Snyder, actually a combination of two. Dr. Snyder, you showed that over 6 or 7 years the use of red cells, platelets, and fresh frozen plasma has been remarkably stable; yet you also told us you are adding programs and doing more things; so my two questions are: 1) do you think your process is bringing down the average utilization; and 2) how come your blood bill is 600,000 dollars a year more?

E.L. Snyder: Well, our audit practices have been not so wonderful I will admit, but that is not why we are over budget; I was raised basically as a haematologist transfusion specialist and I did not go to business school which I am now being held accountable for. Recently at our hospital we added a new childrens hospital, increased the OR-capacity by 20%, started a programme for peripheral stem cells, bone marrow, liver and pancreas transplantations etc. and let helicopters land on our roof, so we are now a class I trauma centre. However, at the time, we did not increase our blood bank budget for blood products as a cost of doing business and I am now being held accountable. That is what the 600,000 dollars came from. We are over our budget and my administrators want me to explain why that is happening. There is a combination of things which I am now beginning to understand; how to go about evaluating that there was an increase in the number of patients transfused so our turnover gets faster, there was an increase in component usage, there is more to it than just some degree of overutilization; some degree of increased need, some degree of increased costs and inflation and expanded services. We have for example a patient with an antibody to FVIII who walked into the hospital and needed porcine factor; there was 95,000 dollars of cost on our budget in it for one month alone; she now will use 200,000 dollars so there is a third of the 600,000 for this year. Those kind of things will require a full court effort on the blood bank's part. We are no longer a simple transfusion service, we are now becoming a quality assurance effort and that is hard for a hospital transfusion service to do but we are going to try; ask me back next year and maybe I will have come up with the answers.

C.Th. Smit Sibinga (Groningen, NL): A question to prof. Vlek, but he unfortunately left. I guess dr. Macpherson might be able at least to comment on what I was going to say. Prof. Vlek, by the end of his presentation came to a list of various aspects in relation to the risk taking and ended up with the donor risk taking and the patient risk taking. Actually the most important in between part is the doctor risk taking. You spoke about that in terms of communication and the patient physicians obligations. Could you dr. Macpherson elaborate a little on what to your opinion should be the elements then of the doctor's risk taking aspects against the background of your considerations in terms of the ethics, because you gave three mechanisms: the paternalism, the autonomy of the patients' wishes and family decision. Now I think there is a fourth one and that is that communication between the patient and the physician as well as the communication on the background between the blood bank and the physician to really put the risk in the right perception before you start counselling.

C. Macpherson (Cincinnati, OH, USA): I think the major problem in most of cases is a lack of understanding of where the family and the patient are coming from and what the attitude of the hospital staff is. I think what needs to be done is to facilitate the interchange between them. An obligation of the blood bank physician would arise only if the blood bank was specifically involved with some procedure. Does that answer your question?

C.Th. Smit Sibinga: More or less, because in the information which I think the physician supposedly is going to provide to the patient to come to the right decision, definitely there is the subjectivity of the doctor's own perception of risk. We come occasionally to the discussion with physicians that their perception of the risk is quite close to the perception of the public by enlarge. So not that far from the left hand side of dr. Holland's model which showed that huge area of wrong perception with relation to the actual safety of blood as compared to the actual risk as it stands at this point of time. That, I think is something to be addressed.

C. Macpherson: The discrepancy between the perception of risk and the reality of risk? I do not have any simple answer to that question. It was much better answered by prof. Vlek who talked about the psychological aspects. I think we, as blood bank physicians, do get into those situations, but unfortunately we are not trained to handle that kind of negotiation with a patient. This is one of the things that we are trying to learn how to do. The perception that there should be zero risk is what we try to correct much of the time. The patient says there should not be any risk, and so does the family. We try to give them the numbers that define what the risk is, but they often do not understand them. We have had a number of patients in that type of setting, and when we have been able to reach some kind of settlement, it has been because some member of the hospital staff has established a relationship with the patient and usually with the family as well. Just by keeping on talking to the patient and family day after day you begin to create the idea that maybe their first perception was not valid. This is not easy to do, nor to explain.

C.Th. Smit Sibinga: Dr. van Epps, I was a bit surprised actually by your scheme for the future. Do you really think the developments in the direction you outlined are supposedly going to happen. Three separate circles: the separate circle of the clinical and the basic scientist investments, the industry in the middle, that is the core, and then you had the blood bank and the cell processing laboratories. I think actually that should be an overlapping trias of circles, because they cannot function separately.

D. van Epps (Roundlake, IL, USA): I agree with you one hundred percent. The depiction of three separate circles is probably more functional for presentation than it is the reality of the way the interaction actually takes place. It is a trias and there have to be close interactions between each of the three groups. Ultimately, the final customer of the blood bank is going to be the clinician. The final customer for the industry is going to be the blood bank. By the time I put all those connecting lines in the diagram became so complex that I tried to make it simple by depicting three groups with interconnecting lines rather than a trias.

C.Th. Smit Sibinga: But after all our perceptions match.

K. Sazama: Dr. ten Duis, it was of interest to see your groups of patients and the different haemoglobin levels at which they were discharged. In at least two of those groups the patients would have been eligible for autologous donations at least in the US. Apparently that is not the usual practice or not a common practice in Europe, in the Netherlands.

H.J. ten Duis (Groningen, NL): Well, it is a very interesting question. The amount of blood that has been lost by those patients is limited, so the amount will vary between 500 ml and may be 1 litre. In my academical thesis[1] 10 years ago I investigated the effect of the aspiration of blood and the shear stresses between the air and blood. You never have a clean field to operate so if you have to aspirate blood with a high velocity enormous shear stresses on your blood cells are encountered. The quality of the blood that you will transfuse in those cases is bad; we measured the survival in these cells which was about 2 or 3 days. So if you want to safe your red cells you have to aspirate them from below the

1. H.J. ten Duis. Intraoperative autotransfusion. The effects on blood elements in dogs. Drukkerij van Denderen BV, Groningen 1982.

surface of a pool of blood like in the peritoneal cavity. Never aspirate from a tissue surface where you have to operate on because you will damage your red cells tremendously.

K. Sazama: But how about normovolaemic haemodilution techniques (you could just deliberately collect the unit of blood at the very onset of the procedure, a unit or two) where you would have no shear stress on the red cells?

H.J. ten Duis: Yes, we do that in our major operations, trauma operations where we expect a blood loss of between 1,5-2 litres. We perform a normal haemodilution procedure and retransfuse the blood at the end of the operation. That is correct, but not in these patients presented.

K. Sazama: Not in the hips?

H.J. ten Duis: Not in the hips. Well, these are very old patients, super eighty's I call them, but we do that in the orthopaedic operations when they are a little bit younger; yes, that is correct.

E.L. Snyder: One brief comment to expand on what dr. Smit Sibinga said. I think the concern I had with the model that dr. van Epps showed was, that it showed the blood bank as separate from the clinician and basic scientist. Our profession is more than just a trade association. In order to survive as we move into the future as dr. van Epps has I think accurately predicted, we need the first circle as well as the third circle. We need the clinicians, we need to get out of the laboratory, out of the transfusion service and get on the ward to interact with the clinicians just to and get on the ward to interact with the clinicians just to survive as an organization. We need to become more clinically oriented and to do more patient care activities, so that we can contribute to industry not just being the beverage distributor, as I refer to transfusion services euphemistically, but actually getting out there and seeing patients. If we want to survive we need to change not just doing pharmaceutical quality control and quality programmes but doing patient care as well.

IV. EVALUATION AND FEED-BACK OF TRANSFUSION POLICIES

EVALUATION OF BEDSIDE TRANSFUSION PRACTICE: BENEFITS VS RISKS

R.S. Eisenstaedt

Introduction

Decisions about blood transfusion are made analogously to those of other medical intervention: benefits are compared to risks; safer alternatives to homologous blood, such as autologous blood or drugs as desmopressin or aprotinin that might reduce the risk of avoiding transfusion are assessed, as well. Such decisions may be analyzed on a global level by public health officials or outcomes assessment experts examining regional or national trends, mean number of transfusions per population, or rates of reported complications [1-4]. Transfusion decisions may also be reviewed by hospital committees studying variation in component use among physicians or the trigger at which different doctors are apt to transfuse patients [5, 6]. But most often transfusion decisions are made and ultimately assessed by doctors at the bedside, working with the short-term data at hand in their effort to interpret benefits and risks of blood administration. In this chapter, that bedside perspective of transfusion decision making will be examined and the biases that might distort the logic reviewed.

Transfusion benefits: RBC

The obvious benefit of red cell transfusion is augmentation of blood oxygen content and, presumably, enhanced oxygen delivery. Several important issues complicate the process. First, the presumption that enhanced oxygen content produces enhanced delivery may not be uniformly correct. During and shortly after transfusion stored red cells are deficient in 2-3 DPG and, thus, less efficient in delivering oxygen to peripheral tissue [7, 8]. Stored erythrocytes are also less deformable and, thus, less efficient in navigating the tortuous microcirculation traversed in delivering oxygen on a tissue or cellular level [9]. Finally, the increased blood viscosity following transfusion may negate the benefit of enhanced oxygen content by slowing circulation. In reality, it is difficult to actually measure oxygen delivery and even more difficult to assess uptake and consumption on a cellular level. Pathophysiological features seen in some sick patients receiving blood further complicate the analysis. Using indirect measures Marik and Sibbald have concluded that splanchnic oxygen delivery in septic patients did not improve following transfusion - in fact, it worsened when blood stored for more than 15 days was transfused [10]. They and others [11] further showed that transfusing red cells did not produce measurable increase in systemic oxygen uptake in patients with sepsis or respiratory failure.

Second, a variety of adaptive responses to anaemia, including increased cardiac output, increased red cell 2-3 DPG, decreased blood viscosity, and vasodilatation serve to protect oxygen delivery despite decreased oxygen content [12-15].

The in vivo relevance of such adaptation is well demonstrated in animals [16] and, less directly, in people. Studies in patients whose religious conviction precluded transfusion [17], pregnant women [18], pediatric patients undergoing heart surgery [19], or patients with bleeding ulcer [20] showed tolerance for moderate to severe anaemia without excess mortality. Though reassuring, these data must be interpreted that:

- many anaemic patients lack the ability to adapt, perhaps because of underlying cardiac disease or because anaemia is occurring too rapidly;
- there are other criteria to consider in interpreting anaemia impact other than mortality, per se. Wound healing, exercise capacity and length of hospital stay are all parameters that could be meaningfully impacted by blood transfusion.

That said, Stehling and Simon in their review suggest that clinical studies to date have not been useful in defining transfusion triggers based on those measures of morbidity [21]. Welch and colleagues have published an excellent review of the physiologic response to anaemia and the role of blood transfusion [22].

The difficulty in translating oxygen content into oxygen delivery and the difficulty in assessing the cut off at which falling oxygen delivery meaningfully impairs tissue or cellular functions have typically led clinicians to discard these parameters in their bedside transfusion practice. Instead, clinicians have tuned to the measure at hand, oxygen content, or more specifically the haemoglobin concentration or haematocrit in making red cell transfusion decisions. In the process they have historically overemphasized the relevance of falling haemoglobin without acknowledging the adaptive response to anaemia and, thus, been too liberal in selecting a haematocrit transfusion trigger that, in reality, did not warrant intervention.

The adagium that patients undergoing general anaesthesia require at least 10 grams of haemoglobin to avoid perioperative morbidity has been disproved. Experts have concluded that many patients will tolerate preoperative haemoglobin concentrations of 7 grams without ill consequence [23]. At the same time, there are select patients who remain transfusion candidates at that 10 gram level and some others who, conceivably, need even higher haemoglobin concentration.

Those patients where anaemia adaption is unlikely to be successful fall into several categories:

- patients whose active bleeding, especially active bleeding that is not readily controlled, may lead to further fall in haemoglobin content steeply enough to overwhelm adaptive compensation;

- patients with myocardial disease unable to increase cardiac output in response to anaemia;
- patients with coronary artery disease, cerebrovascular disease, sepsis and other conditions where the heart, the brain and other vital processes may be more dependent on maintaining adequate oxygen content.

Current practice guidelines discourage making decisions solely on the basis of the haemoglobin and haematocrit and instead interpret that number in the context of other clinical data, including: age, known end organ dysfunction, sepsis, and, with acute or chronic blood loss whether the cause of bleeding is identified and under control or readily able to be controlled. Some investigators have encouraged invasive monitoring to calculate oxygen extraction ratio and mixed venous oxygen tension to assist in determining transfusion needs [24].

When focusing on the haemoglobin concentration and additional supportive clinical data there are actually two relevant transfusion triggers to identify. The first is the ideal haemoglobin concentration to avoid even remotely possible anaemia related morbidity. The second is the minimally acceptable haemoglobin below which adverse outcomes are all too readily predictable. The difference between the two rests with the toxicity or risk of transfusion intervention. Were the transfusion absolutely free of risk the second trigger would rise to become indistinguishable from the first. But, of course, transfusions do have toxicity that compete with their clinical benefit and that must be acknowledged in transfusion decision making.

Transfusion risks: RBC

The complications from blood transfusion can be classified in a variety of ways, but from the perspective of bedside decision making the most logical scheme clarifies acute problems that occur within the same timeframe as the transfusion versus those which are delayed in onset.

Acute transfusion reactions include: ABO incompatibility and acute haemolysis, febrile or other non-red cell directed immune reactions, contamination of the blood leading to acute bacterial infection, and volume overload. A variety of additional adverse reactions have been linked to massively bleeding patients requiring large volumes of blood [25]. These include hypocalcaemia, respiratory distress, coagulopathy, and hypothermia. These latter complications are, with the exception of hypocalcaemia, more related to the underlying problems necessitating massive transfusion than to the blood, per se. The other acute complications of transfusion are either quite rare, i.e. 1:600,000 for ABO incompatibility [26], or generally innocuous, as with febrile transfusion reactions. Thus, doctors gauging transfusion toxicity by what they actually observe during and immediately following the event are likely to be overly reassured of its safety. This "availability" heuristic biases clinical decision making by attaching greater value to most recent experience [27]. At the same time doctors are likely to underestimate the impact of delayed complications. Some of those adverse events may not seem directly linked to the transfusion, as with increased perioperative infection in transfused patients or increased colon cancer recurrence in patients transfused during primary resection [28]. Other complications may not be detected for years or even decades following the transfusion, as with HIV or hepatitis. This lack of appreciation for the magnitude and severity of these delayed problems leads to a flawed bedside assessment of transfusion risks. Like the traditional tendency at the bedside to overestimate the relevance of a falling haemoglobin and undervalue compensatory mechanisms to maintain oxygen delivery, the perception of unimpressive transfusion toxicity when witnessed from the bedside would also lead to excessive transfusion.

There are two additional points of importance in assessing bedside transfusion risks. First is that the blood transfused today is clearly safer than it was a decade ago and, probably, safer than it was in the pre-HIV era [29]. The progress in reducing transfusion HIV through better donor screening and the dramatic steps to decrease the far more common problem of post-transfusion hepatitis (PTH) have undoubtedly modified the decision making algorithm. Assuming that the inherent benefit of transfusion has remained constant, as elusive as that benefit may be to measure, decreased transfusion risks should clearly ratchet upward the transfusion trigger toward that aforementioned idealized haemoglobin level and away from the second, "minimally acceptable" standard. This concept in bedside decision making is important and worth clarifying further.

Consider bedside decision making when transfusing autologous red cells. These products are inherently safer than homologous blood by virtue of their avoiding transmission of virus infection or inciting immunological reactions [30]. Whatever haemoglobin level would trigger intervention when considering homologous blood risks versus benefit in any given patient would clearly be adjusted upward, i.e. earlier transfusion intervention, if that blood component were a safer auto logous unit. At the same time autologous blood transfusion is not devoid of risks. Clerical errors may result in the wrong unit being administered. Volume overload is equally apt to occur with autologous as homologous blood in any given patient. The red cell storage defects of 2-3 DPG and deformability are identical. That some risks remain, albeit at a much lower magnitude than for homologous blood, requires that there still be some space between the ideal haemoglobin concentration and the haemoglobin triggering transfusion, but the difference becomes much smaller as those transfusion risks decrease. That same principle applies whether the transfusion risks decreases at a set time because a safer autologous component is transfused or whether the risk decreases over time because of better donor screening when the same type of component is administered.

A second tenant in assessing transfusion risks involves acknowledging and interpreting the dynamic nature of those complications. That dynamic perspective is similar to how benefits are viewed, changing from patient to patient and, over time, within the same patient. Transfusion complications are traditionally viewed as more fixed events with finite statistical probabilities that may be generically applied. That premise is logical when viewing some complication, like the risk of ABO incompatibility. However, even that seemingly static event is more likely to hurt a patient who is blood type O, A or B than one who is type AB and is, questionably, more apt to occur when any individual patient is transfused in certain settings, an operating room, an ICU, or an emergency room.

The dynamic nature of some other complications is more readily discerned. While volume overload and pulmonary oedema can occur in any transfusion recipient if the I's and O's are imprecisely monitored, it is more likely to occur when chronically anaemic patients with pre-existing heart disease are given blood.

The dynamic features of post-transfusion hepatitis may not, at first glance, be so easily recognized. Indeed, the incidence of post-transfusion hepatitis seems fairly fixed, and it may be that the probabilities of subsequent chronic liver disease and cirrhosis also remain fairly constant. But what is not constant but highly variably is the ultimate impact of this complication in transfusion recipients. That dynamic variable helps to explain one of the most vexing uncertainties in transfusion medicine: the clinical significance of post-transfusion hepatitis. On the one hand the incidence of this complication is appreciable even if dramatically decreased in recent years, 10% in 1980, 1% in 1990, lower still in 1995. At least half of those with initial infection develop chronic hepatitis and most of those with chronic hepatitis have liver pathology that suggests likely progression to cirrhosis [31]. But on the other hand there seems to be far fewer transfusion recipients dying of cirrhosis than the epidemiology would suggest. In the best study to date that has critically examined this issue Seeff and colleagues studies more than 1500 transfused patients, of whom 568 had post-transfusion hepatitis. After 18 years of follow-up, overall survival of those with hepatitis was no different than that of recipients who escaped this complication [32].

Two additional principles help explain the paradox. First, the general population receiving blood products are sick with underlying problems that independent of transfusion limit their survival. The controls in Seeff's study who did not develop hepatitis still died more than a decade prematurely. Second, the cirrhosis that ultimately evolves from chronic PTH is an insidious, slowly progressive problem, requiring 1-2 decades for clinical expression. In that timeframe an 18 year follow-up may be too short to detect a notable impact. Indeed, Seeff did note a significant increase in liver related mortality (3.3 vs. 1.5%, $p = 0.03$) in patients with chronic PTH.

The dynamic nature of PTH should have a major impact on bedside transfusion decision making. In elderly patients or those with serious underlying morbidity not apt to be readily reversed by transfusion or any other therapy there is far less likelihood that they will survive the 10 to 20 years needed for PTH and cirrhosis to influence their lives. The decreased cost of intervention argues for more liberal transfusion trigger intervention. These patients are often the same people whose difficulty in adapting to anaemia pathophysiology likewise justifies a lower transfusion threshold. On the other hand, young patients and especially those whose need for transfusion arises from a reversible problem might anticipate lengthy survival in the absence of additional complications. For these patients death from PTH and cirrhosis 20 years later might still result in many lost years of expected life. The additional weight that should be added to the cost of that complication requires more cautious transfusion intervention. That conservative approach is, again, reinforced by younger and otherwise healthier patients being more tolerant adapting to anaemia.

Transfusion decisions: Platelets

Decision making for platelet transfusion is, at first glance, less complicated than for erythrocytes. The primary indication for platelet transfusion is to restore effective haemostasis and prevent bleeding in patient with thrombocytopenia or, less often, qualitative platelet defects. The difficulty in equating haemoglobin concentration with oxygen delivery and oxygen extraction is no longer an issue, but the 2 analogous challenges are (1) determining what factors beyond the platelet count, per se, contribute to bleeding in an individual patients and (2) assessing whether the witnessed bleeding in a patients is proportionate and directly attributable to tissue trauma or excessive because of faulty platelets. In the bedside assessment of platelet transfusion most scrutiny has been focused on two decisions: platelet support during cardiovascular surgery and prophylactic transfusion in patients at risk of bleeding because of severe thrombocytopenia.

During cardiac surgery the surgeon and anaesthesiologist first try to identify patients at greater risk of requiring platelet support, as there are data showing the routine transfusion of platelets unnecessary [33]. Patients requiring their second open heart procedure will bleed more, and patients with haemostatic defects, are at risk [34]. Perioperative aspirin use causes predictable qualitative platelet injury beyond the expected defect as platelets traverse the extracorporeal oxygenator during bypass. Aspirin use has been shown to lead to subtle, but measurably significant increased blood loss [35]. Furthermore, drugs such as desmopressin [36], or aprotinin [37] that pharmacologically boost platelet function will reduce operative needs in select cardiac surgery patients. Nonetheless, such aspirin use per se has not proved to be a useful predictor of who will need subsequent component support [38].

During a procedure like open-heart surgery where all patients bleed to some extent it may be difficult for the surgeon and anaesthesiologist to determine when that haemorrhage has exceeded the norm. Indeed the definition of that norm is likely to vary from doctor to doctor. This interobserver variability likely explains the wide range in component support observed at differences in physician awareness of platelet toxicity, also play a role is unproven.

Similar uncertainty clouds platelet decision making in other actively bleeding patients. That said, an expert panel has concluded that the bleeding patient with a platelet count of 50,000 per microliter or greater is unlikely to benefit from platelet transfusion in the absence of an additional qualitative defect [39]. Whether that additional qualitative injury can be identified by a prolonged bleeding time alone [39] or whether more precise information is required to identify the defect and assess its relevance [40] remains uncertain.

The second area of debate in bedside platelet transfusion decisions examines how low the platelet count should be to warrant prophylactic intervention. Appropriate decision making, again, looks beyond the number to other issues that suggest increased bleeding likelihood at that degree of thrombocytopenia. Such patient specific features that heighten bleeding risk include: rapidly falling platelet count or additional threats to haemostasis, i.e. underlying vascular or endothelial injury, qualitative platelet defects, clotting factor abnormalities. In patients with haematological malignancy, fever, infection, amphotericin administration, and the nature of the malignancy and its therapy are all useful in predicting bleeding [41].

The risk of platelet transfusion are comparable to those of red cells. While acute haemolysis should not be an issue, bacterial infection is more prevalent because of the room temperature platelet storage. Perhaps febrile reactions are more common. Alloimmunization and refractoriness will occur in a significant number of patients receiving longterm support but is not consistently related to the number of prior platelet transfusions [42].

In assessing benefits and risks most experts conclude that prophylactic support is seldom needed when the platelet count is greater than 20,000 per microliter [43]. More recently others have advised that 5,000 or 10,000 per microliter may be a more realistic trigger [44]. As stated, appropriate bedside decisions should go beyond that single number to assess a variety of other issues that clarify more precisely the benefits and risks of platelet support in an individual patient.

Transfusion decisions: Fresh frozen plasma (FFP)

An analogous process is used to make decisions regarding FFP. These decisions are complicated by similar problems as have been mentioned for red cells and platelets. While an expert panel concluded over a decade ago that FFP should be used to treat a deficiency of multiple clotting factors or for a single clotting factor deficiency for which no more concentrated component exists [45], there is today little data to clarify what degree of coagulopathy warrants intervention.

Prolongation of the prothrombin time (PT) is the major trigger that prompts FFP administration. Although it is logical to conclude that the longer the PT the greater the bleeding risk, the nature of an abnormal PT cutoff where the increased risk is first apparent is unknown, and in several studies there seemed to be little correlation between PT and bleeding [46, 47]. Furthermore, many different combinations and permutations of clotting factor deficiency may give rise to an identically prolonged PT. Whether the pattern of abnormality is important or irrelevant in interpreting that prolonged PT is uncertain. Finally, it may be difficult to separate the therapeutic efficacy of FFP from the Vitamin K which is often given concomitantly.

The risks of FFP are similar to that discussed for red cells or platelets except for certain infections, such as HTLV-I, which are only transmitted by cellular products. Though these risks seem readily assessed, the uncertain benefit has led experts to conclude that almost any "abnormal" PT may be a realistic trigger for intervention.

External factors

While transfusion decisions are actually made of the bedside they are modified by many other factors. The role of the doctor's prior experience, the availability heuristic, has already been mentioned [27]. Other influences include journal articles or other sources of continuing medical education, peer recommendations, feedback, administrative effort, financial incentives and patient attitudes and desires. The effects of these factors have been reviewed in detail [48] and will be summarized here.

In examining the impact of education in modifying bedside decision making, one notes the efforts of locally recognized leaders to be far more influential than outside experts [49]. Feedback which is constructive, timely, and directed toward individuals actually making decisions may reinforce educational efforts to modify transfusion practice [50]. Administrative support from hospital governance can legitimize the worthiness of such education and feedback. More overt administrative obstacles or incentives may have less predictable impact. Financial incentives or penalties have facilitated changing physician behaviour in diverse areas of healthcare but have not been directly studies in modifying transfusion practice. Finally, public perception and the concerns of individual patients in avoiding transfusion HIV have undoubtedly modified transfusion practice at the bedside [51].

Although beyond the scope of this chapter to discuss in detail, recognize that other issues impact on those bedside decisions. In a society where informed consent and patient involvement in their own health care form crucial legal and ethical tenants, the patient should participate in the decision making process. When resources are limited, as is often the case for single donor platelets and less often for other components, a central authority may need to assume triage responsibility overseeing individual decisions. Financial costs need to be acknowledged, as well. Though, for the clinician at the bedside, it is difficult to argue that decisions in which clinical benefit clearly outweighs costs in terms of toxicity should be modified by costs measured solely in financial terms.

Conclusion

The bedside analysis of transfusion benefits and risks require, for starters, physician knowledge of easily retrieved triggers such as the haemoglobin concentration or platelet count. But beyond this readily available data doctors must interpret the pathophysiological consequence of those abnormalities in individual patients. Common themes in the individualized decision making include the following:

- How rapidly has the haemoglobin, platelet count or clotting factor concentration fallen?
- What other pathophysiologic problems increase the patient's sensitivity to that blood count-clotting factor defect?
- Is the basic process that has led to the red cell, platelet, clotting factor

deficiency now under control, expected to soon be under control, or out of control and expected to worsen?
- What are the generalized costs of transfusion intervention?
- Finally, how do those generalized risks dynamically apply to the patient at hand?

References

1. Stehling L, Ellison N, Gotta A, et al. A survey of transfusion practice among anesthesiologists. Vox Sang 1987;52:60-2.
2. Surgenor D, Wallace E, Hale G, et al. Changing patterns of blood transfusions in four sets of United States hospitals, 1980 to 1985. Transfusion 1989;28:513-18.
3. Goodnough LJ, Johnston MFM, Toy PTCY, et al. The variability of transfusion practice in coronary artery bypass surgery. JAMA 1991;265:86-90.
4. Surgenor SM, Wallace EL, Hao SH, Chapman RH. Collection and transfusion of blood in the United States. N Engl J Med 1990;322:1646-51.
5. Soumerai SB, Salem-Schatz S, Avorn J. A controlled trial of educational outreach to improve blood transfusion practices. JAMA 1993;270:961-66.
6. McCullough J, Steeper TA, Connelly DP, et al. Platelet utilization in a university hospital. JAMA 1988;259:2414-18.
7. Apstern CS, Dennis RL, Briggs L, et al. Effect of erythrocyte storage and oxyhemoglobin affinity changes on cardiac function. Am J Phys 1985;285:4508-15.
8. Sugarman HJ, Davidson DT,Vibal S, et al. The basis of defective oxygen delivery from stored blood. Surg Gynecol Obst 1970;131:733-41.
9. Stuart J, Nash GB. Red cell deformability and hematological disorders. Blood Rev 1990;4:141-47.
10. Marik PE, Sibbald WJ. Effect of stored-blood transfusion on oxygen delivery in patients with sepsis. JAMA 1993;269:3024-29.
11. Ronco JJ, Phang PT, Walley KR, et al. Oxygen consumption is independent of changes in oxygen delivery and oxygen uptake in severe adult respiratory distress syndrome. Amer Rev Respir Dis 1991;143:1267-73.
12. Levine E, Rosen A, Sehgal L, et al. Physiologic effects of acute anemia: Implications for reduced transfusion trigger. Transfusion 1990;30:11-19.
13. Woodson RD, Auerbach S. Effect of increased oxygen affinity and anemia on cardiac output and its distribution. J Appl Physiol 1982;53:1299-306.
14. Rodman T, Close HP, Purcell MK. The oxyhemoglobin dissociation curve in anemia. Ann Intern Med 1960;52:295-309.
15. Stehling L, Zander HL. Acute normovolemic hemodilution. Transfusion 1991;31:857-68.
16. Chapler CK, Cain SM. The physiologic reserve in oxygen carrying capacity: Studies in experimental hemodilution. Can J Physiol Pharmacol 1986;64:7-12.
17. Spence RK, Carson JA, Poses R, et al. Elective surgery without transfusion: Influence of preoperative hemoglobin level and blood loss on mortality. Am J Surg 1990;159: 320-24.
18. Fullerton WT, Turner AG. Exchange transfusion in treatment of severe anemia in pregnancy. Lancet 1922;i:75-78.
19. Kawaguchi A, Bergsland J, Subramanim S. Total bloodless open heart surgery in the pediatric age group. Circulation 1984;70(Suppl I):30-34.

20. Alexiu O, Mircea N, Balaban Furtunescu B. Gastrointestinal hemorrhage from peptic ulcer. An evaluation of bloodless transfusion and early surgery. Anaesthesia 1975;30: 609-16.
21. Stehling L, Simon TL. The red blood cell transfusion trigger: Physiology and clinical studies. Arch Pathol Lab Med 1994;11:429-34.
22. Welch HG, Meehan KR. Goodnough LT. Prudent strategies for elective red blood cell transfusion. Ann Int Med 1992;116:393-406.
23. NIH Consensus conference. Perioperative red cell transfusion. JAMA 1988;260: 2700-02.
24. Stehling L, Zauder HL. How low can we go? Is there a way to know. Transfusion 1990;30:1-3.
25. Eisenstaedt RS. Transfusion therapy: Blood components and transfusion complications. In: Rippe JM, Irwin RS, Alpert JS, Fink MP (eds). Intensive care medicine. Boston: Little Brown and Co 1991:1055-61.
26. Linden JV, Kaplan HS. Transfusion errors: Causes and effects. Trans Med Rev 1994;8:169-89.
27. Tversky A, Kahneman D. Judgement under uncertainty: Heuristics and biases. Science 1984;185:1124-31.
28. Blumberg N, Heal JM. Effects of transfusion on immune function: Cancer recurrence and infection. Arch Pathol Lab Med 1994;118:371-79.
29. Donahue JG, Munoz A, Ness PM, et al. The declining risk of post-transfusion hepatitis C infection. N Engl J Med 1992;327:369-73.
30. Aubuchon JP. Minimizing donor exposure in hemotherapy. Arch Pathol Lab Med 1994;118:380-91.
31. Takahasi M, Yamada G, Miyamoto R, et al. Natural course of hepatitis C. Am J Gastroenterol 1993;88:240-43.
32. Seeff LB, Buskell-Boles Z, Wright EC, et al. Long-term mortality after transfusion-associated non-A, non-B hepatitis. N Engl J Med 1992;327:1906-11.
33. National Blood Resource Education Program. Indications for the use of red blood cells, platelets, and fresh frozen plasma. In: Transfusion Alert. Publication no. 9-2974a, Bethesda.
34. Woodman RC, Harker LA. Bleeding complications associated with cardiopulmonary bypass. Blood 1990;76:1680-97.
35. Sethi GK, Copeland JG, Goldman S. Implications of preoperative administration of aspirin in patients undergoing coronary artery bypass grafting. J Am Col Card 1990; 15:15-20.
36. Salzman EW, Weinstein MJ, Weintraub RM, et al. Treatment with desmopressin acetate to reduce blood loss after cardiac surgery. N Engl J Med 1986;314:1402-6.
37. Royston D. High dose aprotinin therapy: A review of the first five years experience. J Cardiothorac Vasc Anesth 1992;6:76-100.
38. Goodnough LT, Johnston MFM, Toy PTCY, et al. The variability of transfusion practice in coronary artery bypass surgery. JAMA 1991;265:86-90.
39. Consensus confernce. Platelet transfusion therapy. JAMA 1987;257:1777-80.
40. Lind SE. The bleeding time does not predict surgical bleeding. Blood 1991;77:2547-52.
41. Schiffer CA. Prophylactic platelet transfusion. Transfusion 1992;32:295-98.
42. Saarinen UM, Kehomak R, Siimes MA, Myllyla G. Effective prophylaxis against platelet refractioness in multitransfused patients by the use of leukocyte-free blood components. Blood 1990;75:512-17.

43. Tomasulo PA, Lenes BA. Platelet transfusion therapy. In: Hemostatic disorders and the blood bank. Arlington, VA: American Association of Blood Banks 1984:63-89.
44. Beutler E. Platelet transfusion: The 20,000/μL trigger. Blood 1993;81:1411-13.
45. Consensus conference. Fresh frozen plasma. Indications and risks. JAMA 1985;253: 551-53.
46. Ewe K. Bleeding after liver biopsy does not correlate with indices of peripheral coagulation. Dig Disease and Sciences 1981;26:388-93.
47. McVay PA, Toy PTCY. Lack of increased bleeding after paracentesis and thoracentesis for patients with mild coagulation abnormalities. Transfusion 1991;31:164-71.
48. Eisenstaedt RS. Transfusion triggers: Development and implementation. In: Aubuchon JP, Issitt PD (eds). Limiting donor exposure in hemotherapy. Behtesda, MD: American Association of Blood Banks 1994:27-44.
49. Soumerai SB, Avorn J. Principles of education outreach ("academic detailing") to improve clinical decision making. JAMA 1990;263:549-56.
50. Greco PJ, Eisenberg JM. Changing physician's practices. N Engl J Med 1993;329: 1271-74.
51. Heaton WAL. Changing patterns of blood use. Transfusion 1994;34:365-67.

THE CLINICAL CONSULTATIVE ROLE OF THE BLOOD BANK IN TRANSFUSION MEDICINE

C.Th. Smit Sibinga

Introduction

In 1991 during one of the consultations organized by the WHO Global Blood Safety Initiative [1], a working definition of Transfusion Medicine was composed and defined in consensus to facilitate communication, evaluation and exchange of information and expertise. The definition reads:

'Transfusion Medicine deals with that part of the Health Care System which undertakes the appropriate provision and use of human blood resources.'

Transfusion Medicine thereby provides the essential scientific and clinical information for transfusion practice and the link between the altruistic blood donor and the patient.

Medicine develops through fundamental and applied science, where new developments are continuously tested and validated. Subsequently these developments become accepted and routine and then require reproducibility to allow standard of practice. This also relates to transfusion medicine and particularly to the developments triggered by the bedside, where there is a specific need for communication between the responsible clinician and the transfusion medicine specialist. Practice in medicine, irrespective of the field should be based on well defined criteria and evidence gained by properly designed and conducted scientific research. However, the quality of the ultimate bedside practice is not exclusively defined by or depending on the individual practitioner. Practice in medicine relates intimately to the appropriate and applicable code of practice, the specifically defined criteria of practice or standards and their implementation and audit. The practice of transfusion medicine, bridging the community (the donor) to the bedside (the patient), covers three distinct operational fields:

1. The blood collection process; donor motivation and management, medical selection and the ultimate collection.
2. The testing and processing of the donation; quality and safety control, processing and preservation, quarantine release and storage.
3. The clinical interface; distribution, clinical indication setting and decision taking, consultative services, compatibility testing and the ultimate administration or transfusion.

Clinical demands

Clinical demands in transfusion medicine seem to depend on many variables, both predictable such as elective transfusion needs and supportive haemotherapy in most non-acute clinical situations, and unpredictable such as in emergency medicine in the surgical and the non-surgical field. Each of these situations demands an appropriate and individual patient oriented approach, tailor-made to the specific clinical circumstances and conditions.

Given the variability from donor to donor and the changes in biological function and behaviour of the various components of the blood over time, it follows that the individual patient's clinical needs seemingly will depend more on the desired clinical outcome of the transfusion than on the pharmaceutical characteristics and assumed uniformity of the component offered by the blood bank.

The demands should never be defined or commanded by the blood bank, whatever high grade of pharmaceutical and GMP controlled quality processing is achieved. Here we deal with a specific clinical responsibility, to which the blood bank could contribute on a consultative basis, provided there is sufficient expertise of the reality aspects of the clinical interface and the bedside situation.

Transfusion policies

Bedside transfusion policies should be based on consensus, on general clinical principles such as the assessment of the real needs, the setting of the indications and the definition of the desired clinical efficacies and outcomes. Tailor-made policies are necessary for each and every clinical situation, although there are certain generalities and rules of thumb. Whatever policy is set, evaluation is needed to determine whether the anticipated clinical outcome meets the desired and expected efficacy. Equally important is to determine whether the calculated and expected benefits do outweigh the anticipated risks. Quite often the policies and related expectations are influenced by strong marketing efforts of the blood bank, advocating in a strongly convincible manner certain advantages of new processing procedures and pharmaceutical innovations such as depletion of leukocytes to the uncountable extreme or additive solutions that allow a better ex vivo storage and related logistics for the blood bank, but are not based on proper and scientific clinical evidence.

Anecdotically it resembles the adorable story (Figure 1) of the couple at the diner table, where the wife serves ordinary chicken prepared in a special way. The husband, recognizing the taste, comments:

"Hey, this is some kind of chicken!"

The lady of the house, however, smiles and responds with pride and satisfaction:

"It is coq au vin!".

The husband, apparently a no-nonsense person, then answers:

"You could have fooled me. It sure tastes like chicken."

Equivocally the story illustrates the historically grown customs and traditions

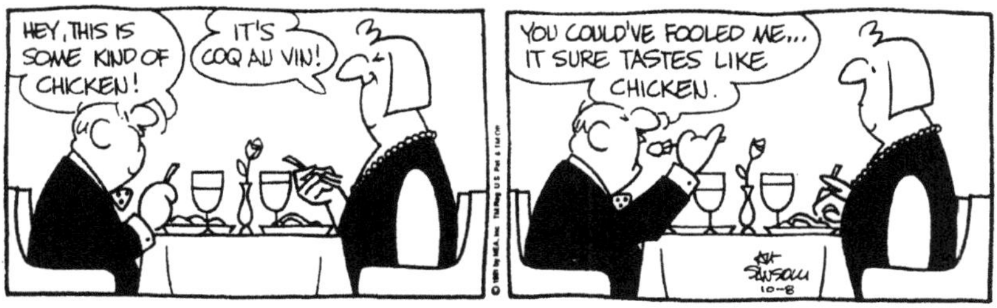

Figure 1.

that are often the underlying justification of current clinical transfusion practices. To evaluate these practices consensus protocols and audits are needed to trigger improvement and optimisation of clinical transfusion policies and practices [2-5].

Transfusion medicine speciality

The goal of clinical transfusion practice is an appropriate, safe and optimal use of human blood and blood resources. With the introduction and implementation of the quality concept [6] and Good Manufacturing Practice principle [7] in blood banking and additionally in transfusion medicine and the clinical practice, there are two major fields of attention and expertise to be distinguished:

1. Transfusion medicine pharmaceutical (technical) field, dealing with:
   - the availability and choice of products whether blood components or plasma derivatives;
   - their functional technical aspects such as serology, virology and immuno-haematology;
   - the compatibility testing, the documentation and traceability.
2. Transfusion medicine medical (clinical) field, the doctors, dealing with
   - the clinical decision taking and indications;
   - the desired supportive haemotherapy and anticipated clinical outcome;
   - the transfusion regime, protocols and evaluation;
   - the treatment of adverse effects and transfusion reactions;
   - the feed-back of results and clinical outcomes as well as the appropriate documentation.

Over the past century, transfusion medicine has shown considerable developments and changes in emphasis, in particular in the blood bank and transfusion laboratory:

– In the traditional concept, the field of expertise is characterised by the dominance of the laboratory oriented serologist, mostly a clinical pathologist with some general medical education, largely part-time involved and committed because of the so many other fields of attention in clinical pathology and laboratory medicine. The transfusion medicine expertise is largely 'self-made' with no or just a limited clinical experience. Here we find a variety of medical and related academical backgrounds, but relatively little professional interest in and attention to donor and recipient.

– The necessary introduction of quality principles and GMP has changed this traditional concept over the last decade. Now the emphasis is predominantly on the technology and documentation of processes and procedures, standardisation and automation. Pharmaceutical principles and approaches have been introduced, through which the blood banks have developed and metamorphosed largely into pharmaceutical production entities [8]. These developments did bring along the supermarket concept based on the availability of good quality products, readily offered to potential customers. Under the public pressure induced by the AIDS epidemic, the many negative accusations and subsequent liability problems, the attitude has become highly defensive. A shift in professional background is the result, changing towards pharmacists and microbiologists, focusing the attention primarily on laboratory defined safety and product characteristics and specifications; the purer the better.

This newer generation of blood bankers has reorganised and re-enforced the traditional castles and ivory towers, ruling the transfusion medicine world without fully realising that the need for clinical evidence prevails over the extrapolated laboratory evidence. The essential question at the bedside indeed is whether the expected clinical outcome of a transfusion will be significantly better and safer in terms of quality adjusted life years (QALY) with 'coq a vin' instead of just 'chicken' [9]. Needless to say that there is also an increasingly important economical cost-effectiveness question to be considered.

– These aspects now lead to an awakening awareness of the importance of clinical transfusion medicine practice. This clinical outcome triggered change underlines the importance of the clinical interface in transfusion medicine, including a strategic reorientation of the field. In many industrialised countries, legislation and governmental regulations now force hospitals to take full responsibility for safe, efficient and cost-effective transfusion practice based on professional hospital transfusion organisations where the clinical interface bridges the bedside practice to the blood bank as a processing laboratory. These recent developments imply a major emphasis to be given to the impact of supportive haemotherapy, both standard and advanced (immunotherapy, stem cells and gene therapy), comprehensive bedside transfusion practice and intercollegial clinical consultative services. These developments should be seen as additional and complementary to the earlier pharmaceutical orientation. It brings along the need for clinically trained and experienced transfusion medicine specialists supported by GMP and product oriented transfusion medicine pharmacists.

Transfusion medicine and clinical consultation

Today the transfusion of blood has become a more prominently integrated, recognised and appreciated part of clinical medicine. Supportive haemotherapy has gained its own share in clinical treatment strategies [10]. However, there is still a fair amount of day-to-day tradition-driven transfusion practice, without sufficient appreciation of the expected clinical outcome. Because the benefits are not always fully discerned, there is still a considerable over- and undertransfusion of patients. Often blood transfusion is the result of an impulsive reaction to an acute clinical situation or a sudden change in the clinical condition of the patient, without serious consideration of the key questions 'Is there a real need?', 'If so, how should the need be defined?' followed by 'What, how much and over what length of time should there be transfused?'. Impulsive reactions seldom allow careful balancing of pro's and con's in the light of the necessary clinical actions to achieve a desired and justified clinical outcome of treatment. Equally uncertain and hazardous are the clinical practices based on assumptions and unrealistic perceptions of risk, overemphasising and exaggerating the negative effects without appreciating the positive contributions to a patient's well-being in a given clinical situation.

As clinical medicine is often complicated and many different but important parts of the diagnostic and treatment strategy have to be given appropriate attention and judged for their correct rank in priority, blood transfusion is not always given the notice it deserves as a transplant with its full immunological implications [11]. These considerations justify the access to a consultative and supportive specialist experienced in the field of blood transfusion. Such a specialist should have a clinical background and training, with sufficient bedside experience. The specialist should be broadly and multi-disciplinary oriented; for instance be sufficiently experienced and knowledgeable in the transfusion dependent areas of neonatology, traumatology, nephrology and neurology, obstetrics, orthopaedics, haemato-oncology and organ transplantation, etc.

The specialist should have adequate and up-to-date practical and scientific knowledge and expertise of the various clinical indications and contra-indications, therapeutic regimes and dosageing as well as potential interactions with other treatment modalities. There should be knowledge and experience of potential adverse effects and risks, the actual bedside practice and the clinical monitoring of blood transfusion. Besides, the specialist should know about possible alternatives to blood transfusion and be experienced in the field of haemapheresis. Such a clinical specialist can only support the clinician, when there is a professional basis of mutual trust and respect. The clinician should be willing to accept the professional expertise provided in a consultation in which the transfusion medicine specialist is given co-responsibility for the patient and is allowed to play an active and participating role in the supportive haemotherapeutic treatment strategy.

Such a clinical relationship can be achieved through regular contact with the clinic; physical visits and rounds, exchange of knowledge and expertise at ward level and in clinical conferences, and active involvement in clinical development.

Conclusion

The clinical consultative role of the Blood Bank in Transfusion Medicine and in particular in the clinical or bedside transfusion practice can best be achieved and instituted through clinically trained transfusion medicine specialists providing the bridge between the technical-pharmaceutical expertise of the Blood Bank and the clinical outcome defined needs at the bedside.

Ultimately the clinical consultative role is determined by the ancient Hippocratic and ever valid adagia 'primum est non nocere' and 'salus donores et aegroti suprema lex'.

References

1. Report of the GBSI informal consultation on Collaboration in Training in Transfusion Medicine. Geneva WHO/LBS/92.7.
2. Consensus Conference: Fresh frozen plasma: Indications and risks. JAMA 1985;253: 551-53.
3. Consensus Conference: Platelet transfusion therapy. JAMA 1985;257:1777-80.
4. Consensus Conference: Leucocyte depletion of blood and blood components. The Royal College of Physicians of Edinburgh, Edinburgh 1993.
5. Consensus statement on red cell transfusion. Trans Med 1994;4:177-78.
6. Quality assurance in blood banking and its clinical impact. Smit Sibinga CTh, Das PC, Taswell HF (eds). Martinus Nijhoff Publ., Boston, The Hague, Dordrecht, Lancaster, 1984.
7. The rules governing medicinal products in the European community. Vol IV. Guide to Good Manufacturing Practice for Medicinal Products. ECSC-EEC-EAEC, 1989.
8. Zuck TF. The Good Manufacturing Practice concept. In: Smit Sibinga CTh, Das PC, Heiniger HJ (eds). Good Manufacturing Practice in Transfusion Medicine. Kluwer Acad. Publ., Dordrecht, Boston, London, 1994:25-34.
9. Bordin JO, Heddle NM, Blajchman MA. The biologic effect of leukocytes present in transfused cellular blood products. Blood 1994;84:1703-21.
10. Supportive therapy in haematology. Das, Smit Sibinga CTh, Halie MR (eds). Martinus Nijhoff Publ., Boston, Dordrecht, Lancaster, 1985.
11. Murphy WG. Factors effecting the clinical efficacy of blood transfusion. In: Smit Sibinga CTh, Das PC, Snijder EL (eds). Trigger factors in transfusion medicine. Kluwer Acad. Publ., Boston, Dordrecht, London, 1996:65-72.

AUDITING IN TRANSFUSION MEDICINE: APPROACHES TO OPTIMIZING TRANSFUSION PRACTICE

C.H. Wallas

Introduction

Since approximately 20 million blood components are transfused each year in the United States alone and since transfusion therapy is not without risks, there have been increasing efforts made to evaluate how blood components are utilized with a view toward improving practice. The Joint Commission on the Accreditation of Healthcare Organizations (JCAHO) has been the group primarily driving this effort from the hospital perspective and the American Association of Blood Banks (AABB) the group promoting this effort from the laboratory perspective. The overall purpose of these initiatives is to achieve continuous improvement in transfusion practices rather than to identify and punish individual physicians. This paper will review the historical perspectives and the current role of the JCAHO and the AABB in this process, the existing practice guidelines, the results of transfusion practice audits as well as several strategies which have been implemented to improve practice.

Background

Historical notes

In 1910, Ernest Codman, M.D. a surgeon at the Massachusetts General Hospital, recommended that each patient be examined one year post-operatively to determine whether symptoms for which they were treated were alleviated [1-3]. These efforts led to formation in 1918 of the American College of Surgeons (ACS) Hospital Standardization Program. This group established Standards, hospital inspections as well as an accreditation programme. In 1951, because of rising costs for accreditation, the ACS decided to join forces with the American Medical Association, the American Hospital Association, the American College of Physicians and the Canadian Medical Association to sponsor the Joint Commission on Accreditation of Hospitals (JCAH). The emphasis of this undertaking was on process and structure rather than on outcome (i.e., signs were required to be posted indicating that oxygen was in use; this approach assumed that meeting this standard automatically resulted in quality care). Between 1960 and 1980, the increasing role of professional accountability coupled with increasing consumer expectations as well as concerns about rising costs resulted in a shift in emphasis toward outcome. In addition, case law increasingly identified the hospital as accountable for acts of its medical staff. These activities culminated in the legislative initiative leading the formation of professional standard review organization. During the 1980s and 1990s, the JCAH and its successor organization, the JCAHO, has increasingly promulgated standards which have emphasized the use of outcome evaluations especially for procedures which are high volume, high risk, and potentially error prone, which transfusion therapy clearly is.

The role of the JCAHO

Since 1985, as a condition for accreditation, the JCAHO has required that all hospitals perform blood usage reviews and have policies and procedures relating to blood utilization [4]. These required the inclusion of the processes for ordering appropriate blood and components; the proper distribution, handling an dispensing of blood and policies for the administration and monitoring of the effects of blood on patients. The latter requirement involves performance of blood usage reviews at least quarterly using predetermined guidelines to evaluate the appropriateness of an adequate number of transfusion cases for all departments and services using blood in order to identify single cases or patterns of cases that require more intensive review. The JCAHO also requires the evaluation of all confirmed significant transfusion complication. Finally, written reports must be developed for each of the activities including conclusions, recommendations, actions taken, and the results of those actions must be maintained and presented at specified intervals to all departments and services.

Quality assurance activities

The role of the Hospital Transfusion Committee

A key initiative for establishing a process for improving the quality of transfusion practice within a hospital is the creation of a working committee [5-8]. This committee can be a freestanding group, typically named the transfusion committee or can function as a subgroup of a broader scope quality assurance committee. In either setting, the group should be constituted with representatives who have overlapping terms of appointment and who come from medical services using the most blood (i.e., anaesthesiology, surgery, haematology-oncology, cardiac surgery, etc.), nursing services, the laboratory services, hospital administrative services as well as from the regional blood supplier. The focus of this group's activities should be to establish policies and procedures relating to: the ordering of appropriate blood components (to include agreements with a blood supplier in order to assure an adequate supply of blood); the distribution and handling of blood (as established by the hospital transfusion service); the administration of blood components (as established by the nursing department including procedures for the use of devices such as blood warmers and pumps); and the monitoring of the effects of transfusion (involving the selection of those specific activities to be audited as well as the development of guidelines to be used during the performance of those audits). These guidelines can be internally developed or can be based partially or entirely on published recommendations. In either case, it is critical that the stakeholder medical service has an opportunity for input and ultimate agreement with the finalized version before implementation of the audit; otherwise if problems in transfusion practice are identified, corrective action will be more difficult or even impossible to implement. In addition, for the work of this group to have the potential for maximum impact on the improvement of transfusion practice, there must be a process established in advance of what consequences exist for any member of the hospital staff who is unwilling to address issues detected during auditing activities.

Table 1. JCAHO monitoring and evaluation model applied to blood usage review.

Task	Activities
– Assign responsibility for review	Select members of QA committee; elect a chair
– Define scope	Define all activities that comprise the transfusion service
– Identify important aspects of care	QA committee develops guidelines for use of RBC, platelets, FPP, etc.; embraced by medical staff
– Identify indicators of care	These may include specific laboratory data (protime, PTT, platelet count), as well as medical information such as cardiovascular status, pulmonary status, related diseases, etc.
– Establish thresholds related to these indicators	These may include thresholds for laboratory data (i.e., platelet count $<50\times10^9$/L; PT >18 seconds) and medical information (i.e., EKG abnormalities)
– Collect and analyze data	Collect data about transfusion usage and associated lab and medical information. Identify "potential outlyers"
– Evaluate care when thresholds are exceeded	Refer "outlyers" to QA committee for further evaluation
– Take action to improve care	Develop education strategies to address defined problems
– Assess effectiveness of actions instituted to improve care	Reaudit function defined originally as "outlyer"
– Communicate information	Distribute findings to medical staff

In general, the formation and the audit activities of the transfusion committee should follow the format outlined in Table 1 with the specific areas selected for each audit depending upon the healthcare setting; thus an audit of an OB/GYN department may focus on the timely administration of Rh immunoglobulin, an orthopaedic service on the use of intraoperative and post operative blood salvage; and a haematology-oncology department on the incidence of refractoriness to platelet transfusions and strategies to overcome this including the use of HLA matched or crossmatched single donor platelets. In addition, the committee would usually evaluate other activities which are based on evaluations of trend analyses such as the use if single units of red cells, the crossmatch/ transfusion ratio, complications of transfusions, outdate rates as well as parameters which are based on peer group statistics such as the over-utilization of a particular blood component. The ultimate goal of these activities will be to identify problems, assist in designing corrective action and implementing a process for follow-up to assess the effectiveness of the process.

An example of an audit performed to evaluate blood wastage in a community hospital was published by Clark and Ayoub [10]. Prior to initiation of their study, it as found that of 13,368 units of blood transfused in a 12 month period, 412 (3.08%) were wasted. As a result of this evaluation, letters were sent to the physician of record for each of these incidents; and the personnel involved in each situation involving blood wastage was provided an inservice session aimed at improving practice. The following year when 11,930 transfusions were audited, as a result of these activities, only 98 (0.8%) components were found to be wasted.

Table 2. An example of audit criteria used to flag RBC transfusions as potentially inappropriate [Adapted from reference 11].

- RBC transfusion flagged as a potential "outlyer" if:
  - PCV before transfusion ≥ 30% *unless* ≥ 6% decrease in previous 24 hours
  - PCV before transfusion between 24% and 30% unless:
    - ≥ 6% decrease in previous 24 hours
    - angina within previous 24 hours
    - MI within previous 6 months
    - EKG changes indicating ischemia/infarct
    - blood loss ≥ 1000 ml before transfusion
- RBC transfusion acceptable if PCV < 24%

Table 3. An example of audit criteria used to qualify RBC transfusions as acceptable [Adapted from reference 12].

- Presence of symptomatic anemia in a normal volume patient
- Acute blood loss ≥ 15% estimated blood volume
- Acute blood loss < 15% estimated blood volume but with evidence of hypoxia
- Preoperative haemoglobin ≤ 80 gm/dl when > 1000 ml blood loss anticipated during surgery
- Haemoglobin level < 90 gm/dl when chronic transfusions are required

Table 4. NIH consensus conference on the indications for the use of fresh frozen plasma [Adapted from reference 15].

- Replacement of isolated deficiencies of Factors II, V, VII, IX, X and XI when specific component therapy is neither available nor appropriate
- Replacement of the functional vitamin K-dependent coagulation Factors II, VII, IX and X, as well as proteins C and S in patients who are anticoagulated with warfarin and are actively bleeding or require emergency surgery
- Reversal of haemostatic disorders in patients who have recieved massive blood transfusions (greater than one blood volume within several hours) and in whom factor deficiencies are presumed to be the sole or principal derangement
- In conjunction with therapeutic plasma exchange for the treatment of thrombotic thrombocytopenic purpura
- Replacement of antithrombin III in patients who are deficient in this inhibitor and are undergoing surgery or who require heparin for treatment of thrombosis
- Replacement of immunoglobulines in infants with immunodeficiency secondary to severe protein-losing enteropathy in whom total parenteral nutrition is ineffectual and in children and adults with humoral immunodeficiency

Existing Practice Guidelines

Red blood cells (RBC): There are numerous examples of RBC transfusion audit criteria. For several reasons, most of these have been applied retrospectively (days or weeks after the blood has been administered) rather than prospectively (prior to release of blood) or concurrently (within hours of the transfusion): RBC transfusions are usually high volume, making it difficult to audit use in advance; such audits could interfere with patient care when the patient is actively bleeding; and laboratory data used to assess these transfusions often do not accurately reflect the patient's RBC mass during active bleeding. On the other hand, retrospective analyses also have significant limitations since the decision to transfuse is usually based on estimates (anticipated blood loss, an unknown; the patient's blood volume, estimated blood loss, usually a guess, and the haematocrit; and the cardio-pulmonary status and related symptoms); and the reviewer's conclusion about appropriateness is based on hindsight analysis. These limitations aside, it is still usually productive to apply guidelines to the performance of retrospective audits of RBC usage, an example of which is displayed in Table 2. Other useful sets of criteria can be found in Stehling et al [12] (see Table 3) as well as in papers by Welch et al [13] and Audet and Goodnough [14].

Fresh frozen plasma (FFP): The most widely recognized indications for the use of FFP were published as a result of an NIH Consensus Conference held in 1984. These are listed in Table 4. The NIH consensus panel agreed that there was no justification for the use of FFP as a source of nutrients or as a volume expander. Rather they emphasized that the uses of FFP are in fact specific and should be targeted to replacement of multiple deficiencies of coagulation factors when

Table 5. NIH consensus conference on the indications for platelet transfusions [Adapted from reference 15].

- Platelet transfusions are indicated for treatment of actively bleeding patients with thrombocytopenia or thrombocytopathy or both if the platelet disorder is likely to be causing or contributing to the bleeding
- Platelet transfusions are indicated for patients with documented thrombocytopenia following massive transfusion (greater than one blood volume transfused within several hours) and who are experiencing clinically abnormal bleeding
- Prophylactic platelet transfusions may benefit patients with severe thrombocytopenia, particularly when it is consequent to myelosuppressive therapy
- Prophylactic platelet transfusion may be required to prepare patients with thrombocytopenia or thrombocytopathy for invasive procedures, especially those in which haemostasis cannot be assessed by direct observation or in patients threatened with haemorrhage in the central nervous system or other sites in which a small amount of bleeding could be critical. Such patients include those with associated disorders of coagulation or platelet function that cannot be completely corrected (example, advanced hepatic or renal insufficiency)
- Platelet transfusions are unlikely to be effective in controlling bleeding in a patient with a platelet count of greater than or equal to 50×10^9/L if thrombocytopenia is the sole abnormality
- Platelet transfusions are unlikely to control bleeding in a patient with a bleeding time of less than twice the upper limit of normal unless there are other conditions that interfere with haemostasis
- Routine prophylactic platelet transfusions are generally not required to treat patients with chronic thrombocytopenia caused by impaired platelet production (example, aplastic anaemia, myelodysplastic disorders)
- Prophylactic platelet transfusions are rarely indicated for patients with accelerated destruction but active production of platelets (example, idiopathic thrombocytopenia purpura)
- There is no justification for prophylactic platelet administration in patients undergoing open-heart surgery

Table 6. Indications for platelet transfusion [Adapted from reference 12].

- Platelet count < $10\text{-}20\times10^9$/L in a nonbleeding patient with failure of platelet production
- Platelet count < 50×10^9/L and impending surgery or invasive procedure
- Diffuse microvascular bleeding in a patient with documented disseminated intravascular coagulation or transfusion ≥ 1 blood volume and platelet count < 50×10^9/L or laboratory values not yet available
- Diffuse microvascular bleeding following cardiopulmonary bypass or with intra-aortic balloon pump and platelet count not yet available or < 100×10^9/L
- Bleeding in a patient with a qualitative platelet defect, regardless of platelet count

a concentrate did not exist as well as for selected patients being massively transfused who exhibited excessive bleeding associated with abnormalities in coagulation screening tests. Transfusion of FFP was also felt to be appropriate for the patient with thrombotic thrombocytopenic purpura. Several of the other recommendations in Table 4 are now considered to be outdated with the availability of intravenous immunoglobulin and antithrombin III. More recently developed guidelines can be found in a paper by Stehling et al [12]; these guidelines consider the use of FFP appropriate if the protime (PT) and/or partial thromboplastin time (PTT) is greater than 1.5 times the normal value in a nonbleeding patient scheduled for surgery; if diffuse microvascular bleeding is occurring in a patient given more than 1 blood volume replacement and the PT and/or PTT is greater than 1.5 times baseline or not yet available; or if there is evidence of excessive coumarin therapy associated with major bleeding or impending surgery.

Once agreed upon by the hospital QA Committee and the medical staff, these guidelines can be instituted by the hospital transfusion service in a prospective manner, since unlike RBC usage, requests for FFP are much less frequent and usually only involve 1-2 units requested at any given time. Nonetheless it is often quite difficult to evaluate many of the requests for FFP prospectively since most are for patients undergoing surgery where the emotions of the moment run high and the opportunities for successful use of science based rationales to improve practice quite slim at that time. If that is also the case in your institution, retrospective analysis remains a major tool for evaluating and improving practice, though again the importance of obtaining buy-in of audit criteria by all of the potential users of FFP before these guidelines are applied cannot be overemphasized; otherwise improvement in practice will be quite difficult to implement.

Platelets: In 1986, the NIH, following on the footsteps of the successful consensus conference on FFP utilization, convened another group to examine the indications for platelet transfusion [15]. The recommendations resulting from this conference are summarized in Table 5. The panel agreed that platelet transfusions are indicated for treatment of actively bleeding patients with thrombocytopenia or thrombocytopathy or both if contributing to bleeding. Specifically such transfusions would be indicated in patients with thrombocytopenia and active bleeding during the marrow recovery phase following chemotherapy or in a massively transfused patient. Conversely, such transfusions are not likely to be effective in controlling bleeding in a patient with a platelet count greater than $50x10^9/L$ in the absence of a platelet function defect. Prophylactic platelet transfusions were felt to benefit patients with severe thrombocytopenia even in the absence of bleeding especially when it follows myelosuppressive therapy or to prepare patients with thrombocytopenia or thrombocytopathy for invasive procedures but may not be useful in patients with chronic thrombocytopenia caused by impaired platelet production (i.e., aplastic anaemia), accelerated platelet destruction states associated with accelerated production (i.e., ITP) or in patients undergoing open heart surgery. Finally the conference concluded that HLA-matched, single donor platelets are most effective in patients refractory to unselected single- or multiple-donor platelets but not in patients who have not been alloimmunized. Guidelines which were published in 1994 by the AABB [12] are summarized in Table 6; additional guidelines have been developed by several hospitals and are reviewed by Simpson [16].

Implementation of QA activities: patterns of component utilization

Personal observation

While being the medical director of the hospital bank at Vanderbilt University, the laboratory information systems group developed a computer-assisted review programme which allowed me to review rapidly and retrospectively approximately 35,000 transfusions given to 6,000 patients each 12 month period. Used in conjunction with prospective application of guidelines, the programme printed monthly reports summarizing transfusion therapy for individual patients and correlated therapy with selected laboratory data. Each month these reports were reviewed, and charts were selected to be evaluated by the hospital QA committee using transfusion audit criteria developed in conjunction with the medical staff.

In each case where criteria were not met, charts were referred to the appropriate attending physician so that additional information could be provided about the specific transfusion question. For purpose of whole blood (WB) and RBC review, the report consisted of a list of selected patients who received WB/RBC and were discharged with a haematocryt or PCV > 35%. For purpose of FFP and platelet review, the report consisted of a list of all patients who received FFP and/or platelets with relevant laboratory data, including the PT, PTT and platelet count. During a recent 9 month period, the data base included 25,577 products. Of these, 11,800 units were red cells which had been given to 3,788 patients (3.1 units/patient); 96 of these (0.8%) had been given to 64 patients (1.7%) in whom the PCV was greater 35%. On further review, it was found that only one unit had only rarely been given; rather the extra and unnecessary unit(s) were part of a series of transfusions in which 1 or 2 units could have been avoided if the PCV had been more frequently measured. There were 1,967 units of FFP transfused to 385 patients (5.1 units/patient) of which 237 units (12.0%) had been given to 44 patients with normal coagulation data, for a total of 370 units (18.8%) potentially inappropriately being given to 155 patients (40.2%) (2.38 units/patient). Finally there were 11,810 units of platelets transfused to 575 patients (20.5 units/patient) of which 352 units (3.0%) had been given to 51 patients with no platelet count and 173 units (1.5%) to 24 patients with normal platelet count for a total of 525 units (4.5%) potentially inappropriately being given to 75 patients (13.0%) (7.0 units/patient). In all, the computer audit identified 991 potentially inappropriate units being given to 294 patients, representing 3.9% of all units given. Approximately 50% of these were ultimately identified as inappropriate when peer review of each patient's chart was completed. In each case written notifications were sent to all attending physicians appraising them of the audit findings. A similar approach was described by Hamoudi et al [17] and Lepage et al [18].

Survey by the College of American Pathologists (CAP)

In 1995 the CAP [19] published the results of a questionnaire completed by 552 member hospitals in 1993 which was designed to provide information about what these hospitals were doing to audit transfusion practice. These hospitals had transfused 753,880 components into 193,409 patients; of this number, 473,503 transfusions given to 128,496 patients had been audited. On initial review, 34,500 components (7%) transfused to 10,313 patients (8%) were deemed inappropriate; when subjected to peer review, 7,332 components (1.5%) transfused to 2,246 patients (1.7%) were viewed to be inappropriate. Based on more subjective criteria, 2.5% of the units FFP transfused were not given according to establish criteria, while RBC, "whole blood" platelets and apheresis platelets were virtually never given inappropriately. While this is certainly not a perfect record, it is an excellent one and demonstrates that transfusion practice is currently being provided according to well defined audit criteria. It would now be useful to review published information about the usage patterns for RBC, FFP and platelets to place current practice into perspective.

Additional observations

Red blood cells: Because of the marked increase in the use of RBC transfusions, several studies have been performed to define usage patterns and appropriateness of utilization based on audit criteria. Tartter and Barron [20] evaluated 288 patients, 177 of whom (60%) received 448 units of blood (2.5 units/patient). Transfusion was viewed as unnecessary if the preoperative PCV exceeded 36% or the intraoperative or postoperative/discharge PCV exceeded 33%. On this basis 112 patients (2/3 of those transfused) were viewed to have received at least 1 unit of unnecessary blood (i.e., approximately 25% of blood used was unnecessary). This was felt to have occurred because the PCV was not measured with each unit given to the patient preoperatively (i.e. patients were transfused with at least two units of blood before additional PCV measurements were made). As a result, these authors recommended measuring the PCV before each unit is given. Additional published studies tended to confirm these observations, showing that the numbers of patients receiving RBC transfusions which met pre-established audit criteria ranged from 57-88% [21-23]. A more recent study by Goodnough et al [24] showed, as would be expected, that the percentage of transfusions meeting audit criteria depended on the stringency of those criteria. Thus, using the discharge PCV and the amount of blood lost during surgery, as the percent of the blood volume which had been lost in order to justify a transfusion increased from 10 to 20 to 30 percent, the percent of patients transfused appropriately decreased from 70% down to 40%. Of additional interest, women were inappropriately transfused more frequently than men (26% vs 13%) and patients who had predeposited autologous units were more frequently inappropriately transfused than those who had not (25% vs 11%). The result of all of these studies are summarized in Table 7 and provide guidance for the development of educational strategies to improve practice.

Table 7. Results of studies evaluating the appropriateness of RBC transfusions.

Reference	Number of patients	Percent of transfusions meeting audit criteria
Tartter and Barron (1985) [20]	217	48
Stehling and Esposito (1987) [21]	520	81
Brien et al. (1989) [22]	297	88
Mozes et al (1989) [23]	269	57
Goodnough et al. (1992) [24]	525	40-75

Fresh frozen plasma (FFP): As the usage of FFP increased during the past two decades, attention has been directed at defining transfusion patterns. One of the earliest studies was performed by Shaikh et al [25] who evaluated the transfusion of 364 units during a 4 month period. Approximately 33% if these were given for blood pressure support predominately during surgical procedures (of which 75% were given with RBCs); 35% were given for clotting support, usually while the patients were not in the operating room; and 14% of units were given for both indications. These results were confirmed by a subsequent study by Snyder et al [26] who evaluated FFP usage in 9 area hospitals in Milwaukee. They noted that the cardiovascular service used 42% of the FFP transfused. In addition, although 60% was given for coagulation factor replacement, 33% did not meet NIH consensus criteria. Moreover, 25% was given for volume expansion during surgery, 65% were given with RBCs, and in only 10% of the cases was written justification present in the patient's medical record. In general these authors concluded that physicians assume that FFP benefits all bleeding patients, nonbleeding patients with abnormal coagulation data and volume depleted patients. The results of these and other studies are summarized in Table 8 and tend to support the assumption that FFP is being transfused in many cases as a substitute for whole blood which has become practically extinct since FFP and platelets have become available. As with RBC usage, these studies provide a framework for developing strategies to improve transfusion practice.

Table 8. Results of studies evaluating the appropriateness of FFP transfusions.

Reference	Number of patients	Percent of transfusions meeting audit criteria
Shaikh et al. (1985) [25]	68	70
Blumberg et al. (1986) [27]	135	27
Snyder et al. (1986) [26]	345	60
Stehling and Esposito (1987) [21]	79	31
Brient et al. (1989) [22]	83	92
Mozes et al. (1989) [23]	63	18

Platelets: Platelets have played an increasingly important role in transfusion therapy since the late 1970s. The patterns of usage appear to depend primarily on the focus of care in a given hospital, emphasizing that audit criteria and strategies to improve practice must be developed for each hospital. For example, Menitove et al [28] who studied platelets usage in several Wisconsin hospitals from 1979 to 1981 found that 41% of platelets were used for open heart surgery while 43% were used to support oncology patients. A similar observation was published by Silver et al [29] who audited practice in Canada, finding that 38% of platelets were used for oncology patients while 28% were used in cardiovascular surgery. McCullough et al [30] who reported usage patterns in Minnesota in 1988 noted that 86% of their platelets were used for oncology patients while only 2% were used during heart surgery, reflecting the patient care emphasis in that hospital. While only 22% of patients receiving prophylactic platelets transfusion therapy had a count less than $20x10^9/L$, at least one risk factor for bleeding was present in the 72% of patients who had counts greater that this level.

Implementation of QA activities: strategies to improve practice

This activity is a continuation of the processes outlined above: based on the results of an audit, strategies are developed in order to improve a specific practice. Once implemented, a follow-up audit is performed to evaluate whether additional corrective strategies need to be implemented; if so, once implemented, another audit is performed, and so on. A number of studies describing strategies to improve practice have been published [30-42]. A synopsis of these studies is summarized in Table 9. Most of the strategies employed depend primarily on an intensive education-based approach which appears to be most effective if targeted toward attending physicians [43].

An issue contributing to the risk of transfusion of all blood components was evaluated by Shulman et al [42], who used a concurrent education approach to reduce error rates in patient identification from 50% to less than 1%. In addition to this important general approach, several strategies have been described which have attempted to target the transfusion of all components. In another described by Renner et al [32], a review was undertaken of all 16,000 transfusions given in a 12 month period (2,858 episodes). To initiate the process, criteria were developed along with screening worksheets keyed to those parameters in order to assess the appropriateness of each transfusion. Pathology residents reviewed all clinical records daily (chart, housestaff notes, laboratory data) and prepared written summaries when a transfusion appeared not to meet criteria. These summaries were then sent to physician peers for further review. The results of this study are tabulated in Table 10 and demonstrate a significant reduction as the study progressed from 3.6% to 0.3% in the number of transfusions not meeting criteria. Tomasulo et al [31] utilized pathology residents who automatically reviewed any transfusion request when they matched certain criteria; some of those criteria are listed in Table 11. This approach was felt to have a positive im-

Table 9. Strategies to improve transfusion practice.

Reference	Component / process	Strategy	Pre-strategy	Post strategy
Tomasulo et al. (1986) [31]	All components	Automatic case consulation	Unknown	
Renner (1987) [32]	All components	Daily review; peer review	3.6% inappropriate	0.3% inappropriate
Lichtiger et al. (1988) [33]	RBC platelets FFP	Prospective	28,242 units/yr 27,048 units/yr 7,892 units/yr	22,990 units/yr 19,311 units/yr
Finkle (1992) [34]	All components	Justification codes entered on requisition		
Silver et al. (1992) [35]	All components	Immediate review of all requests		Orders for 114 patients cancelled; orders for 51 patients changed
Rosen et al. (1993) [36]	All components	Justification entered into computer; retrospective review		Decrease in donor exposure of 42,072 during 3 year period
Giovanetti et al. (1988) [37]	Red cells	Audit team visited wards daily to teach	37% (85/230) inappropriate	10% (34/345) inappropriate
Shanberge (1987) [38]	FFP	Daily review; peer review	214 units/month	50 units/month
Solomon et al. (1988) [39]	FFP	Retrospective/ prospective review; monthly talks; FFP request form prospective	189 units/month	90 units/month
Barnette et al. (1990) [40]	FFP	Lectures/follow-up/ questionnaires	53% cases (17/32 inappropriate use)	22% cases (4/18 inappropriate use)
Simpsom (1987) [41]	Platelets	Prospective	520 units/month	230 units/month
McCullough (1988) [30}	Platelets	Retrospective; prospective	72,793 units/yr	62,379 units/yr
Shulman et al. (1994) [42]	Patient ID	Concurrent; review; education	50% with variance	< 1% with variance

pact on improving transfusion practice by increasing communication and trust between the blood bank and the primary care physicians, ultimately increasing the opportunities for the blood bank to be involved more routinely in transfusion decisions. Silver et al [35] used a concurrent review process for component requests which resulted in orders for 114 patients being cancelled and for 51 patients being changed; while Lichtiger [33] using a prospective approach reported a significant reduction in the use of all components being used. Finally, Rosen et al [36] and Finkle [34] described a justification system utilizing predeveloped codes which were required to be used when requesting components; using this approach, Rosen reported a 42,072 unit decrease in donor exposures during a 3 years period.

Table 10. Impact of strategies to improve practice on appropriateness of transfusion. [Adapted from reference 32]

Results	Quarter				
Transfusion	**1st**	**2nd**	**3rd**	**4th**	**Total**
Number of episodes	701	749	678	730	2858
Number not meeting criteria (%)	25 (3.6)	21 (2.8)	5 (0.7)	2 (0.3)	53 (1.9)

Table 11. Examples of situations requiring automatic consultation. [Adapted from reference 31]

- Any request for the emergency release of uncrossmatched blood
- An adult patient's red cell transfusions exceed 8 units in 8 hours
- Inventory dictates that Rh-negative patients receive Rh-positive blood or platelets
- Blood less than 7 days old is requested for an adult patient
- A patient receives more than 6 units of fresh-frozen plasma in 24 hours
- A patient receives platelet transfusions on 3 consecutive days
- Fewer than 3 or more than 12 units of platelets is requested for an adult patient
- More than 2 units of platelets are requested for a newborn
- Cryoprecipitate is requested for a patient who does not have haemophilia A or von Willebrand's disease

A number of studies have also been published which have attempted to target the transfusion of a single blood component. Giovanetti et al [37] focused on RBC usage; an audit team visited patient wards daily to review utilization and to teach the physicians providing care about transfusion practice. During the period of study, the inappropriate use of RBC decreased from 37% to 10%. Several authors used similar approaches to reduce the inappropriate transfusion of FFP [38-40] and platelets [30, 41]. In each instance inappropriate transfusions of the audited component significantly decreased from baseline data.

Conclusion

The process for improving transfusion practice is both critically important as well as continuous. In US hospitals inspected by the JCAHO, these activities are required. The focus for these activities should be an appointed QA committee with members representative of the medical and surgical services using the most blood. This committee should be responsible for adopting guidelines for practice which are embraced by the entire medical staff; for monitoring blood usage and assessing whether transfusion practice complies with those guidelines; for assisting in the development of strategies to improve noncompliant practices; and for reevaluating those audited activities in order to define improvement.

Although many approaches rely on the use of retrospective audit, the use of prospective or even concurrent audit which are more desirable approaches, should be more readily implemented as sophisticated computer systems are introduced into laboratory operations. Such systems allow immediate correlation to be made between the component being requested and relevant laboratory data. The availability of such information has the potential for focusing the attention of the transfusion service medical team on those requests which require additional information to assess the transfusion request. Through such a process of review coupled with patient consultations and educational programmes, the level of transfusion practice can be raised. While we continuously seek to add new strategies and tests to qualify blood donors in order to improve the safety of the blood supply, the reduction in the inappropriate use of blood components is as important a strategy to increase the safety of blood transfusions.

Acknowledgements

The author would like to recognize the outstanding technical support provided by Denise McAvaney.

References

1. Roberts JS, Coale JG, Redman RR. A history of the joint commission on accreditation of hospitals. JAMA 1987;258:936-40.
2. McLendon WW, Ernest A, Codman MD (1869-1940). The end result idea, and The Product of a Hospital. Arch Pathol Lab Med 1990;114:1101-4.
3. Codman EA. The product of a hospital. Arch Pathol Lab Med 1990;114:1106-11.
4. Accreditation manual for hospitals, 1994. Oakbrook Terrace, IL: Joint Commission on Accreditation of Healthcare Organizations, 1993.
5. Grindon AJ, Tomasulo PS, Bergin JJ, Klein HG, Miller JD, Mintz PD. The hospital transfusion committee: Guidelines for improving practice. JAMA 1985;253:540-43.
6. Silberstein LE, Kruskall MS, Stehling LC, Johnston MFM, Rutman RC. Strategies for the review of transfusion practices. JAMA 1989;262:1993-97.
7. Nicholls MD. Quality assurance of hospital transfusion practice. Med J Aust 1993;158: 295-97.
8. Renner SW. Blood usage monitors and desired improvement. CAP Today 1990;4:26-27.
9. Hoeltge GA. Peer review of transfusion practices. In: Summers SH, Smith DM, Agranenko VA (eds). Transfusion therapy: Guidelines for practice. Arlington, VA: American Association of Blood Banks, 1990:157-75.
10. Clark JA, Ayoub MM. Blood and component wastage report: A quality assurance function of the hospital transfusion committee. Transfusion 1989;29:139-42.

11. Avorn J, Soumerai SB, Salem SR, Popovsky M. Documenting and correcting inappropriate use of blood components. In: Kurtz SR, Summers S (eds). Improving transfusion practice: The role of quality assurance. Arlington, VA: American Association of Blood Banks, 1989:21-30.
12. Stehling L, Luban NLC, Anderson KC, et al. Guidelines for blood utilization review. Transfusion 1994;34:438-48.
13. Welch HG, Meehan KR, Goodnough LT. Prudent strategies for elective red blood cell transfusion. Ann Intern Med 1992;116:393-402.
14. Audet AM, Goodnough LT. Practice strategies for elective red blood cell transfusion. Ann Intern Med 1992;116:403-6.
15. Scott EP. Fresh frozen plasma and platelets: Impact of transfusion guidelines on transfusion practice. In: Kurtz SR, Summers S, Kruskall MS (eds). Improving transfusion practice: The role of quality assurance. Arlington, VA: American Association of Blood Banks, 1989:31-51.
16. Simpson MB. The clinical use of platelet preparations. In: Summers SH, Smith DM, Agranenko VA (eds). Transfusion therapy: Guidelines for practice. Arlington, VA: American Association of Blood Banks, 1990:27-51.
17. Hamoudi AC, Cecalupo AJ, Wolf ML, Coe SA, Menke JA. The use of LIS for blood usage review: Experience in a children's hospital. Amer J Clin Path 1991;95:389-92.
18. Lepage EF, Gardner RM, Laub RM, Golubjatnikov OK. Improving blood transfusion practice: Role of a computerized hospital information system. Transfusion; 1992;32: 253-59.
19. Ringel M. Lab assesses transfusions. CAP Today 1995;9:1-16.
20. Tartter PI, Barron DM. Unnecessary blood transfusions in elective colorectal cancer surgery. Transfusion 1985;25:113-15.
21. Stehling LC, Esposito B. Appropriate intraoperative blood utilization. Transfusion 1987;27:545(abstract).
22. Brien WF, Butler RJ, Inwood MJ. An audit of blood component therapy in a Canadian general teaching hospital. Can Med Assoc J 1989;140:812-15.
23. Mozes B, Epstein M, Ben-Bassat I, Modan B, Halkin H. Evaluation of the appropriateness of blood and blood product transfusion using present criteria. Transfusion 1989;29:473-76.
24. Goodnough LT, Verbrugge D, Vizmeg K, Riddell J. Identifying elective orthopedic surgical patients transfused with amounts of blood in excess of need: The transfusion trigger revisited. Transfsuion 1992;32:648-53.
25. Shaikh BS, Wagar D, Lau PM, Campbell EW. Transfusion pattern of fresh frozen plasma in a medical school hospital. Vox Sang 1985;48:366-69.
26. Snyder AJ, Gottschall JL, Menitove JE. Why is fresh-frozen plasma transfused? Transfusion 1986;26:107-12.
27. Blumberg N, Laczin J, McMican A, Heal J, Arvan D. A critical survey of fresh-frozen plasma use. Transfusion 1986;26:511-13.
28. Menitove JE, McElligott MC, Aster RH. Where have all the platelets gone? A strategy for monitoring platelet usage. Wisc Med J 1982;81:11-13.
29. Silver SS, Rock G, Decary F, et al. Use of platelet concentrates in eastern Ontario. Can Med Assoc J 1987;137:128-32.
30. McCullough, Steepter TA, Connelly DP. Platelet utilization in a university hospital. JAMA 1988;259:2414-18.
31. Tomasulo PA, Lenes BA, Noto TA, Klein HG, Menitove JE. Automatic special case consultations in transfusion medicine. Transfusion 1986;26:186-93.

32. Renner SW. Quarterly Review Bulletin 1987,March;13:76-80.
33. Lichtiger B, Fisher HE, Huh Yo. Screening of transfusion service requests by the blood bank pathologist: Impact on cost containment. Lab Med 1988;19:228-30.
34. Finkle HI. A prospective blood utilization review system. Transfusion 1992;32: 787(letter).
35. Silver H, Tahhan HR, Anderson J, Lachman M. A non-computer-dependent prospective review of blood and blood component utilization. Transfusion 1992;32:260-65.
36. Rosen NR, Bates LH, Herod G. Transfusion therapy: Improved patient care and resource utilization. Transfusion 1993;33:341-47.
37. Giovanetti AM, Parravicini A, Baroni L, et al. Quality assessment of transfusion practice in elective surgery. Transfusion 1988;28:166-69.
38. Shanberge JN. Reduction of fresh-frozen plasma use through a daily survey and education program. Transfusion 1987;27:226-27.
39. Solomon RR, Clifford JS, Gutman SI. The use of laboratory intervention to stem the flow of fresh frozen plasma. Am J Clin Pathol 1988;89:518-21.
40. Barnette RE, Fish DJ, Eisenstaedt RS. Modification of fresh-frozen plasma transfusion practices through educational intervention. Transfusion 1990;30:253-57.
41. Simpson MB. Prospective-concurrent audits and medical consultation for platelet transfusions. Transfusion 1987;27:192-95.
42. Shulman IA, Lohr K, Derdiarian AK, Picukaric JM. Monitoring transfusionist practices: A strategy for improving transfusion safety. Transfusion 1994;34:11-15.
43. Salem-Schatz SR, Avorn J, Soumerai SB. Influence of clinical knowledge, organizational context, and practice style on transfusion decision making. JAMA 1990;264: 476-83.

LÈGISLATIVE AND REGULATORY IMPACT ON TRANSFUSION MEDICINE PRACTICE

K. Sazama

Introduction

The hysteria that continues to accompany the AIDS epidemic is unequalled in modern times for its medical, social, societal, ethical, legal and governemental impact. Globally, in transfusion medicine, highly respected physicians have been sent to jail, governments have altered longstanding legal protection afforded to blood banks, huge blood collecting organizations have been subjected to regulatory sanctions and the rights of individuals are stridently advocated. In the US where healthcare is not fully government-subsidized, the impact of transfusion-transmitted HIV is being played out with threats of huge monetary rewards in civil suits in the courtroom as well as through focused criticism of the government [1].

The events triggering increased governmental involvement stem from global concerns about blood safety and encompass actions such as changing policies and practices regarding national collection activities to achieve self-sufficiency, standardizing blood collection and transfusion processes and changing the emphasis of accreditation to focus on quality practices (Table 1). Paralleling these actions are the reviews of actual medical practice targeted to concerns over appropriateness and use of blood components for specific patient categories. In Europe, in particular, the policy statements requiring national self-sufficiency issued in 1992 and 1993 resulted from recognition that some of the safety problems in European countries stemmed directly from longstanding reliance on US plasma which contributed to transfusion-transmitted AIDS in haemophilia and other patients.

Safety of blood

While the likelihood of receiving a unit of blood containing human immunodeficiency virus (HIV) was probably as high as 1 in 100 in San Francisco in 1983 [2] current statistics suggest that the US risk is now less than 1:400,000 [3]. (In some parts of Africa, the risk may still be 1:100 or even higher.) The early recognition of HIV in US transfusion recipients provided an impetus to unravel the mystery and develop strategies to minimize the harm, but did not prevent

Table 1. Legislation and regulation: Triggering events.

Safety: Policy Decisions	
– HIV testing: When, what, handling inventory	Donor issues: Deferral questions
– Manufacturing choices: Discard, withdrawal	Transfusion: Fewer exposures
Self-sufficiency:	
– US, EU, other countries	
Standardization:	
– Forming the European Community/Union	
– ISO: The QUALITY movement	
Appropriateness:	
– Consensus statements	
– Clinical pathways/practice guidelines	
Accreditation:	
– Inspection to assessment	

the global distribution of what has retrospectively been recognized as HIV-infected plasma from US donors. Even after the possibility of HIV infection transmissible by these US plasma products was identified, a number of European countries continued to use them in manufacturing, in part, because of concerns over unavailability of life-saving therapies if such "raw materials" were discarded.

There were (and still are) significant differences in the safety of blood for transfusion (and further manufacturing) in countries around the world. In Japan, for example, only 36 (out of 6,610,484) units of blood have reportedly been found to be test positive for HIV since screening began in 1986 [4]. The Canadian Red Cross, on advice of Canada's Commission of Inquiry on the Safety of the Blood Supply, announced in May 1995 that it will close clinics where blood supplies have higher than normal HIV infection rate [5]. Italian health authorities are reportedly planning to exert tighter control over Italy's blood transfusion services following labelling and donor suitability violations [6]. However, during the mid-1980s (after testing first became available), variance in policies between collection facilities and between countries clearly contributed significantly to the safety of blood components. (Table 2).

Table 2. Policy variances that affected blood safety.

Donation process:	AIDS education, confrontational questioning
HIV Testing:	Prospective, inventory, handling of reactive unites
Donor Deferrals:	Repeat reactive, confirmed, reported to whom
Manufacturing practices:	Market withdrawal of all, viral inactivation
Transfusion practices:	Limiting donor exposures, autologous/directed, transfusion "trigger" change, cryo not concentrate
Other:	"Surrogate" testing, donor payment

AIDS education of donors

Blood collection organizations in the US rapidly adopted the 1983 federal requirements for donor education about the source and risks for acquiring AIDS. That these efforts were succesful in diverting unsuitable donors is now established. Subsequent changes in interviewing techniques and improved information continued to contribute to US blood safety. These measures were incorporated into some, but not all, blood centres in Europe, but not in endemic areas of Africa where most donors would obviously be deferred.

The effect of confrontational questioning of donors may explain in part the increasingly alarming reports of blood shortages, not only in the US, but also in Australia [7] and Russia [8].

HIV testing

Both before and after a specific HIV test was devised by US and French scientists, policies critical to possible reduction in subsequent disease transmission resulted in deametrically opposed practices. Even answers to obvious questions such as when and what to test for HIV (once testing was available) were different: some collection facilities tested only blood collected subsequent to receipt of test kits, some tested inventory as well; some facilites "swapped out" test positive inventory (all components), some swapped only short-date components; some facilities began testing and "swap out" within several days of receiving testing equipment, others delayed for several weeks to permit adequate training and quality control measures to be established. Perhaps what is less well appreciated is that, even though anti-HTLV-III (now anti-HIV 1) testing was available and recommended for use by blood and plasma collecting facilities in the US as early as March 1985, it was NOT fully implemented until fall of 1985 or even later.

Donor deferral practices

Even today in most states in the US, it is possible for a donor deferred by one blood or plasma collection facility to donate in another one. There is no national donor deferral registry and no standard system of donor registration throughout the collecting facilities in the US. In those states in which a donor deferral must be reported, the "rules" of reporting vary such that, e.g., in California, a plasma centre donor deferral report is likely to differ from reporting by a blood centre. The American National Red Cross is attempting to establish a national donor deferral registry, but it collects only half or less of all whole blood collected in the US and only a minor quantity of plasma. The remaining non-Red Cross collection activities are the responsibiliy of other community blood centres, the military blood programme, hospital-based collection activities and numerous commercial plasma centres, none of which communicate their donor deferral information to each other or to the Red Cross.

Manufacturing pracitices: market withdrawal and viral inactivation

National policies for discarding test positive plasma also varied during the early years of testing. Although the US Food and Drug Administration insisted that US manufacturers discard and incinerate plasma in inventory as well as fully manufactured components when known infected units were implicated, other countries did not have the resources to require similar practices. The significant shortages of factor concentrates in the later 1980s in the US and Canada were directly attributable to the regulatory requirements for quarantine, discard or significant re-manufacturing. Unfortunately, plasma brokers in the US may not have been as rigorous as US manufacturers in eliminating the potentially contaminated units from distribution outside the US.

Manufacturing changes were also not standardized. Some methods, e.g., heat treating, differed between manufacturers; others, e.g. chemical disinfection, were proprietary. The timing and application of additional viral inactivation methods to plasma components impacted safety in the US and abroad. Because of the long history of regulation of blood in the US, the opportunity to address these safety concerns existed when the epidemic began. The agency's response to the challenge provides lessons for future improvements.

Transfusion Practices

Strategies for reducing number of donor exposures to lessen the possibility of AIDS transmission by transfusion were effected before any regulatory requirement was drafted. These actions included implementing directed plasma donations for preparing cryoprecipitate for newly diagnosed haemophilia in infants and small children, an upsurge in autologous and directed whole blood collections, renewed interest in whole blood (rather than component preparation) for recipients requiring both red cells and plasma components, and consensus development on lowering the "transfusion trigger" for transfusion at all. The effectiveness of these practices in the US has been demonstrated. Studies are just now underway in other countries to evaluate policies then and now in place regarding appropriateness and number of blood components transfused in various recipient groups.

Other

The debate over "surrogate" testing has nearly run its course in US courts with the overwhelming consensus that there was no single surrogate that would have improved safety of US blood for transfusion in the year or two between when HIV transmission was thought to be transfusion-transmitted until a specific test for antibody to HIV was available. Some testing, e.g., CD4 counts, is still not routinely available due to its complexity.

Self-sufficiency in blood collection

The United States has traditionally supplied numerous other countries (Europe, Japan, others) with plasma for manufacturing but depends in part on importation of red blood cells from European collectors. Both practices are regulated by the US Food and Drug Administration (FDA) as well as by the differing regulations of individual countries. Because the US compensates plasma donors in cash and the US regulations permit frequent, large volume collections of plasma, surplus plasma from US donors in exportable. In 1992, the Council of Europe resolved to achieve self-sufficiency in plasma [9]. A similar resolution for blood self-sufficiency was passed by the EC in 1993 [10].

Standardization

The changing focus of the US Food and Drug Administration

Quality systems activities have not gone unrecognized in the legislative and regulatory bodies of various countries. While US regulations regarding blood articulated the need for "safety, purity, potency and efficacy" of the component being transfused (using terminology analogous to its longstanding regulation of drugs), the federal agency responsible for blood safety, the Food and Drug Administration (FDA), looks beyond the manufacturing steps leading to a final product ready for a consumer. In the first blood regulations, published in 1975 [11], the US FDA extended its interest to activities traditionally considered to be part of transfusion medicine, namely, compatibility of blood with individual recipients, criteria for proper storage temperatures and expirations, errors or accidents involving recipients and fatality reporting. Recent emphasis by the US FDA on quality assurance [12] that specifically encompasses the application of current good manufacturing practices for drugs and pharmaceuticals to blood and blood components is a relatively late recognition of similar efforts that resulted in the 1987 publication of the ISO 9000 series by the European Union [13].

In retrospective reviews of their decisions made during the early years of the AIDS epidemic, some public officials in Europe have been tried and sentenced to jail, some in Canada are under threat of similar actions and some governments have taken what can be considered rather draconian measures (e.g., in the UK, governmental protection against strict liability for blood used in transfusions was removed in 1991 [14]. In US courts, a few practitioners heve sustained huge fines because juries have found there was no need for transfusion and that recipients were not properly informed of risks. Consumers have demanded legislative mandates for choice of autologous and directed donors and several states, including California and New Jersey, mandate appropriate informed consent for transfusion. More urgently today, legislators at all levels are being urged to make blood safe [1].

The quality movement previously limited to manufacturing and defense activities exploded into the worldwide health care arena in the 1990's. Even though many US physicians may still be only partially aware of "Total Quality Management" (TQM), the concern for quality is voiced whenever cost-containment activities are described. The US Congress has grilled Dr. Kessler, the FDA Commissioner, regarding lapses in regulatory control and an unseemly collegial relationship between the governmental agency and the "regulated industry" as the public has demanded answers and redress for harm resulting from transfusions. The 15 years of worldwide AIDS hysteria has culminated in numerous restrospective evaluations, including a recently released report from the Institute of Medicine, from which legislators are likely to create additional requirements [1] (Table 3).

Table 3. Recommendations for responding to the "next" crisis; US Institute of Medicine 1995.

Public Health Service: Coordination	Blood safety "CZAR" Blood safety council
Centers for Disease Control and prevention: Assessment of risk	Surveillance system Assessment prevails
Food and Drug Administration: Risk management	Implement partial solutions Periodic review of decisions Distinguish regulations/guidelines Revamp advisory committee
Consider legislation: "No fault" compensation	

The pressures to contain health care costs as they soar byond 18% of the US GNP will likely result in as many changes in transfusion medicine practices as will the quality movement. Increased attention to the collection and distribution of blood for transfusion is apprarent in governmental efforts worldwide to apply pharmaceutical and medical device quality standards to all aspects of blood banking and transfusion medicine. Such efforts should not ignore the substantive regulatory actions that curtailed the US AIDS epidemic early on (Table 4).

Table 4. Time line of specific actions: US.

1983	Change donor screening
1985	HIV test approved
1986	Donor screening
1988	HIV regulation
1993	QA Guide
1995	JCAHO: Informed consent

The Eurpean Union

In Europe, the BSI drafted the first set of voluntary standards for quality assurance known as BS 5750 in 1979. These standards were adopted virtually unchanged in 1987 as the ISO 9000 series of standards. The European Union (now comprised of Austria, Belgium, Denmark, Finland, France, Germany, Greece, Ireland, Italy, Luxembourg, the Netherlands, Portugal, Spain, Sweden and the United Kingdom) have encouraged adoption of the ISO 9000 in their efforts to unify these countries into a single internal market. By 1995, 80 countries have adopted the ISO 9000 series as a national standard.

How transfusion medicine will fare as part of these unification efforts has not yet been fully resolved. A number of recently published guidelines [15, 16] should assist in effecting standardization. Standardization globally has focused principally

Table 5. Standard-setting organizations.

AABB	American Association of Blood Banks (Bethesda, MD)
ANSI	American National Standards Institute (Washington, DC)
BSI	British Standards Institute
CEN	European Committee for Standardization
CENELEC	European Committee for Electrotechnical Standardization
DIN	German Institute for Standardization
FDA	Food en Drug Administration (Washington, DC)
ISO	International Organization for Standardization (Geneva)
JCAHO	Joint Commission on Accreditation of Healthcare Organizations

Table 6. Some specific actions: European Union.

1993	Belgium	Minors may refuse transfusion
1985	Spain	Blood donation regulation
1993	Netherlands	Individual Health Care Act (BIG)
1993	Spain	Minors may NOT donate blood
1995	Italy	Tighter control
1995	EU	Proposed directive for medical devices

in the technical arena, with less progress in professional and functional standardization or in effecting legal and regulatory harmony [17]. The professional standards can be considered as voluntary or private standards, such as those used by the JCAHO for accrediting healthcare organizations in the US and Canada, while legal and regulatory standards are mandatory. Various organizators are engaged in standard-setting activities in transfusion medicine. (Table 5) The forum to harmonize these activities is not completely defined. Legal systems differ between countries of the EU as well as between the EU, the US, Japan and other nations. However, continuing efforts to address safety are evidenced by specific legal and regulatory changes in a number of countries (Table 6).

Appropriateness/utilization

Transfusion medicine has been overtly recognized as a new discipline of clinical practice in the US in the past decade [18]. This "NEW" discipline is defined similarly with the European model where transfusion medicine is comprised of physicians whose practice experience relates to collection, processing, storage and distribution of blood components as well as devising responsible transfusion practices for patients in their institutions, all consistent with pertinent regulatory requirements. The decisions about whether, when and what to transfuse patients remain primarily the responsibility of the attending physician (not that of the transfusion medicine specialist). However, even these "medical" choices (which, before AIDS, were considered in general to be a matter of medical judgment except for the US use of MSBOS [19] to guide transfusion during surgery) have come into question. Adverse decisions in transfusion-transmitted AIDS litigation in the US have successfully raised questions of whether transfusions were indicated and the adequacy of informed consent. The changing economy of healthcare affects informed consent doctrine in other countries as well [20].

Particularly in the US and Canada where peer review of transfusion practices has long been mandated by private accreditating organizations such as the Joint Commission on Accreditation of Healthcare Organization (JCAHO) and the College of American Pathologists (CAP), but also increasingly in the UK and other European countries [21] every aspect of blood transfusion ordering and administration practices is currently undergoing intense scrutiny [22]. The development of consensus statements for appropriate use of components including albumin, platelets, red blood cell use and plasma has occurred during the past 20 years in the US [23, 24] and, within the past decade, in the Caribbean [25], the UK [26 - 28] and the Netherlands [29] as well as by the World Health Organization [30]. The development of US clinical practice guidelines specifically targeted to appropriate use of each type of blood component is also well underway [31]. It should come as no surprise that data derived from actual practices is being used successfully to determine compensation.

In a recently published (1994) study of selected transfusion practices in 10 EU member countries that was conducted between January 1990 and July 1992, it was readily apparent to the participants that wide disparities of practice exist. These differences included when and how much blood to transfuse, when and which other fluids or drugs are used, the use of autologous blood, and other factors. Any interesting divergence was that some similarities were noted between the data from the SANGUIS study and several published US studies of blood use during coronary artery bypass graft procedures [32, 33]. However, by far, the intersection of quality systems standards, current good manufacturing practices and the practice of transfusion medicine is the new frontier for the '90's, particularly as the US healthcare system transitions from a fee-for-service to a managed care system.

Accreditation

Accreditation by authorized organizations is fundamental to access to US federal payments for healthcare for targeted members of society. The regulations that permit payment require that organizations have a third party certification based on compliance with compulsory and voluntary standards, from JCAHO or state sources. While the EU functions somewhat differently, it is safe to predict that the focus of future inspection and accreditation evaluations in transfusion medicine will no longer stop outside the patient's door, but will reach into the operating room and continue to expand into new arenas such as haematopoietic stem and progenitor cell reconstitution from bone marrow and peripheral and cord blood infusions. The philosphy of accreditation is refocusing from in-depth inspection to discover mistakes to reliance on quality assessments [34] of ongoing audits and other evaluations that provide the institution with some basis for demonstrating quality processes [39].

In general, the ISO 9000 standards as well as those originating with the AABB, JCAHO and other certifying bodies are viewed as providing a standard of practice which is persuasive in legal situations. Regulations are viewed by US courts as minimal standards which help to provide a framework for evaluation practices. The specific legal and regulatory requirements for individual EU members are found in both legislative and judicial records [36]. Transfusion medicine specialists in the future will be as knowledgeable about good manufacturing practices, quality management, certification standards, accreditation requirements and legal and regulatory decisions as they currently are about good medical practices and peer review activities.

References

1. HIV and the blood supply: An analysis of crisis decisionmaking. Institute of Medicine, Washington, DC, 1995.
2. Samson S, Busch M, Ward J, et al. Identification of HIV-infected transfusion recipients: The utility of crossreferencing previous donor records with AIDS case reports. Transfusion 1990;30:214-18.
3. Dodd RY. Viral contamination of blood components and approaches for reduction of infectivity. Immunol Invest 1995;24:25-48.
4. News Summaries. AABB Blood Bank Week, August 4, 1995:4.
5. Business Briefs. International Blood and Plasma News, May 1995:136.
6. Business Briefs. International Blood and Plasma News, May 1995:137.
7. Business Briefs. International Blood and Plasma News, January 1995:77.
8. Business Briefs. International Blood and Plasma News, January 1995:76.
9. Council of Europe. Plasma products and European self-sufficiency: Collection, preparation and use, ISBN 92-871-1925-2, Strassbourg (France), Council of Europe Press, 1992.
10. Commission of the European Communities. Blood self-sufficiency in the European Community, Luxembourg, Office for Official Publications of the European Communities, 1993.
11. Federal Register, Volume 40, No. 223, Tuesday, November 18, 1975. Human blood and blood products, collection, storage and processing, 53532-53544.
12. Guideline for Quality Assurance in Blood Establishments, US Food and Drug Administration, Rockville, MD, July 11, 1995.
13. Peach RW (ed). The ISO 9000 Handbook, 2nd ed, CEEM Information Services, Fairfax, VA, 1995.
14. Harvey E, Hewison C, Nevalainen DE, Lloyd HL. Maintaining quality in blood banking. Blood Rev 1995;9:15-24.
15. Stivala JFA, Wagstaff W. Quality assurance in blood transfusion. Vox Sang 1994;67(Suppl 5):37-42.
16. Guidelines for Quality Assurance Programmes in Blood Transfusion Services. Geneva, World Health Organization, 1993.
17. Moran RF. Setting standards: A global mission. Advance/laboratory 1995;4:17-21.
18. Klein HG. Transfusion medicine. The evolution of a new discipline. JAMA

1987;258:2108-9.
19. Mintz PD, Laurenstein K, Hume J, Henry JB. Expected hemotherapy in elective surgery. A follow-up. JAMA 1978;239:623-25.
20. Annas GJ, Miller FH. The empire of death: How culture and economics affect informed consent in the US, the UK and Japan. Am J Law Med 1994;20:357-94.
21. European Parliament. Joint motion for a resolution on safe blood transfusions and of blood derivatives, 17 November 1993.
22. Safe and Good Use of Blood in Surgery (SANGUIS), Sirchia G, Giovanetti AM, McClelland RBL, Fracchia GN (eds). European Commission, IV Medical and Health Research Programme, Luxembourg, 1994.
23. National Institutes of Health Consensus Development Conference Statement, 1984. Fresh frozen plasma indications and risks. National Heart, Lung and Blood Institute. Bethesda, MD. JAMA 1984;253:551-53.
24. National Institutes of Health Consensus Development Conference, 1988. Perioperative red cell transfusion. National Heart, Lung and Blood Institute, Bethesda, MD. JAMA 1988;260:2700-3.
25. Gibbs WN, Green M. Clinical aspects of blood transfusion in adults. Vox Sang 1994;67(Suppl 5):43-49.
26. Davies SC, Kinsey SE. Clinical aspects of paediatric blood transfusion: Cellular components. Vox Sang 1994;67(Suppl 5):50-53.
27. Chalmers EA, Gibson BES. Clinical aspects of paediatric and perinatal transfusion: Plasma products. Vox Sang 1994;67(Suppl 5):54-58.
28. British Committee for Standards in Haematology Blood Transfusion Task Force. Guidelines for administration of blood products: Transfusion of infants and neonates. Transfusion Med 1994;4:63-69.
29. De Wolf JThM. Consensus protocols for supportive hemotherapy. In: Smit Sibinga CTh, Das PC, Heiniger HJ (eds). Good Manufacturing Practice in Transfusion Medicine, Kluwer Acad Publ., Dordrecht, Boston, London, 1994:263-67.
30. LAB/89.9. Guidelines for the appropriate use of blood; WHO Geneva, 1993. Guidelines for quality assurance programs for blood transfusion services.
31. Welch G, Meehan KR, Goodnough LT. Prudent strategies for elective red blood cell transfusion. Ann Intern Med 1992;116:393-402.
32. Goodnough LT, Johnston MFM, Toy PTC and the Transfusion Medicine Academic Award Group. The variability of transfusion practice in coronary artery bypass surgery. JAMA 1991;265:86-90.
33. Surgenor DM, Wallace EL, Churchill WH, et al. Red cell transfusions in coronary artery bypass surgery (DRGs 106 and 107). Transfusion 1992;32:458-64.
34. Quality Plan. American Association of blood Banks, Bethesda, MD, 1994.
35. Sazama K (ed). Accreditations Requirements Manual, 6th edition. American Association of Blood Banks, Bethesda, MD, 1995.
36. Nys H (ed). Medical Law. In: Blanpain R (ed). International Encyclopaedia of Laws. Kluwer Law and Taxation Publishers, Deventer, the Netherlands, 1994.

DISCUSSION

C.Th. Smit Sibinga and E.L. Snijder – moderators

P.V. Holland (Sacramento, CA, USA): First of all I want to compliment all the speakers for a dynamic and exciting programme this morning. Dr. Smit Sibinga, I would like to ask you where you got your definition of "standard of practice". I like it very much and I would like to ask if it is indeed the standard of practice in the Netherlands or in Europe.

C.Th. Smit Sibinga (Groningen, NL): The definition actually emerged out of a discussion which was fundamental to an informal report of WHO, but which is available[1]. In 1991 at WHO in Geneva we specifically spoke about the need for communication and consultative services, we set down and tried to define what we were really talking about. Subsequently it was taken as a fundamental definition of transfusion medicine and transfusion practice for the symposium which we held in 1991 on facts and fictions in transfusion medicine[2]. If you want to discriminate between the facts and fictions you have to know what you talk about, that is how we got to the definition.

H.J.C. de Wit (Leeuwarden, NL): Dr. Smit Sibinga, you said in your lecture that changes over time in blood products are important, not to be neglected and not part of the pharmaceutical properties. Perhaps it would be an idea to specify more strictly these properties of blood products we use in clinical trials, also in terms of age. Perhaps we could solve a little bit of the problem by making the blood products a bit purer, because what we give now is a cocktail of cells, plasma constituents, with age differences, amounts of biological response modifies like interleukins etcetera. We transfuse dying or anergic white cells in different amounts and the effect of the white cells might be even influenced by plasticisers or maybe diet of the donors. Could not we make better clinical trials if we define better the products that we use in those trials?

---

1. Report of the GBSI informal consultation on Collaboration in Training in Transfusion Medicine. Geneva, WHO/LBS/92.7.
2. Transfusion medicine: Fact and fiction. Smit Sibinga CTh, Das PC, Cash JD (eds). Kluwer Academic Publishers. Boston, Dordrecht, London, 1992.

C.Th. Smit Sibinga: I think I agree with your last point, but this actually echoes the discussion of yesterday morning where based on the presentations in the morning it became evident that there is a great lack of uniformity in what at least is written up in the literature. Therefore the possibilities for comparison of actual outcomes is limited. We came to the conclusion that for instance the ages of the blood components used in the trials are usually not given; that is to say more precise characteristics are not given. Yet we judge and we come to the conclusion that more concise studies are needed to really know whether the clinical outcome significantly improves or deteriorates or remains the same as compared to previous practices in studies to be achieved. Dr. de Wolf can give you a formula on how that should actually be calculated statistically to know how large the study should be to really get to that point. Such an approach is definitely needed; you need to define the products and that is where your pharmaceutical expertise is needed for.

H.P. Olthuis (Nijmegen, NL): Dr. Sazama, I would like to stress the point of no-fault compensation system, which is an item in the Netherlands at the moment. Personally I believe that it is useful to give a compensation to patients that have been infected by blood transfusion where the fault is not with the transfusion centre, but I wonder if this is going to be a regular system, a no-fault compensation system. What will be the consequences for other fields of medicine where also compensation will be asked for damage where no fault is made.

K. Sazama (Philadelphia, PA, USA): Yes, you ask a very important question, and it is a fundamental change in thinking. In the United States, there is already a model for a different type of injury compensation. About ten years ago the Congress enacted the legislation called the National Childhood Vaccine Act which provides exactly the kind of compensation that is the model that could be used. It is basically recognition that some children will be injured while many more benefit from vaccination. I think your point is how would one define the limits of which kinds of injuries you want to compensate. It is easy when you talk about well-defined small groups of people or relatively small options. I think there will be a lot of discussion and debate about that.

H.P. Olthuis: Dr. Eisenstaedt, you mentioned with a question mark the directed donation. I should like to know the recent opinions in the United States about the risk of directed donations and I will combine this to the before mentioned point of a no-fault compensation. How is for instance that directed donation perhaps to be related to a no-fault compensation if a directed donor gets an infection or is the reason for the infection.

R.S. Eisenstaedt (Philadelphia, PA, USA): I am not sure if I can quote the party line under directed donation, but I think that most official organizations still say that it is no safer than blood which is donated altruistically by the community. My own opinion is that there are certain instances where directed donation is uniquivally safer, for example if you have a monogamous couple beyond the childbearing age and one needs transfusion it seems to me that the partner has got to be a safer donor than the donor that would come from the community. There are communities where the prevalence of HIV is much higher than in other communities. We have heard just recently about efforts to close down donor centres in some of those areas. So it seems again to me that designated donations from those areas would be safer. But most fundamentally what I learnt yesterday from prof. Vlek is that the reason people want those directed donations deals with this issue of trust and control and whether or not it is safer.

K. Sazama: As to the possibility of how a no-fault compensation might work it would be difficult to imagine why we would treat differently than any other donation, I mean, other than personal feelings like guilt or remorse or whatever. I do not think the system would permit a different result for the victim. No-fault is really intended to try to compensate the person who is harmed and not to place blame.

C.H. Wallas (Charlotte, NC, USA): To say something about directed donations, I actually think in my own view that there are some data that suggest that that may be less safe. So my concern would be that in fact if we provide these components for use and provide the service, they are not to be crossed over in the blood supply. Because, I think emotions are driving this process not science. We take the view at least in our blood centre region that these are in fact designated for a specific recipient and if not used, like autologous blood, would not be used for other patients. So, I really believe that we should work to limit these components and that if we do collect them that we recognize we are collecting them to support an emotional need and not cross them over.

M. Blajchman (Hamilton, C): Dr. Eisenstaedt, during your interesting presentation you talked about communication to recipients of risks and benefits. It is relatively easy to communicate risks. You can give a number 1 in 50,000, 1 in a 1,000, whatever, what in my experience is not easy is communication of benefit. You can talk about cost benefit or quality additional life years. How would you propose to communicate benefit in order to balance the equation between risk and benefit. I think this needs some attention and I like to hear your thoughts on this matter.

R.S. Eisenstaedt: It is extremely difficult to quantitate those benefits in terms of numbers, statistics, ratios whatever you like. On the other hand I do not think it makes any difference that you cannot do that because patients do not understand that information. They do not react to in a logical manner based upon the statistics that you are giving them. So I think you can be much more qualitative in describing that benefit in saying "this is going to help you, this is going to make you feel better, this is going to do something to protect against problems". The important part of these informed consent processes is at least the importance of information that you are giving to the patient, is hearing from the patient what their concerns are and recognizing that their concerns may be way out of line, but the precise statistics that you are going to attach to those risks will generate a different perception.

M. Blajchman: But, as you know those risks rather than those benefits are coloured by the press considerably. The things that get attention are what recently has been described as the Bobbitt phenomenon. The Bobbitt phenomenon, for those of you who do not remember, is the man who had his penis severed; that got a lot of attention and caused concern among some individuals, which is far out of range of the attention it should have deserved.

R.S. Eisenstaedt: I think that there are going to be some instances where the patient will overreact to the psychological issues, such that they may refuse lifesaving transfusion support. In most instances I think it does not make that much difference whether you give the unit or do not give the unit. Those decisions are sort of a close enough call that you can listen to patient's preferences as part of the informed choice process and do not need to worry much about the precise statistics.

M. Blajchman: Dr. Sazama, one of the concerning things to me is the expectation that all over the world good decisions be made on limited information. Nowhere in the recent IOM report, for example, is there any indication that we should enhance the information gathering system. I wonder if you have any thoughts about how we should obtain appropriate information in the current climate. There needs to be a greater emphasis on gathering information that is to do proper studies, in order to be able to make good decisions.

K. Sazama: Dr. Blajchman, I think you make a very good point. I think the troubling aspect to me as you heard in discussing the IOM report and also in the practices that you are going to be seeing as well out of the Klever Commission report, is that what the public is telling us is they do not want science; that in fact science is an enigma to many people and is perceived (I believe) in a way that dr. Holland depicted in terms of what their world looks like. I think the recent verdict in the O.J. Simpson case is another reflection of disdain for the entire scientific attitude that we have. I think it is really a reaction of that strongly held value that we have, which says facts have to support decisions. I think what prof. Vlek helped us all to think about again is that facts are different for different people and what the public is telling us is we cannot hide behind a scientifically correct position in order to move forward. We cannot use that as a shield, as a means by which we deflect the responsibility. They are really saying "pay attention to these other values", and the values we have do not depend on having the exact scientific information.

T. Smith (Girvan, UK): I am both a medical practitioner and a journalist, so that I am part of the media that has been criticised in the last few days. In the United Kingdom we have since 1977 the Medical Journalists' Association (MJA), members of which have been working hard with leading doctors to put a more balanced view of medicine across to the British public. I write a Sunday "health page" for a Scottish newspaper that reaches half the population – is to keep medical scare stories, or stories that have been blown up out of all proportion, out of my newspaper. As the paper's doctor I am contacted about any medical stories for my opinion on whether they are correct or, frankly, rubbish, and the journalists almost always take my advice on their suitability for publication. Most newspapers have people like me on their staff or available on the end of a telephone. Nowadays they are almost always members of the MJA. Half of the MJA membership are qualified doctors, and the others usually have university degrees (not necessarily scientific) and have special interest in medical matters. The MJA runs regular meetings and visits to hospitals and research institutes, and is a good training ground for journalists without scientific or medical backgrounds. In particular it allows non-medically trained journalists to meet with those like myself who know the pitfalls and problems of medical research and the results of wrong and scaremongering publicity. I do not know whether such an association of medical writers exists in the United States. If it does not, I would strongly advise American doctors in research and in practice to get in touch with people who write lay press medical columns with a view to getting them to band together in this way. If the British can get their media to change (and I think the MJA has done much to improve coverage of medical matters in the British press), then the same could be done in the United States.

J. Emmanuel (Geneva, CH): Before asking my question I would like to thank the organizers dr. Smit Sibinga, mr. de Wit and dr. Das for hosting this meeting and inviting WHO. I would like to inform the people here who are not aware of it that the Groningen Centre is a WHO Collaborating Centre. The centre carries out a vital service not only at the cutting edge of science, but also in developing countries, training staff and improving blood transfusion. From WHO's point of view the Groningen Centre is performing a very valuable collaboration.

Dr. Sazama, you have been talking about the question of whether there should have been less collaboration between the AABB, the FDA and various other organizations without involving the Red Cross. I wonder if you could expand a little on that because WHO is trying to promote a task force of interested parties of the major organizations and institutions involved in blood safety to harmonize and to improve global blood safety through a better exchange of information, to improve technologies and guidelines and bring everybody together to discuss these issues. That seems to be in contradiction to what the IOM is saying and as there will be representation from the FDA at this meeting I would appreciate some explanation.

K. Sazama: Let me see if I can characterize that a little bit more. I think that the critisism of the IOM was that the FDA relied too heavily on the regulated group, namely the blood collecting and transfusion organizations. Neither the FDA nor any other government agency can have all the expertise residing within public servants; you just do not have enough people of the right background and there is no one who serves in public service in the United States, who regularly practices medicine as well. I think it is really a reaction to a few people again, a very vocal group of people, the haemophiliacs, who have been the most adversely affected. We all acknowledge that there is truth in insisting that another mechanism should have been put in place. I do not think the government, I do not think the institute of medicine knows what it is what they said and I am not sure that there is any solution other than the one that has always been in place namely that there is liaison relationships between the regulatories and the regulatees with an exchange of information; that is extremely important. But I do think what they are saying is what we have just been discussing, which is there was not sufficient representation of the non-scientific recipient group of people who were affected by all these decisions, whose voice was not heard or was perceived not to have been heard. I think the message perhaps is that, although the scientific and medical and technological input is extremely important, there ought to be representation of the potential beneficiaries of those actions in sufficient numbers for their interest also to be represented. So, I believe the ultimate goal of this recommendation is not to simply provide total separation of the regulators and the regulatees but to pay closer attention to the balance of the interests that are present in the discussions that are going on. Any discussion, such as the important decisions that WHO is undertaking and perhaps the message from the IOM, should ensure that haemophiliacs, chronically transfused patients, recipients, people who undergo surgery have elective transfusions, etcetera, are also at the table during such discussions.

J. Emmanuel: Yes, the point is taken. The difficulty is that they will be represented through organizations, but how do you represent all the recipients of even the blood donors? I think the message is that they were critical of the collaboration and maybe they were critical of the limitations of the collaboration.

C.H. Wallas: There is perhaps another issue. There is one joint statement issue. Organizations got together and wrote joint statements. They were being accused of being in collision with each other to try to prevent any dialogue from occurring and so not only was it the issue of the organization dealing with the regulators but perhaps being too tightly bound to each other and I am not sure if that is one of the issues that is being addressed to you.

K. Sazama: Dr. Wallas, you are absolutely right. I think it is again the distrust of the scientific process. We would all agree that what was intended by a joint statement was to prepare a single consensus position so as to minimize any additional confusion that could arise. What benefit would it have been for the public to have three different positions that varied by three or four sentences; what kind of confusion or what kind of distrust would have ensued? I know that the consensus statement resulted from the good faith effort of reputable people who took all the information we had and tried to make some coherent sense out of it. I do not think we should retreat from that position. The suspicions that there was a conspiracy to suppress information has not been proven and there is no basis for believing. The facts were shared as they were given: all of the issues were out on the table. There is a transcript, so you can know whatever was discussed. The transcript is available to the public and always has been. Discussions were held in open, not closed meetings. The media were there, all voices were heard. The suspicion that vital information was withheld is unfounded.

INDEX

α-interferon 95
ABO incompatibility 203, 204
absolute risk reduction 59, 61
acceptance 115
acquired immune deficiency syndrome, *see* AIDS
AIDS 19, 21, 94, 97, 152, 161, 188, 216, 237–239, 242
ALARA principle 125
albumin 177
allogeneic stem cell transplantation 183
alloimmunization 65, 74, 75, 88, 207
altruism 128
amegakaryocytic thrombocytopenia 87
anti-HCV 92, 93
anti-HIV 1 and 2 92
anti-HIV 237
antithrombin III 223, 225
aplastic anaemia 87, 224, 225
ASA scores 140, 141
audit 143, 144, 148, 153, 156–158, 215, 219, 221–223, 225, 226, 227, 229, 243
Audit Review Committee 154
autologous blood transfusion programmes 14, 66, 68
autologous donor 170
autologous stem cell transplantation 183, 186
autologous transfusion (AT) 20, 26

beneficence 172
blood salvage 222
bone marrow transplantation 79, 183

CD34 184
CD34 selection 184
$CD34^+$ cells 184–186, 188
CD4 97, 238
cell-mediated immunity 76
CFU-GM 186
chronic non-cirrhotic hepatitis 94
cirrhosis 94, 95
clinical interface 213, 214, 216
colloid osmotic pressure 139, 143
computer audit 226
concurrent audit 152, 153, 155, 232
congenital CMV infection 149
cord blood 242
cord blood banks 187
cost-benefit analysis, 172
crossmatch/ transfusion ratio 222
current good clinical practice (cGCP) 158
current good manufacturing practice, *see* GMP
cytomegalovirus (CMV) 79, 92, 148–151

decision-making 115, 116, 120, 121, 125–127
2-3 DPG 201, 202, 204
dysmyelopoeitic syndrome 87

EBV 92
erythropoietin (EPO) 26, 68, 178
Ethics Committee 173, 174
ex vivo cell therapies 178, 179, 181, 188

Factor IX 91, 98
Factor VIII 91, 95–98, 177

febrile non-haemolytic transfusion reactions (FNHTR) 62, 73, 74, 80, 150, 151
fibrin glue 91

G-CSF 148, 178, 186
GBV-C 95
gene therapy 179, 180, 182, 183, 185, 196, 216
gene transfer 185
GM-CSF 148, 178, 186
GMP 3, 214–216, 242. 243
graft-versus-host disease (GvHD) 73, 150, 151, 183, 188
growth-promoting effect 78

haematopoietic stem cell 242
haemophilia 91, 95, 98, 177, 235
haemophilia B 98
HAV 93
HBsAg 92
hepatitis A 93, 99
hepatitis B 171
hepatitis C virus (HCV) 93–95
hepatitis G virus 95
hepatocellular carcinoma (HCC) 94, 95
high-risk donors 169
HIV 19, 94, 95, 97, 98, 149, 169, 204, 208, 235, 237, 238
HIV-1 79
HLA 89, 222
HLA-alloimmunization 61, 62, 75, 150, 161
Hospital Transfusion Committee 220
human immunodeficiency virus (HIV), *see* HIV
hypofibrinogenaemia 146

idiopathic thrombocytopenic purpura (ITP) 89, 224, 225
immunoglobulin 177
immunomodulation 73, 76, 79, 80
immunotherapy 216
indication equivalence 68, 69
informed consent 17–19, 21, 22, 67, 239
inhibitors 95, 96
intraoperative blood salvage 133, 138, 146
intrauterine transfusion 150
intravenous immunoglobulin 225
ISO 9000 series 239, 240
isovolaemic haemodilution 133

Kaposi sarcoma 92

LAK (lymphokine activated killer cells) 183

MHC 76
multi-drug resistance gene 180

national donor deferral registry 237
neoantigens 96
NK cell 76
non-maleficence 171, 172

oxygen carrying capacity 143
oxygen transport capacity 136, 137, 139

p24 antigen 169
paradoxical splanchnic ischaemia 68
parvovirus 92, 93, 99
PCR 94
peripheral blood stem cell transplantation 15, 178, 179
plasma exchange 145
platelet refractoriness 74–76, 80, 146, 151
porcine Factor VIII 98
post-operative bacterial infection 78
post-storage leukodepletion 74, 78
post-transfusion hepatitis (PTH) 204, 205
pre-storage leukodepletion 74, 76, 78, 80, 150
preoperative donation 133
preoperative haemodilution 138
progenitor cell 242
progenitor cell expansion 185
prospective audit 152, 153, 155

QA committee 225, 226, 231
quality adjusted life years (QALY) 216
quality assurance 154, 239, 240
quality assurance committee 220
quality management 243
quality systems 5, 9, 239, 242

Quality Plan 158

recombinant Factor VIII 95, 96, 99
recombinant Factor VIIa 99
refractoriness 75, 207, 222
relative risk reduction (RRR) 59, 60
retrospective audit 152, 153, 155, 223, 232
risk acceptance 115, 116, 120, 123, 125, 127
risk assessment 115, 116, 120, 121, 125, 126
risk communication 115, 126–128
risk control 115, 116, 120, 121, 126, 127
risk decision-making 116
risk limitation 125
risk management 116, 120, 121, 127, 128
risk perception 115

safety management 115, 116, 126, 127
self-sufficiency 235, 239
serum free culture system 186
sickle cell anaemia 154
social responsibility 128
somatic cell therapy 179
stem cells 216
supportive haemotherapy 13, 59, 62, 216, 217
surrogate equivalence 68, 69

TGF B 97
Thrombopoietin (TPO) 178
thrombotic thrombocytopenic purpura (TTP) 69, 145, 155, 223, 225
TIL (tumor infiltrating lymphocytes) cell therapies 183
total quality management (TQM) 128, 239
transfusion algorithms 37, 40, 41, 42
transfusion consent 18, 19
transfusion medicine specialist 241, 243
transfusion risk communication 127
Transfusion Committee 153–155
transfusion-associated AIDS (TAA) 19, 21
transfusion-associated graft-versus-host disease (GvHD) 150
transfusion-induced death 67
transfusion-related acute lung injury (TRALI) 152, 157
transfusion-transmitted AIDS 235, 242
transfusion-transmitted CMV infection 148, 149
transfusion-transmitted HIV 235
transfusion-transmitted infection 79, 80
tumor necrosis factor (TNF) 74

unit equivalence 68

viral vectors 189
von Willebrand's disease 145

DEVELOPMENTS IN HEMATOLOGY AND IMMUNOLOGY

1. H.R. Lijnen, D. Collen and M. Verstraete (eds.): *Synthetic Substrates in Clinical Blood Coagulation Assays*. 1980 ISBN 90-247-2409-0
2. C.Th. Smit Sibinga, P.C. Das and J.O. Forfar (eds.): *Paediatrics and Blood Transfusion*. Proceedings of the 5th Annual Symposium on Blood Transfusion, organized by the Red Cross Bloodbank Groningen-Drenthe, The Netherlands (1980). 1982 ISBN 90-247-2619-0
3. N. Fabris (ed.): *Immunology and Ageing*. 1982 ISBN 90-247-2640-9
4. G. Hornstra: *Dietary Fats, Prostanoids and Arterial Thrombosis*. With an Introductory Chapter by A. Bleakley Chandler. 1982 ISBN 90-247-2667-0
5. C.Th. Smit Sibinga, P.C. Das and J.J. van Loghem (eds.): *Blood Transfusion and Problems of Bleeding*. Proceedings of the 6th Annual Symposium on Blood Transfusion, organized by the Red Cross Bloodbank Groningen-Drenthe (1981). 1982 ISBN 90-247-3058-9
6. J. Dormandy (ed.): *Red Cell Deformability and Filterability*. 1983 ISBN 0-89838-578-4
7. C.Th. Smit Sibinga, P.C. Das and H.F. Taswell (eds.): *Quality Assurance in Blood Banking and Its Clinical Impact*. Proceedings of the 7th Annual Symposium on Blood Transfusion, organized by the Red Cross Bloodbank Groningen-Drenthe (1982). 1984 ISBN 0-89838-618-7
8. A.M.H.P. van den Besselaar, H.R. Gralnick and S.M. Lewis (eds.): *Thromboplastin Calibration and Oral Anticoagulant Control*. 1984 ISBN 0-89838-637-3
9. P. Fondu and O. Thijs (eds.): *Haemostatic Failure in Liver Disease*. 1984 ISBN 0-89838-640-3
10. C.Th. Smit Sibinga, P.C. Das and G. Opelz (eds.): *Transplantation and Blood Transfusion*. Proceedings of the 8th Annual Symposium on Blood Transfusion, organized by the Red Cross Bloodbank Groningen-Drenthe (1983). 1984 ISBN 0-89838-686-1
11. H. Schmid-Schönbein, L.J. Wurzinger and R.E. Zimmerman (eds.): *Enzyme Activation in Blood-perfused Artificial Organs*. 1985 ISBN 0-89838-704-3
12. J. Dormandy (ed.): *Blood Filtration and Blood Cell Deformability*. 1985 ISBN 0-89838-714-0
13. C.Th. Smit Sibinga, P.C. Das and E. Seidl (eds.): *Plasma Fractionation and Blood Transfusion*. Proceedings of the 9th Annual Symposium on Blood Transfusion, organized by the Red Cross Bloodbank Groningen-Drenthe (1984). 1985 ISBN 0-89838-761-2
14. S. Dawids and A. Bantjes (eds.): *Blood Compatible Materials and their Testing*. 1986 ISBN 0-89838-813-9
15. C.Th. Smit Sibinga, P.C. Das and T.J. Greenwalt (eds.): *Future Developments in Blood Banking*. Proceedings of the 10th Annual Symposium on Blood Transfusion, organized by the Red Cross Bloodbank Groningen-Drenthe (1985). 1986 ISBN 0-89838-824-4
16. A. Berlin, J. Dean, M.H. Draper, E.M.B. Smith and F. Spreafico (eds.): *Immunotoxicology*. Proceedings of the International Seminar on the Immunological System as a Target for Toxic Damage – Present Status, Open Problems and Future Perspectives, in collaboration with the UNEP-ILO-WHO IPCS and the Commission of the European Communities. 1987 ISBN 0-89838-843-0

DEVELOPMENTS IN HEMATOLOGY AND IMMUNOLOGY

17. T. Ottenhoff and R. de Vries: *Recognition of M. leprae Antigens*. 1987
ISBN 0-89838-887-2
18. J.-L. Touraine, R.P. Gale and V. Kochupillai (eds.): *Fetal Liver Transplantation*. 1987
ISBN 0-89838-975-5
19. C.Th. Smit Sibinga P.C. Das and C.P. Engelfriet (eds.): *White Cells and Platelets in Blood Transfusion*. Proceedings of the 11th Annual Symposium on Blood Transfusion, organized by the Red Cross Bloodbank Groningen-Drenthe (1986). 1987
ISBN 0-89838-976-3
20. C.F.M. Hendriksen: *Laboratory Animals in Vaccine Production and Control*. 1988
ISBN 0-89838-398-6
21. C.Th. Smit Sibinga, P.C. Das and L.R. Overby (eds.): *Biotechnology in Blood Transfusion*. Proceedings of the 12th Annual Symposium on Blood Transfusion, organized by the Red Cross Bloodbank Groningen-Drenthe (1987). 1988
ISBN 0-89838-404-4
22. C.Th. Smit Sibinga, P.C. Das and C.F. Högman (eds.): *Automation in Blood Transfusion*. Proceedings of the 13th Annual Symposium on Blood Transfusion, organized by the Red Cross Bloodbank Groningen-Drenthe (1988). 1989
ISBN 0-7923-0488-8
23. S. Dawids (ed.): *Polymers: Their Properties and Blood Compatibility*. 1989
ISBN 0-7923-0491-8
24. C.Th. Smit Sibinga, P.C. Das and H.T. Meryman (eds.): *Cryopreservation and Low Temperature Biology in Blood Transfusion*. Proceedings of the 14th Annual Symposium on Blood Transfusion, organized by the Red Cross Bloodbank Groningen-Drenthe (1989). 1990 ISBN 0-7923-0908-1
25. C.Th. Smit Sibinga and L. Kater (eds.): *Advances in Haemapheresis*. Proceedings of the 3rd International Congress of the World Apheresis Association (Amsterdam, The Netherlands, 1990). 1991 ISBN 0-7923-1312-7
26. C.Th. Smit Sibinga, P.C. Das and P.M. Mannucci (eds.): *Coagulation and Blood Transfusion*. Proceedings of the 15th Annual Symposium on Blood Transfusion, organized by the Red Cross Bloodbank Groningen-Drenthe (1990). 1991
ISBN 0-7923-1331-3
27. C.Th. Smit Sibinga, P.C. Das and J.D. Cash (eds.): *Transfusion Medicine: Fact and Fiction*. Proceedings of the 16th International Symposium on Blood Transfusion, organized by the Red Cross Bloodbank Groningen-Drenthe (1991). 1992
ISBN 0-7923-1732-7
28. C.Th. Smit Sibinga, P.C. Das and T.H. The (eds.): *Immunology and Blood Transfusion*. Proceedings of the 17th International Symposium on Blood Transfusion, organized by the Red Cross Bloodbank Groningen-Drenthe (1992). 1993
ISBN 0-7923-2380-7
29. C.Th. Smit Sibinga, P.C. Das and H.J. Heiniger (eds.): *Good Manufacturing Practice in Transfusion Medicine*. Proceedings of the 18th International Symposium on Blood Transfusion, organized by the Red Cross Blood Bank Groningen-Drenthe (1993). 1994 ISBN 0-7923-3009-9

DEVELOPMENTS IN HEMATOLOGY AND IMMUNOLOGY

30. C.Th. Smit Sibinga, P.C. Das and E. Briët (eds.): *Hereditary Diseases and Blood Transfusion.* Proceedings of the 19th International Symposium on Blood Transfusion, organized by the Red Cross Blood Bank Groningen-Drenthe (1994). 1995
ISBN 0-7923-3694-1
31. C.Th. Smit Sibinga, P.C. Das and E.L. Snyder (eds.): *Trigger Factors in Transfusion Medicine.* Proceedings of the 20th International Symposium on Blood Transfusion, organized by the Red Cross Blood Bank Noord-Nederland (1995). 1996
ISBN 0-7923-4225-0

KLUWER ACADEMIC PUBLISHERS – DORDRECHT / BOSTON / LONDON

www.ingramcontent.com/pod-product-compliance
Ingram Content Group UK Ltd.
Pitfield, Milton Keynes, MK11 3LW, UK
UKHW020250290926
15470UKWH00002B/839
* 9 7 8 0 7 9 2 3 4 2 5 5 7 *